MW01199612

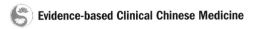
Evidence-based Clinical Chinese Medicine

Volume 6

Herpes Zoster and Post-herpetic Neuralgia

Evidence-based Clinical Chinese Medicine

Print ISSN: 2529-7562
Online ISSN: 2529-7554

Series Co Editors-in-Chief

Charlie Changli Xue *(RMIT University, Australia)*
Chuanjian Lu *(Guangdong Provincial Hospital of Chinese Medicine, China)*

Published

Vol. 8   *Alzheimer's Disease*
         Lead Authors: Brian May & Mei Feng

Vol. 7   *Insomnia*
         Lead Authors: Johannah Shergis & Xiaojia Ni

Vol. 6   *Herpes Zoster and Post-herpetic Neuralgia*
         Lead Authors: Meaghan Coyle & Haiying Liang

Vol. 5   *Allergic Rhinitis*
         Lead Authors: Claire Shuiqing Zhang & Qiulan Luo

Vol. 4   *Adult Asthma*
         Lead Authors: Johannah Shergis & Lei Wu

Vol. 3   *Chronic Urticaria*
         Lead Authors: Meaghan Coyle & Jingjie Yu

Vol. 2   *Psoriasis Vulgaris*
         Lead Authors: Claire Shuiqing Zhang & Jingjie Yu

Vol. 1   *Chronic Obstructive Pulmonary Disease*
         by Charlie Changli Xue & Chuanjian Lu

Forthcoming

Vol. 10 *Diabetic Kidney Disease*
         Lead Authors: Johannah Shergis & Lihong Yang

Vol. 11 *Acne Vulgaris*
         Lead Authors: Meaghan Coyle & Haiying Liang

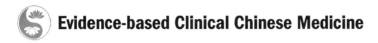
Evidence-based Clinical Chinese Medicine

Co Editors-in-Chief

Charlie Changli Xue
RMIT University, Australia

Chuanjian Lu
Guangdong Provincial Hospital of Chinese Medicine, China

Volume 6
Herpes Zoster and Post-herpetic Neuralgia

Lead Authors

Meaghan Coyle

Haiying Liang

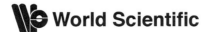
World Scientific

NEW JERSEY · LONDON · SINGAPORE · BEIJING · SHANGHAI · HONG KONG · TAIPEI · CHENNAI · TOKYO

Published by

World Scientific Publishing Co. Pte. Ltd.

5 Toh Tuck Link, Singapore 596224

USA office: 27 Warren Street, Suite 401-402, Hackensack, NJ 07601

UK office: 57 Shelton Street, Covent Garden, London WC2H 9HE

Library of Congress Cataloging-in-Publication Data

Names: Xue, Charlie Changli, author. | Lu, Chuan-jian, 1964–   author.

Title: Evidence-based clinical Chinese medicine / Charlie Changli Xue, Chuanjian Lu.

Description: New Jersey : World Scientific, 2016. | Includes bibliographical references and index.

Identifiers: LCCN 2015030389| ISBN 9789814723084 (v. 1 : hardcover : alk. paper) |

   ISBN 9789814723091 (v. 1 : paperback : alk. paper) |

   ISBN 9789814723121 (v. 2 : hardcover : alk. paper) |

   ISBN 9789814723138 (v. 2 : paperback : alk. paper) |

   ISBN 9789814759045 (v. 3 : hardcover : alk. paper) |

   ISBN 9789814759052 (v. 3 : paperback : alk. paper)

Subjects: | MESH: Medicine, Chinese Traditional--methods. | Clinical Medicine--methods. |

   Evidence-Based Medicine--methods. | Psoriasis. | Pulmonary Disease, Chronic Obstructive.

Classification: LCC RC81 | NLM WB 55.C4 | DDC 616--dc23

LC record available at http://lccn.loc.gov/2015030389

Volume 6: Herpes Zoster and Post-herpetic Neuralgia

ISBN 978-981-3209-66-4

ISBN 978-981-3209-67-1 (pbk)

British Library Cataloguing-in-Publication Data

A catalogue record for this book is available from the British Library.

For any available supplementary material, please visit
https://www.worldscientific.com/worldscibooks/10.1142/10438#t=suppl

Printed in Singapore

Disclaimer

The information in this monograph is based on systematic analyses of the best available evidence for Chinese medicine interventions both historical and contemporary. Every effort has been made to ensure accuracy and completeness of the data of this publication. This book is intended for clinicians, researchers, and educators. The practice of evidence-based medicine must consider the best available evidence, practitioners' clinical experience and judgment, and patients' preferences. Not all interventions are acceptable in all countries. It is important to note that some of the substances mentioned in this book may no longer be in use, may be toxic, or may be prohibited or restricted under the provisions of the Convention on International Trade in Endangered Species of Wild Fauna and Flora (CITES). Practitioners, researchers, and educators are advised to comply with the relevant regulations in their country and with the restrictions imposed on the trade of species included in CITES appendices I, II, and III. This book is not intended as a guide for self-medication. Patients should seek professional advice from their qualified Chinese medicine practitioners.

Foreword

Since the late 20th century, Chinese medicine, including acupuncture and herbal medicine, has been increasingly used throughout the world. The parallel development and spread of evidence-based medicine has provided challenges and opportunities for Chinese medicine.

The opportunities manifest in the form of evidence-based medicine's emphasis on the effective use of the best available clinical evidence and incorporating clinicians' clinical experience subject to patients' preference. Such practices are patient-oriented which reflects the historical nature of Chinese medicine practice. However, the challenges are also significant due to the fact that, despite the long-term development of a rich literature that has accumulated over 2,000 years, there is an overall lack of high level clinical evidence for many of the interventions used in Chinese medicine.

To address this knowledge gap, we need to generate high quality clinical findings through rigorous clinical studies and evaluate these findings to enable the effective use of such available evidence to support and promote evidence-based Chinese medicine practice.

Modern Chinese medicine is rooted in the classical literature and the legacies of ancient doctors, grounded in the practice of expert clinicians, and increasingly informed by clinical and experimental research efforts. In recognition of the unique features of Chinese medicine, for each of the conditions examined in this series, a 'whole evidence' approach is used to provide a synthesis of the different types and levels of evidence to enable practitioners to make clinical decisions informed by the current best evidence.

There are four main components underlying the 'whole evidence' approach. First, we present current approaches to the diagnosis, differentiation, and treatment of each condition based on expert consensus on textbooks and clinical guidelines. This provides an overview of how the condition is currently managed. The second section provides an analysis of the condition in historical context based on systematic searches of the *Encyclopedia of Traditional Chinese Medicine* (*Zhong Hua Yi Dian*) which includes the full texts of more than 1,000 classical medical books. These analyses provide objective views on how the condition has been treated over two millennia, reveal continuities and discontinuities between traditional and modern practice, and suggest avenues for future research.

The third component is the assessment of evidence derived from modern clinical studies of Chinese medicine interventions. The methods established by the *Cochrane Collaboration* are used for conducting systematic reviews and undertaking meta-analyses of outcome data for randomised controlled trials. In addition, the clinical relevance of meta-analysis data is enhanced by examining the herbal formulas, individual herbs, and acupuncture treatments that were assessed in the randomised controlled trials while the evidence base is broadened by the inclusion of data from non-randomised, controlled clinical trials and non-controlled studies. The fourth component is to determine how the herbal medicine interventions may achieve the effects indicated by the clinical trials. Thus, for each of the most frequently used herbs, we provide reviews of their effects in pre-clinical models and their likely mechanisms of action.

For each condition, this 'whole evidence' approach links clinical expertise, historical precedents, clinical research data, and experimental research to provide the reader with assessments of the current evidence for the efficacy and safety of Chinese medicine interventions using herbal medicines, acupuncture and moxibustion, and other health care practices such as *taichi*.

Since these books are available in Chinese and English, they can benefit patients, practitioners, and educators internationally and enable practitioners to make clinical decisions informed by the current best evidence.

These publications represent a major milestone in the progress of Chinese medicine and contribute significantly to the development of evidence-based Chinese medicine globally.

Co-Editors-in-Chief

Professor Charlie Changli Xue, RMIT University, Australia
Professor Chuanjian Lu, Guangdong Provincial Hospital of Chinese Medicine, China

Purpose of the Monograph

This book is intended for clinicians, researchers, and educators. It can be used to inform tertiary education and clinical practice by providing systematic, multi-dimensional assessments of the best available evidence for using Chinese medicine to manage each common clinical condition.

How to use this monograph

Some definitions

A glossary is included which contains terms and definitions that frequently appear in the book. It also describes the definitions of statistical tests, methodological terms, evaluation tools, and interventions. For example, in this book, Integrative Medicine refers to the combined use of a Chinese medicine treatment with conventional medical management, and that combination therapies refer to two or more Chinese medicines from different therapy groups (Chinese herbal medicine, acupuncture, or other Chinese medicine therapies) administered together.

Data analysis and interpretation of results

In order to synthesise the clinical evidence, a range of statistical analysis approaches are used. In general, the effect size for dichotomous data is reported as a risk ratio with 95% confidence intervals, and for continuous data, they are reported as mean difference with 95% confidence intervals. Statistically significant effects are indicated with an asterisk.* Readers should note that statistical significance does not necessarily correspond with clinical importance. Interpretation of results should take into consideration the clinical significance, quality (expressed as high, low, or unclear risk of bias in this book), and statistical heterogeneity amongst the studies. Tests for heterogeneity are conducted using the I^2 statistic. An I^2 score greater than 50% may indicate substantial heterogeneity.

Use of evidence in practice

The Grading of Recommendations Assessment, Development, and Evaluation (GRADE) approach was used to summarise the quality and strength of the evidence for critical comparisons and outcomes. Due to the diverse nature of Chinese medicine practice, treatment recommendations are not included with the summary-of-findings tables. Therefore, readers will need to interpret the evidence with reference to the local practice environment.

Limitations

Readers should note some of the methodological limitations of the classical literature and clinical evidence.

- Terms that were used to search the *Zhong Hua Yi Dian* database may not include all the terms that have been used for the condition and this may alter the findings.
- Chinese language has changed over time. Citations have been interpreted based on subjective judgment for analysis, and such interpretations may be subject to disagreement.
- Chinese medicine theory has evolved over time. As such, concepts described in the classical Chinese medical literature may no longer be found in contemporary works.
- Symptoms described in citations may be common to many conditions and a judgment was required to determine the likelihood of the citation being related to the condition. This may have introduced some bias due to the subjective nature of the judgment.

- The vast majority of the clinical evidence for Chinese medicine treatments has come from China. The applicability of the findings to other populations and other countries requires further assessment.
- Many studies included participants with varying disease severity. Where possible, subgroup analyses were undertaken to examine the effects in different sub-populations. As this was not always possible, the findings may be limited to the population included and not to sub-populations.
- The potential risk of bias found in many included studies indicates methodological limitations. The findings for GRADE assessments based on studies of very low to moderate quality evidence should be interpreted accordingly.
- Nine major English and Chinese language databases were searched to identify clinical studies in addition to clinical trial registers. Other studies may exist which were not identified through these searches and may alter the findings.
- The calculation of the frequency of herbal formulas used was based on formula names only. It is possible that some studies evaluated herbal treatments with the same or similar herb ingredients but gave these herbal treatments different formula names. Due to the complexity of herbal formulas, it was considered not appropriate to make a judgment on the similarity of formulas for analysis. As such, the frequency of formulas reported in Chapter 5 may be underestimated.
- The most frequently used herbs that may have contributed to observed treatment effects have been described in Chapter 5. These herbs may provide leads for further exploration. Determining which herbs have potential benefits is based on the frequency of formulas reported in the studies and does not take into consideration the clinical implications and functions of every herb in a formula.

Authors and Contributors

Co-Editors-in-Chief

Prof. Charlie Changli Xue (*RMIT University, Australia*)
Prof. Chuanjian Lu (*Guangdong Provincial Hospital of Chinese Medicine, China*)

Co-Deputy Editors-in-Chief

Assoc. Prof. Anthony Lin Zhang (*RMIT University, Australia*)
Dr. Brian H. May (*RMIT University, Australia*)
Prof. Xinfeng Guo (*Guangdong Provincial Hospital of Chinese Medicine, China*)
Prof. Zehuai Wen (*Guangdong Provincial Hospital of Chinese Medicine, China*)

Lead Authors

Dr. Meaghan Coyle (*RMIT University, Australia*)
Dr. Haiying Liang (*Guangdong Provincial Hospital of Chinese Medicine, China*)

Co-Authors

RMIT University (Australia):
Dr. Kaiyi Wang
Assoc. Prof. Anthony Lin Zhang
Prof. Charlie Changli Xue

Guangdong Provincial Hospital of Chinese Medicine (China):

Prof. Hongyi Li

Members of Advisory Committee and Panel

Co-Chairs of Project Planning Committee
Prof. Peter J. Coloe (*RMIT University, Australia*)
Prof. Yubo Lyu (*Guangdong Provincial Hospital of Chinese Medicine, China*)
Prof. Dacan Chen (*Guangdong Provincial Hospital of Chinese Medicine, China*)

Centre Advisory Committee (Alphabetical order)
Prof. Keji Chen (*The Chinese Academy of Sciences, China*)
Prof. Aiping Lu (*Hong Kong Baptist University, China*)
Prof. Caroline Smith (*University of Western Sydney, Australia*)
Prof. David F. Story (*RMIT University, Australia*)

Methodology Expert Advisory Panel (Alphabetical order)
Prof. Zhaoxiang Bian (*Hong Kong Baptist University, China*)
The late Prof. George Lewith (*University of Southampton, United Kingdom*)
Prof. Jianping Liu (*Beijing University of Chinese Medicine, China*)
Prof. Frank Thien (*Monash University, Australia*)
Prof. Jialiang Wang (*Sichuan University, China*)

Content Expert Advisory Panel (Alphabetical order)
Prof. Johannes Fleckenstein (*University of Bern, Switzerland*)
Prof. Aimin Liu (*Henan Province Hospital of Traditional Chinese Medicine, China*)

Professor Charlie Changli Xue, PhD

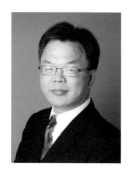

Professor Charlie Changli Xue holds a Bachelor of Medicine (majoring in Chinese Medicine) from Guangzhou University of Chinese Medicine, China (1987) and a PhD from RMIT University, Australia (2000). He has been an academic, researcher, regulator, and practitioner for almost three decades. Prof. Xue has made significant contributions to evidence-based educational development, clinical research, regulatory framework and policy development, as well as the provision of high quality clinical care to the community. Prof. Xue is recognised internationally as an expert in evidence-based traditional medicine and integrative healthcare.

Prof. Xue is the Inaugural National Chair of the Chinese Medicine Board of Australia as appointed by the Australian Health Workforce Ministerial Council (in 2011), and he was reappointed for the second term in 2014. Since 2007, he has been a Member of the World Health Organization (WHO) Expert Advisory Panel for Traditional and Complementary Medicine, Geneva. Prof. Xue is also Honorary Senior Principal Research Fellow at the Guangdong Provincial Academy of Chinese Medical Sciences, China.

At RMIT, Prof. Xue is the Executive Dean of the School of Health and Biomedical Sciences. He is also Director of the World Health Organization (WHO) Collaborating Centre for Traditional Medicine.

Between 1995 and 2010, Prof. Xue was Discipline Head of Chinese Medicine at RMIT University. He leads the development of five successful undergraduate and postgraduate degree programs in

Chinese Medicine at RMIT University which is now a global leader in Chinese medicine education and research.

Prof. Xue's research has been supported by research grants worth over AU$15 million including six project grants from the Australian Government's National Health and Medical Research Council and two Australian Research Council grants. He has contributed over 200 publications and has been frequently invited as a keynote speaker for numerous national and international conferences. Prof. Xue has contributed to over 300 media interviews on issues related to complementary medicine education, research, regulation, and practice.

Professor Chuanjian Lu, MD

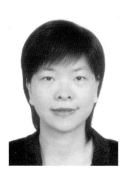

Professor Chuanjian Lu, Doctor of Medicine, is the Vice President of Guangdong Provincial Hospital of Chinese Medicine (Guangdong Provincial Academy of Chinese Medical Sciences, Second Clinical Medical College of Guangzhou University of Chinese Medicine). She is also the Chair of the Guangdong Traditional Chinese Medicine (TCM) Standardisation Technical Committee and the Vice-chair of the Immunity Specialty Committee of the World Federation of Chinese Medicine Societies.

Prof. Lu has engaged in scientific research into TCM, clinical practice, and teaching for some 25 years. Her research has been devoted to integrating traditional and western medicine. She has edited and published 12 monographs and 120 academic research articles with over 30 articles being included in SCI journals.

Prof. Lu has received widespread recognition for her achievements with awards such as 'Excellent Teacher of South China', 'National Outstanding Women TCM Doctor', and 'National Outstanding Young Doctor of TCM'. She also received 'The Science and Technology Star of the Association of Chinese Medicine', the 'National Excellent Science and Technology Workers of China Award', and the 'Five-Continent Women's Scientific Awards of China Medical Women's Association'.

Prof. Lu has won the Award of Science and Technology Progress over 10 times from Guangdong Provincial Government, China Association of Chinese Medicine and Chinese Hospital Association.

Acknowledgments

The authors and contributors would like to acknowledge the valuable contributions of Dr. Ziyang He, Dr. Shefton Parker, Dr. Iris Wenyu Zhou, Dr. Liang Zhang, and Dr. Neil Owens who assisted with database searches, data extraction, data screening, data assessment, translation of documents, editing, and/or administrative tasks.

Contents

Contents

List of Figures

List of Tables

1

Introduction to Herpes Zoster

OVERVIEW

Herpes zoster is a painful skin rash that develops in individuals who have been previously exposed to the varicella zoster virus. The rash is usually limited to the dermatome of the affected nerve. In young people and those with competent immune systems, herpes zoster usually resolves without any need for treatment. For older patients, antiviral therapies are recommended to aid recovery and inhibit the development of post-herpetic neuralgia. This chapter describes the characteristics, identified risk factors, pathological processes, and current management of herpes zoster.

Definition of Herpes Zoster

Herpes zoster, commonly known as shingles, is a painful skin rash caused by a reactivation of the latent varicella zoster virus.[1] Primary infection of the varicella zoster virus results in chickenpox.[2,3] The varicella zoster vaccine has been shown to be moderately effective in preventing primary infection of the varicella zoster virus,[4] although it does not prevent all cases. Once the initial infection has resolved, the virus lies dormant in the dorsal root and cranial nerve ganglia.[2] Herpes zoster can occur at any age[5] and the virus can lie dormant for several decades.[1] Factors such as age, immune suppression, or immunodeficiency can lead to a reactivation of the virus,[1] and the virus spreads along sensory ganglia to the neural tissue of the affected segment, resulting in localised skin eruptions.[1,3]

Three clinical stages are usually seen in herpes zoster: the prodromal phase, acute phase, and healing phase.[6] The prodromal phase occurs in 70–80% of patients[2] and can last from one day[6] to more than 10 days.[2] The length of the prodromal phase usually relates to the amount of time the virus takes to travel from the dorsal ganglia to the cutaneous nerves and replicate in the skin.[2] Symptoms of the prodromal phase include pain or abnormal skin sensations, malaise, headache, and nausea.[2,3,6]

During the acute phase, development of a painful, unilateral, and erythematous rash,[6] typically in areas innervated by the thoracic, cervical, and trigeminal sensory nerves, is observed.[7] Pain is usually described as burning, throbbing, or stabbing.[2] Small macules and papules appear in clusters which develop into vesicles after one to two days.[2] New vesicles can appear for a further three to five days.[3] Pustulation occurs within one week of rash development, after which ulceration and crustation occurs.[2] Healing time can vary from two to four weeks in immunocompetent patients.[1,3]

Presentation can be atypical in patients with a compromised immune system.[1] The rash may involve more than one dermatome and be of longer duration.[1] Patients with compromised immunity are at greater risk of disseminated and visceral zoster.[2]

While the disease is self-limiting,[6] between 10% and 21% of people with herpes zoster go on to experience post-herpetic neuralgia (PHN).[5,6,8,9] Dubinsky *et al.*[8] emphasised that there is no agreed definition of PHN, with definitions ranging from one month to six months after the rash has resolved. The definition provided by Dubinsky *et al.*[8, p959] that PHN is the "persistence of the pain of herpes zoster more than 3 months after resolution of the rash" is generally accepted for clinical diagnosis and research. Pain arises due to sensory nerve damage, can be intermittent, and may be accompanied by allodynia (pain from stimuli that would not normally produce pain).

Complications of herpes zoster are not uncommon, and are grouped according to four categories: cutaneous, visceral, neurological, and ocular.[7] PHN is the most common complication, affecting up to 21% of people with herpes zoster.[6] Other common complications include opthalmic zoster, Ramsay Hunt syndrome (involving the geniculate ganglion of the facial nerve),[2] zoster encephalitis, dissemi-nated zoster (defined as 20 or more lesions in a secondary dermatome),[10] and visceral involvement. Further, bacterial infection of the rash may require antibiotic treatment.[11] For an extensive list of herpes zoster complications, see Volpi *et al.*[6]

Epidemiology

A global epidemiological review of herpes zoster found that the median incidence was 4–4.5 per 1,000 person-years.[12] Incidence has been reported to be higher in Germany (5.3–5.5 per 1,000 person-years)[13] and in immunocompetent patients aged 50 years or older in Italy (6.31 per 1,000 person-years).[14] Incidence of herpes zoster increases with age. The mean age of onset of herpes zoster is 59.4 years, with over two thirds of cases (68%) occurring in people aged 50 years or older.[15] An early epidemiological peak at between 30–34 years was noted by Gialloreti *et al.*[14], with a second peak at 75–79 years. Women are more likely to develop herpes zoster than men;[13,16] the age-adjusted inci-dence is 3.9 per 1,000 person-years for females and 3.2 per 1,000 person-years for males.[15]

Burden

Herpes zoster has a significant impact on health-related quality of life (HRQoL). Comparison with other chronic diseases showed that herpes zoster has a greater impact on the domain 'role limitations due to physical problems' of the Medical Outcome Study 36-item Short Form Health Survey (SF36; a HRQoL questionnaire) compared to hypertension, congestive heart failure, diabetes mellitus, myocar-dial infarction, and depression.[17] Herpes zoster also led to poor quality of life (that is, a score of less than 50 out of 100) in infected individuals for four out of eight domains of the SF36.[17] Herpes zoster has also been shown to be a risk factor for development of depressive disorders.[18]

HRQoL in acute stage herpes zoster decreases with increasing pain levels,[19] and pain associated with PHN has a higher impact on

HRQoL than pain due to herpes zoster in the acute stage.[20] The impact of herpes zoster on HRQoL can be felt long after the resolution of skin rash, with research showing that HRQoL was lower than baseline levels for up to 180 days of follow up.[21] In addition to its impact on HRQoL, data from the European World Health Organization database shows that herpes zoster-related mortality ranged from 0 to >0.07 per 100,000.[22] Herpes zoster-related mortality was higher in older women than men.[22,23]

The economic burden of herpes zoster and PHN is considerable. The estimated total annual cost burden of herpes zoster and PHN in Europe ranges from €26.97 million in Sweden to €271.21 million in the UK.[23] Outpatient management costs are higher for PHN than herpes zoster.[23] This is likely related to the increased utilisation of health care resources for extended periods of time. In the UK, mean direct cost per herpes zoster patient was £103, compared with £341 and £397 per episode for PHN using one-month and three-month definitions, respectively.[24] Similar findings were seen in Singapore.[25] The mean number of visits to general practitioners was higher in patients with PHN (11.9–12.0) compared with herpes zoster (1.9),[14] and the mean direct cost for outpatient management increases with pain severity.[24]

Like other aspects of herpes zoster and PHN, costs increase with age. Annual incidence of general practitioner visits in the Netherlands were 32.8 per 10,000 in those aged less than 60 years, and this number increased to 93.1 and 113.2 per 10,000 in those aged 60–64 and >65, respectively.[26] Direct costs were higher in older patients while indirect costs (for example, work absenteeism) were higher in younger patients.[23] Females have been reported to be at greater risk of hospitalisation.[27]

Risk Factors

Age is the main risk factor for developing herpes zoster.[1] Other risk factors include immunosuppression, sex (with females generally being at higher risk, although research provides conflicting results), ethnicity (with Caucasians being at higher risk),[7] mechanical trauma,[28] family history,[29,30] and diabetes.[31] Recent psychological stress has also been proposed as a risk factor,[32,33] as has depression, family history of herpes zoster, sleep disturbance, and recent weight loss.[33]

Several risk factors have been identified that increase the likelihood of developing PHN including older age, female gender, presence of prodromal phase and significant prodromal pain,[34,35] cranial or sacral involvement,[34,36] and greater severity of rash and pain during the acute stage.[6,34,35] Immune status is not a factor for developing PHN.[6]

Pathological Processes

Varicella zoster virus is one of eight human herpes viruses.[37] While other herpes viruses such as herpes simplex viruses can reactivate multiple times, the varicella zoster virus usually reactivates once after initial infection,[1] although multiple recurrences have been reported with incidence rates similar to first occurrence.[12] The varicella zoster virus is highly infectious and transmits via the respiratory tract.[7]

On primary infection, the virus replicates rapidly and spreads from lymphoid tissues to circulating T lymphocytes.[2,7] The incubation period ranges from 10–21 days,[7] during which the virus travels to the skin. Replication of the virus occurs in epithelial cells, aided by down-regulation of interferon (IFN)-α and inhibition of adhesion molecules.[2]

Three key components are involved in the immune response to varicella zoster virus. These include innate immunity (a non-specific defense mechanism activated by chemical properties of the pathogen), humoral immunity (which neutralises the cell-free virus), and cell-mediated immunity (CMI; T-cell-mediated immunity removes pathogens from inside the cell).[7] CMI is regarded as more crucial than humoral immunity.[37] With the immune defenses lowered, vesicles appear.[2] The varicella zoster virus spreads in two ways. Specifically, in the superficial epidermis, the cell-free virus is shed from cells and the virus particles spread, while in the basal epidermis, the virus spreads via cell-to-cell contact.[7]

The varicella zoster virus establishes latency in order to further spread to new hosts. Two main hypotheses have been proposed for how the varicella zoster virus accesses the dorsal and cranial root ganglia. The first hypothesis proposes that the cell-free varicella zoster virus infects intra-epidermal projections of sensory neurons, travelling to the cell body by retrograde transport and establishing latency.[7] The second hypothesis proposes that the virus travels to the dorsal and cranial root ganglion inside infected T cells during the primary infection.[7] The infected T cells infect the neuronal cell body after fusing with the neuron. The virus then begins proliferation in the cell body. Cell death is prevented, proliferation stops, and latency is established.

Reactivation may be triggered by expression of the ORF61 protein from the cell body or by mediators of inflammation, and this process is associated with a decline in CMI.[7] When reactivation occurs, the varicella zoster virus travels along microtubules in sensory axons to epithelial cells where infection occurs.[7] The characteristic herpes zoster rash appears in the dermatome of the infected sensory nerve. Inflammation and cell death also occurs in the affected ganglion[7] and is likely to be the origin of the prodromal pain.[2]

Diagnosis

During the prodromal phase where pain is present and lesions have not yet developed, diagnosis can be challenging and may spur the investigation of other diseases relevant to the affected dermatome.[2] Once the lesions develop, the cause of prodromal pain becomes obvious. Herpes zoster usually presents as an asymmetrical skin rash mostly limited to one dermatome with segmental pain.[1] The main features considered important for making a clinical diagnosis include painful prodrome, lesions distributed predominantly within one dermatome, clustered vesicles, multiple sites within the dermatome, no previous history of a similar rash in the same location, and pain and allodynia in the vicinity of the rash.[2] Due to the distinctive appearance of herpes zoster, clinical diagnosis is usually accurate.[3]

Polymerase chain reaction (PCR) can be used to detect the varicella zoster virus in swabs of skin lesions[1,2,10] but is expensive and can take more than one day to obtain results.[2] An immunohistochemical analysis of lesion scrapings in the vesicular phase is inexpensive and sensitive,[2] and immunofluourescence can also be used to detect the varicella zoster virus.[1] Blood tests may also be used to detect varicella zoster virus-specific immunoglobulins (IgG, IgM, and IgA).[1]

If the disease is in the prodromal or early acute phase with only erythematous skin lesions present, diagnosis may be problematic.[1] Similarly, the less common zoster sine herpete (absence of skin lesions) may be difficult to diagnose. In this case, PCR should be used to confirm the diagnosis. Similarly, atypical presentations, varicella zoster virus infections in pregnant women and newborn babies, and suspected infection of the central nervous system should be confirmed using laboratory methods.[1] Viral detection is not possible by serological tests once lesion healing has completed.[1]

Differential diagnoses of herpes zoster include zosteriform herpes simplex, contact dermatitis, bullous dermatoses, and insect bites.[1,2] Zoster sine herpete, a sub-type of herpes zoster, presents with pain in the absence of skin lesions.

Management

Vaccination

Prevention of herpes zoster in those who are most vulnerable can be achieved by vaccination.[38] The vaccine has been found to reduce the incidence of herpes zoster by 51.3% compared with placebo.[39] The vaccine stimulates CMI to reduce the frequency and severity of herpes zoster.[39] The live attenuated vaccine Oka/Merck strain (Zostavax, manufactured by Merck Sharp and Dohme) was introduced in the US in 1995.[6] In 2006, the USA Advisory Committee for Immunization Practices recommended the vaccine for people aged 60 years and older, and Australia followed suit in 2009.[40] The USA Food and Drug Administration (FDA) extended the licensure to include people aged 50–59 years.[41] The use of the vaccine in the UK and other European countries is targeted toward high risk individuals.[6]

The herpes zoster vaccine is effective, especially in the 60–69 year age group, and is well-tolerated.[42] Uptake of the vaccine has been reported to be low.[38] This may reflect production shortfalls[41] or high cost of the vaccine when not subsidised.[10]

Pharmacological Management

Clinical management of the acute stage of herpes zoster is focused on alleviating pain, promoting rash healing, and reducing complications and PHN.[1,2,43, 44] In immunocompromised patients, inhibition of viral replication is important.[2] Patients with opthalmic zoster should be referred for specialist ophthalmic management to prevent complications.[1,2]

At least four clinical practice guidelines exist which describe the clinical management of herpes zoster.[1,2,44,45] The guidelines of the German Dermatology Society[1], the European consensus-based (S2k) guidelines by Werner *et al.*,[44] and the evidence-based treatment recommendations developed by Dworkin *et al.*[2] have informed the discussions that follow in this chapter as they are the most current available guidelines on the management of herpes zoster. Further, discussion has been focused most specifically on management of herpes zoster in immunocompetent individuals.

As herpes zoster is a self-limiting disease, zoster on the thoracic region and extremities in otherwise healthy young people will generally heal without complications.[1] Antiviral therapy can hasten the healing process and is recommended in patients 50 years and older, immunocompromised patients, and patients with malignant disease, cranial nerve involvement, or involvement of more than one dermatome.[1] Dworkin *et al.*[2] and Werner *et al.*[44] add that systematic antiviral therapy should be considered as first-line therapy for immunocompetent patients meeting the following criteria: over 50 years, with moderate to severe pain, with moderate to severe rash, or with non-truncal involvement. In addition, antiviral therapy is indicated for people with severe atopic dermatitis and eczema[1,44] as well as children and adolescents using salicylic acid and corticosteroids long-term.[44]

There is a lack of evidence for topical antiviral therapies and thus they are not recommended for herpes zoster.[2] Systemic antiviral therapy reduces virus replication and new lesion formation, promotes rash healing, and reduces the severity and duration of pain.[2] Four antiviral therapies have been found to be effective in clinical trials, namely acyclovir, famciclovir, valacyclovir, and brivudin (see Table 1.1). Brivudin has not yet been approved by the FDA.[46] Based on results from clinical trials, brivudin, famciclovir, and valacyclovir were more efficacious than acyclovir.[2]

The success of antiviral therapy depends on when it is initiated. Initiation is recommended to commence within 72 hours of rash onset,[1] although it is acknowledged that this is an arbitrary inclusion criterion for clinical trials and does not necessarily reflect cessation of viral replication.[2] Dworkin *et al.*[2] stress that evidence is lacking on the effectiveness of antiviral therapy in people under 50 years and those with less severe disease. Patients under 50 years with low risk of complications may still benefit from antiviral therapy in reducing the risk of PHN, although findings from a Cochrane review showed that oral acyclovir was not effective in reducing the incidence of PHN.[47] Further, despite the suggested initiation of antiviral therapy within 72 hours, the extent of treatment effectiveness when initiated after 72 hours is still unknown.[2] Despite this, the low safety profile may mean that antiviral therapies are worth considering.

Table 1.1   Guideline-recommended Antiviral Therapies for Herpes Zoster

Drug Name	Recommended Dosage
Acyclovir	800 mg, 5 times daily for 7–10 days
Famciclovir	500 mg, 3 times daily for 7 days (approved dose in USA); 250 mg, 3 times daily (approved dose in some countries outside the USA)
Valacyclovir	1000 mg, 3 times daily for 7 days
Brivudin	125 mg once daily for 7 days

Adapted from Dworkin *et al.*[2]

Antiviral therapies are very well-tolerated with the most common side effects being nausea and headache.[2]

In order to alleviate acute pain and possibly reduce the risk of PHN, analgesics may be used if pain is not sufficiently controlled by antiviral therapy. According to Dworkin *et al.*,[2] selection of analgesic therapy should consider pain severity, underlying conditions, and previous experience with analgesic therapy. A stepped-care approach is recommended for analgesic therapy,[1,6,44] starting with paracetamol (acetaminophen) and then progressing through codeine to strong opioid analgesics (see Table 1.2). Other treatment options include tricyclic antidepressants and anticonvulsant medications for significant pain.[6] As the severity of pain can vary with time, ongoing and regular assessment is needed to ensure that pain relief is maintained.[2] Analgesic therapies should be prescribed to ensure continuous pain relief rather than as-needed use.

Table 1.2   Guideline-recommended Analgesic Therapies for Herpes Zoster

Analgesic Therapy Class	Drug Name	Initial Dose
Simple analgesics and antipyretics	Paracetamol (acetaminophen)	1 g every 4–6 hours as required; maximum 4 g daily[40]
Nonsteroidal anti-inflammatory drugs (NSAIDs)	(Various)	None stated
Corticosteroids	(Various)	Prednisone: 60 mg daily for 7 days, tapering over 2 weeks[2]
Opioid analgesics	Morphine	None stated
	Oxycodone	5 mg every 4 hours[2]
Opioid-like analgesics	Tramadol	50 mg once or twice daily[2]
Tricyclic antidepressants	Amitriptyline	10–25 mg at night[40]
	Nortriptyline	25 mg at night[2]
	Despiramine	None stated
Anticonvulsants	Gabapentin	300 mg at night, or 100–300 mg 3 times daily[2]
	Pregabalin	75 mg at night, or 75 mg twice daily[2]

Adapted from Dworkin *et al.*[2]

There are few studies that have evaluated the use of simple analgesics or NSAIDS for acute herpes zoster pain.[17] Corticosteroid therapy as an adjunct to antiviral therapy may shorten the duration of pain but does not reduce the chance of PHN.[1] If pain relief is not attained with opioid analgesics, guidelines recommend the addition of either anticonvulsants (gabapentin or pregabalin), tricyclic antidepressants (nortriptyline is preferred to others as it is better tolerated), or corticosteroids.[2] Steroids are not recommended in patients at risk of corticosteroid-induced toxicity.[3]

There is conflicting advice on the potential value of neural blockades. Dworkin *et al.*[2] reported that the long-term benefits have not been evaluated while Johnson[48] stated that there is consistent evidence from controlled trials. Another treatment for which there is limited evidence is topical capsaicin.[1,2]

While antiviral and analgesic therapies are effective and antiviral therapies are well-tolerated, a recent study found that they do not meet the expectations of patients.[19] The Treatment Satisfaction with Medication questionnaire was administered to patients with acute herpes zoster and PHN. Irrespective of the medication received (that is, antiviral only, antiviral plus level one analgesic, or antiviral plus level two or three analgesic), the aspect of treatment that patients were most satisfied with was side effects experienced while patients were least satisfied with the effectiveness of the intervention. The authors suggest there is an unmet need in terms of patient expectations of herpes zoster therapies.

Non-pharmacological Management

Patient education, which includes information about the risk of transmission of the virus to unexposed individuals, proposed treatment plans, advice on quality of life, wound care, and reassurance, is important.[2] Patients should be informed to keep the rash clean and dry to reduce likelihood of infection and to avoid topical antibiotics and adhesive dressings.[1,2] The discomfort from lesions may be alleviated with sterile wet dressings,[2] lotio alba (emollient with varying formulas; may include zinc oxide, zinc sulphate, lead subacetate solution, sulphurated potassa, glycerin, lime water, and rose water),[49] vioform zinc mixture, or crust removal.[1] A wet compress applied for 15–30 minutes, 5–10 times per day, can assist in breaking the vesicle and remove serum and crust.[50]

Patients should be advised to use loose clothing made from natural fibres so as not to irritate lesions.[6] Guidelines also describe transcutaneous/percutaneous electrical nerve stimulation as another treatment option for herpes zoster, although evidence is limited.[2]

Prognosis

Patients can be assured that herpes zoster is a self-limiting disease. If antiviral therapy is administered early, the severity and impact of herpes zoster can be reduced and the incidence of PHN can potentially be inhibited. Antiviral therapy is effective and many analgesic therapies have also demonstrated positive effects.

The most common complication of herpes zoster is PHN. While other complications can occur, many are rare. Major complications include encephalitis, opthalmic zoster (alone or with delayed contralateral hemiparesis resulting from stroke), retinitis, and post-herpetic itch.[2] Other complications are grouped according to the body system involved and include cutaneous, visceral, neurological, and ocular complications.[1,7,51] A comprehensive list of other herpes zoster complications can be found in Gershon *et al.*[7] and Gross *et al.*[1]

References

1. Gross G, Schofer H, Wassilew S, *et al.* Herpes zoster guideline of the German Dermatology Society (DDG). *J Clin Virol.* 2003; **26**(3): 277–89; discussion 91–3.
2. Dworkin RH, Johnson RW, Breuer J, *et al.* Recommendations for the management of herpes zoster. *Clin Infect Dis.* 2007; **44**(Suppl 1):S1–26.
3. Gnann JW, Jr., Whitley RJ. Clinical practice. Herpes zoster. *N Engl J Med.* 2002; **347**(5):340–6.
4. Marin M, Marti M, Kambhampati A, *et al.* Global Varicella Vaccine Effectiveness: A Meta-analysis. *Pediatrics* 2016; **137**(3): e20153741.

5. Sampathkumar P, Drage LA, Martin DP. Herpes zoster (shingles) and postherpetic neuralgia. *Mayo Clin Proc.* 2009; **84**(3):274–80.

6. Volpi A, Gross G, Hercogova J, Johnson RW. Current management of herpes zoster: The European view. *Am J Clin Dermatol.* 2005; **6**(5): 317–25.

7. Gershon AA, Gershon MD, Breuer J, *et al.* Advances in the understanding of the pathogenesis and epidemiology of herpes zoster. *J Clin Virol.* 2010; **48**(Suppl 1):S2–7.

8. Dubinsky RM, Kabbani H, El-Chami Z, Boutwell C, Ali H. Practice parameter: Treatment of postherpetic neuralgia: An evidence-based report of the Quality Standards Subcommittee of the American Academy of Neurology. *Neurology.* 2004; **63**(6):959–65.

9. Kawai K, Rampakakis E, Tsai TF, *et al.* Predictors of postherpetic neuralgia in patients with herpes zoster: A pooled analysis of prospective cohort studies from North and Latin America and Asia. *Int J Infect Dis.* 2015; **34**:126–31.

10. Wehrhahn M, Dwyer D. Herpes zoster: Epidemiology, clinical features, treatment and prevention. *Australian Prescriber.* 2012; **35**(5):143–7.

11. Johnson RW, Whitton TL. Management of herpes zoster (shingles) and postherpetic neuralgia. *Expert Opin Pharmacother.* 2004; **5**(3):551–9.

12. Yawn BP, Wollan PC, Kurland MJ, St Sauver JL, Saddier P. Herpes zoster recurrences more frequent than previously reported. *Mayo Clin Proc.* 2011; **86**(2):88–93.

13. Hillebrand K, Bricout H, Schulze-Rath R, Schink T, Garbe E. Incidence of herpes zoster and its complications in Germany, 2005–2009. *J Infect.* 2015; **70**(2):178–86.

14. Gialloreti LE, Merito M, Pezzotti P, *et al.* Epidemiology and economic burden of herpes zoster and post-herpetic neuralgia in Italy: A retrospective, population-based study. *BMC Infect Dis.* 2010; **10**:230.

15. Yawn BP, Gilden D. The global epidemiology of herpes zoster. *Neurology.* 2013; **81**(10):928–30.

16. Johnson B, Gatwood J, Palmer L, *et al.* Annual incidence rates of herpes zoster among an immunocompetent population in the United States. ISPOR 20th Annual International Meeting; Philadelphia PA, USA 2015.

17. Johnson RW, Bouhassira D, Kassianos G, *et al.* The impact of herpes zoster and post-herpetic neuralgia on quality-of-life. *BMC Med.* 2010; **8**:37.

18. Chen MH, Wei HT, Su TP, *et al.* Risk of depressive disorder among patients with herpes zoster: A nationwide population-based prospective study. *Psychosom Med.* 2014; **76**(4):285–91.

19. Gater A, Abetz-Webb L, Carroll S, *et al.* Burden of herpes zoster in the UK: Findings from the zoster quality of life (ZQOL) study. *BMC Infect Dis.* 2014; **14**:402.
20. Lukas K, Edte A, Bertrand I. The impact of herpes zoster and post-herpetic neuralgia on quality of life: Patient-reported outcomes in six European countries. *Z Gesundh Wiss.* 2012; **20**(4):441–51.
21. Song H, Lee J, Lee M, *et al.* Burden of illness, quality of life, and health-care utilization among patients with herpes zoster in South Korea: A prospective clinical-epidemiological study. *Int J Infect Dis.* 2014; **20**: 23–30.
22. Bricout H, Haugh M, Olatunde O, Prieto RG. Herpes zoster-associated mortality in Europe: A systematic review. *BMC Public Health.* 2015; **15**:466.
23. Gater A, Uhart M, McCool R, Preaud E. The humanistic, economic and societal burden of herpes zoster in Europe: A critical review. *BMC Public Health.* 2015; 15:193.
24. Gauthier A, Breuer J, Carrington D, Martin M, Remy V. Epidemiology and cost of herpes zoster and post-herpetic neuralgia in the United Kingdom. *Epidemiol Infect.* 2009; **137**(1):38–47.
25. Chen Q, Hsu T-Y, Chan R, *et al.* Clinical and economic burden of herpes zoster and postherpetic neuralgia in patients from the National Skin Centre, Singapore. *Dermatologica Sinica.* 2015; In press:doi:10.1016/j.dsi.2015.04.002.
26. Pierik JG, Gumbs PD, Fortanier SA, Van Steenwijk PC, Postma MJ. Epidemiological characteristics and societal burden of varicella zoster virus in the Netherlands. *BMC Infect Dis.* 2012; **12**:110.
27. Studahl M, Petzold M, Cassel T. Disease burden of herpes zoster in Sweden — predominance in the elderly and in women — a register based study. *BMC Infect Dis.* 2013; **13**:586.
28. Thomas SL, Hall AJ. What does epidemiology tell us about risk factors for herpes zoster? *Lancet Infect Dis.* 2004; **4**(1):26–33.
29. Ansar A, Farshchian M, Ghasemzadeh M, Sobhan MR. Association between family history and herpes zoster: A case-control study. *J Res Health Sci.* 2014; **14**(2):111–4.
30. Hicks LD, Cook-Norris RH, Mendoza N, *et al.* Family history as a risk factor for herpes zoster: A case-control study. *Arch Dermatol.* 2008; **144**(5):603–8.
31. Heymann AD, Chodick G, Karpati T, *et al.* Diabetes as a risk factor for herpes zoster infection: Results of a population-based study in Israel. *Infection.* 2008; **36**(3):226–30.

32. Schmader KE. Epidemiology and impact on quality of life of postherpetic neuralgia and painful diabetic neuropathy. *Clin J Pain.* 2002; **18**(6):350–4.

33. Marin M, Harpaz R, Zhang J, Wollan PC, Bialek SR, Yawn BP. Risk factors for herpes zoster among adults. *Open Forum Infectious Diseases.* 2016; **3**(3):ofw119.

34. Forbes HJ, Thomas SL, Smeeth L, *et al.* A systematic review and meta-analysis of risk factors for postherpetic neuralgia. *Pain.* 2016; **157**(1):30–54.

35. Jung BF, Johnson RW, Griffin DR, Dworkin RH. Risk factors for postherpetic neuralgia in patients with herpes zoster. *Neurology.* 2004; **62**(9):1545–51.

36. Meister W, Neiss A, Gross G, *et al.* A prognostic score for postherpetic neuralgia in ambulatory patients. *Infection.* 1998; **26**(6):359–63.

37. Cunningham AL, Breuer J, Dwyer DE, *et al.* The prevention and management of herpes zoster. *Med J Aust.* 2008; **188**(3):171–6.

38. Van Epps P, Schmader KE, Canaday DH. Herpes zoster vaccination: Controversies and common clinical questions. *Gerontology.* 2016; **62**(2):150–4.

39. Gabutti G, Valente N, Sulcaj N, Stefanati A. Evaluation of efficacy and effectiveness of live attenuated zoster vaccine. *J Prev Med Hyg.* 2014; **55**(4):130–6.

40. eTG complete [internet],. Melbourne: Therapeutic Guidelines Limited; 2014.

41. Update on herpes zoster vaccine: licensure for persons aged 50 through 59 years. *MMWR Morb Mortal Wkly Rep.* 2011; **60**(44):1528.

42. Gagliardi Anna MZ, Gomes Silva Brenda N, Torloni Maria R, Soares Bernardo GO. Vaccines for preventing herpes zoster in older adults. *Cochrane Database of Systematic Reviews.* 2012 (10).

43. Whitley RJ, Volpi A, McKendrick M, Wijck A, Oaklander AL. Management of herpes zoster and post-herpetic neuralgia now and in the future. *J Clin Virol.* 2010; **48**(Suppl 1):S20–8.

44. Werner RN, Nikkels AF, Marinovic B, *et al.* European consensus-based (S2k) Guideline on the Management of Herpes Zoster — guided by the European Dermatology Forum (EDF) in cooperation with the European Academy of Dermatology and Venereology (EADV), Part 2: Treatment. *J Eur Acad Dermatol Venereol.* 2017; **31**(1):20–9.

45. Johnson R, Mandal B, Bowsher D, *et al.* Guidelines for the management of shingles: Report of a working group of the British Society for the Study of Infection (BSSI). *J Infect.* 1995; **30**(3):193–200.

46. Cohen JI. Herpes zoster. *N Engl J Med.* 2013; **369**(18):1766–7.
47. Chen N, Li Q, Yang J, *et al.* Antiviral treatment for preventing postherpetic neuralgia. *Cochrane Database of Systematic Reviews.* 2014 (2).
48. Johnson R. Zoster-associated pain: What is known, who is at risk and how can it be managed. *Herpes.* 2007; **14**(Suppl 2):30A-4A.
49. Raubenheimer O. Lotio alba. *Journal of the American Pharmaceutical Association.* 1914; **3**(5):692–5.
50. Ferri F. *Ferri's Clinical Advisor 2016.* London: Elsevier; 2016.
51. Volpi A. Severe complications of herpes zoster. *Herpes.* 2007; **14**(Suppl 2):35A–9A.

2

Herpes Zoster in Chinese Medicine

OVERVIEW

This chapter describes the aetiology, pathogenesis, syndrome differentiation, and treatments recommended in key Chinese medicine clinical textbooks and guidelines. In Chinese medicine, *she chuan chuang* 蛇串疮 is the main term used in contemporary texts to refer to herpes zoster. Herpes zoster is caused by pathogenic fire resulting from Liver *qi* stagnation or emotional disturbance. Obstruction in the channels can turn to heat which pushes outwards toward the skin. In addition, underlying Spleen deficiency can lead to dampness, which also obstructs the free flow of *qi*. Treatments are determined according to syndrome differentiation.

Introduction

Symptoms of herpes zoster have been described in the classical Chinese medicine (CM) literature, although diversity in the terms used to describe the condition means that the earliest citations referring to herpes zoster is difficult to identify. Some authors suggest that *zeng dai chuang* 甑带疮 was the first term for herpes zoster.[1] Many records have been noted in the classical literature which describe symptoms similar to those of herpes zoster as well as other similar skin diseases.

Chinese names for herpes zoster have been based on two common clinical features (that is, the formation of blisters and distribution around the belt or waist area) and include *zeng dai chuang* 甑带疮, *chan yao long* 缠腰龙, *huo dai chuang* 火带疮, *zhi zhu chuang* 蜘蛛疮, *chan yao huo dan* 缠腰火丹, *she chuan chuang* 蛇串疮, and *she ke chuang* 蛇窠疮. Other names which have been used historically include *she chan* 蛇缠, *she chan chuang* 蛇缠疮, *she dan chuang* 蛇丹疮, *chan she chuang* 缠蛇疮, *chan yao hu dai* 缠腰虎带, *chan she dan du* 缠蛇丹毒, *long chan chuang du* 龙缠疮毒, *bai she chan chuang* 白蛇缠疮, and *bai she chan yao* 白蛇缠腰. This variety of terms has led to confusion in the understanding of herpes zoster in CM and made disease recognition challenging.

In order to standardise the diagnosis of herpes zoster in CM, Professor Bingnan Zhao proposed *she chuan chuang* 蛇串疮 to be the official name for herpes zoster. This was adopted as the official name in the *Guidelines for Diagnosis and Treatment of Common Diseases of Dermatology in Traditional Chinese Medicine* 中医皮肤科常见病诊疗指南, published by the China Association of Chinese Medicine in 2012.[2]

Aetiology and Pathogenesis

In CM, emotional disturbance of any of the seven emotions or pathogenic fire directed outward to the skin as a result of stagnation of Liver *qi* are considered the two main causes of herpes zoster. Emotional disturbance hinders the Liver function of enabling the free-flow of *qi* and emotions, leading to Liver *qi* stagnation.[3] *Qi* stagnation can turn to fire, which blazes outwards to the skin. This results in the characteristic red skin lesions.

Internal fire may also arise from a Spleen deficiency. Spleen deficiency usually results from improper diet, especially excess consumption of cold, raw, or oily foods. When Spleen *qi* is deficient, the function of transformation and transportation of *qi* and fluids is impaired, leading to the formation of dampness-heat. Dampness-heat accumulates and may transform into fire, lead to *qi* stagnation and Blood stasis,[4] or move outward toward the skin producing fluid-filled vesicles.[5] Herpes zoster may also arise due to exogenous pathogenic toxins on the skin. Residual toxins become trapped in the channels and vessels and obstruct *qi* movement, leading to *qi* stagnation and Blood stasis.[5] Syndromes may exist in isolation or may co-exist in the acute stage.

After dampness-heat has resolved, the patient may develop or continue to present with the syndrome of *qi* stagnation and Blood stasis. This syndrome can present in the recovery stage and may continue beyond the resolution of the rash.

Syndrome Differentiation and Treatments

In contemporary CM literature, the treatment principle for herpes zoster is related to the manifesting syndrome. The three main syndromes which are generally accepted to be present in cases of herpes zoster include: 1) stagnated heat in the Liver meridian, 2) Spleen deficiency syndrome with damp retention, and 3) *qi* stagnation and Blood stasis. These syndromes are described in the *Criteria of Diagnosis and Therapeutic Effect of Diseases and Syndromes in Traditional Chinese Medicine* 中医病证诊断疗效标准, published by the State Administration of Traditional Chinese Medicine of the People's Republic of China in 1994,[6] and the *Guidelines for Diagnosis and Treatment of Common Diseases of Dermatology in Traditional Chinese Medicine* 中医皮肤科常见病诊疗指南 published by the Chinese Medical Association in 2012.[2] Both guidelines were used as references for the following section, in addition to other key textbooks and practice guidelines. Syndrome names were referenced to the standard terminologies published by the World Health Organisation.[7]

The use of some herbs may be restricted in some countries. In addition, some herbs are restricted under the provisions of the Convention on International Trade in Endangered Species of Wild Fauna and Flora (CITES). Readers are advised to comply with relevant regulations.

Oral Chinese Herbal Medicine Treatment Based on Syndrome Differentiation

Stagnated Heat in the Liver Meridian or Dampness and Heat in the Liver and Gallbladder

Clinical manifestations: Light skin rash, clustered blisters with tense surface, or haemorrhagic or gangrenous skin damage and sharp pain in severe cases. Other symptoms include bitter mouth, dry throat, irritability, sticky stool, and dark yellow urine; red tongue with yellow and thin (or thick or sticky) coating, taut, smooth and rapid pulse.[8–10]

Treatment principle: Subdue pathogenic fire in Liver, promote *qi* and Blood circulation, and clear dampness-heat and toxins.[2]

Formula: Modified *Long dan xie gan tang* 龙胆泻肝汤 (加减).[2]

Herbs: *Long dan cao* 龙胆草, *zhi zi* 栀子, *huang qin* 黄芩, *chai hu* 柴胡, *di huang* 地黄, *che qian zi* 车前子, *tong cao* 通草, *dang gui* 当归, *ban lan gen* 板蓝根, *mu dan pi* 牡丹皮, *chi shao* 赤芍, *zi cao* 紫草, etc. (for modifications).

Main actions of the herbs: *Long dan cao* 龙胆草, *zhi zi* 栀子, *huang qin* 黄芩, and *ban lan gen* 板蓝根 clear heat. *Mu dan pi* 牡丹皮, *zi cao* 紫草, *di huang* 地黄, and *chi shao* 赤芍 clear heat and regulate Blood. *Che qian zi* 车前子 and *tong cao* 通草 drain dampness. *Chai hu* 柴胡 releases the exterior. *Dang gui* 当归 tonifies the Blood.

Manufactured medicines: *Long dan xie gan wan* 龙胆泻肝丸, *Xin huang pian* 新癀片, *Liu shen wan* 六神丸, *Ji de sheng she yao pian* 季德胜蛇药片, *Qing kai ling kou fu ye* 清开灵口服液, and *Ban lan gen ke li* 板蓝根颗粒.[2,10,11]

Spleen Deficiency Syndrome with Damp Retention

Clinical manifestations: Pale skin rash, blisters with soft surface which are easily broken with inflammatory exudate, and mild to severe pain. Other symptoms include decreased thirst, loss of appetite, abdominal distension, and diarrhoea; pale, tender, soft and enlarged tongue with pale moss coating, slow and deep pulse, or slippery and soft pulse.[8–10]

Treatment principle: Invigorate the Spleen to eliminate dampness and clear heat and toxins.[2]

Formula: Modified *Chu shi wei ling tang* 除湿胃苓汤 (加减).[2]

Herbs: *Cang zhu* 苍术, *hou pu* 厚朴, *chen pi* 陈皮, *fu ling* 茯苓, *ze xie* 泽泻, *bai zhu* 白术, *zhi zi* 栀子, *gan cao* 甘草, *yi yi ren* 薏苡仁, *zhi ke* 枳壳, *bi xie* 萆薢, *tu fu ling* 土茯苓, etc. (for modifications).

Main actions of the herbs: *Cang zhu* 苍术 and *hou pu* 厚朴 transform dampness. *Ze xie* 泽泻, *fu ling* 茯苓, *yi yi ren* 薏苡仁, and *bi xie* 萆薢 drain dampness. *Chen pi* 陈皮 and *zhi ke* 枳壳 regulate *qi*. *Zhi zi* 栀子 clears heat. *Bai zhu* 白术 tonifies the Spleen and drains dampness. *Gan cao* 甘草 harmonises each herb.

Manufactured medicines: *Shen ling bai zhu wan* 参苓白术丸.[11]

Qi Stagnation and Blood Stasis

Clinical manifestations: Rash and blisters resolve, leaving purple macules on the skin. Burning and pain is felt in the local and nearby skin area and the pain can last for several months in severe cases, which usually occurs in older people. Other symptoms include dizziness, fatigue, irritability, restlessness, and constipation; dark-purple tongue or with petechia or spots, with white coating, and taut and unsmooth pulse.[8-10]

Treatment principle: Regulate *qi* and promote Blood circulation, and activate meridians to stop pain.[8]

Formula: Modified *Chai hu shu gan san* 柴胡疏肝散 plus *Tao hong si wu tang* 桃红四物汤 (加减)[8-10] and modified *Xue fu zhu yu tang* 血府逐瘀汤 plus *Jin ling zi san* 金铃子散 (加减).[2]

Herbs: *Chai hu shu gan san* 柴胡疏肝散 plus *Tao hong si wu tang* 桃红四物汤: *chai hu* 柴胡, *chi shao* 赤芍, *chuan xiong* 川芎, *zhi ke* 枳壳, *chen pi* 陈皮, *xiang fu* 香附, *gan cao* 甘草, *tao ren* 桃仁, *hong hua* 红花, *sheng di* 生地, *dang gui* 当归, *bai shao* 白芍, etc. (for modifications).

Xue fu zhu yu tang 血府逐瘀汤 plus *Jin ling zi san* 金铃子散: *tao ren* 桃仁, *hong hua* 红花, *dang gui* 当归, *chuan xiong* 川芎, *bai shao* 白芍, *dan shen* 丹参, *yu jin* 郁金, *wang bu liu xing* 王不留行, *yan hu suo* 延胡索, *chuan lian zi* 川楝子, *xiang fu* 香附, *chai hu* 柴胡, *chen pi* 陈皮, *zhi ke* 枳壳, *gan cao* 甘草, etc. (for modifications).

Main actions of the herbs: *Chen pi* 陈皮, *xiang fu* 香附, *zhi ke* 枳壳, *chuan lian zi* 川楝子 and *jin ling zi* 金铃子 regulate *qi*. *Chi shao* 赤芍, *chuan xiong* 川芎, *dan shen* 丹参, *hong hua* 红花, *niu xi*

牛膝, *tao ren* 桃仁, *yan hu suo* 延胡索, and *yu jin* 郁金 regulate Blood. *Dang gui* 当归 and *bai shao* 白芍 tonify Blood. *Chai hu* 柴胡 releases the exterior. *Sheng di* 生地 clears heat. *Jie geng* 桔梗 transforms phlegm. *Gan cao* 甘草 harmonises each herb.

Manufactured medicines: *Xin huang pian* 新癀片, *Xue fu zhu yu pian* 血府逐瘀片, *Da huang zhe chong wan* 大黄蛰虫丸, and *Yuan hu zhi tong jiao nang* 元胡止痛胶囊.[2,11]

Topical Chinese Herbal Medicine Treatment

Topical application of Chinese herbal medicine (CHM) can be used to aid healing of lesions and includes ointments, lotions, and liquids. Treatments vary according to the lesion stage.

Early lesions and unbroken blisters: Topical treatment with *Qing dai gao* 青黛膏 (ointment), *Yu lu gao* 玉露膏 (ointment), *Qing liang ru ji* 清凉乳剂 (lotion), *San huang xi ji* 三黄洗剂 (lotion), *Shuang bai san* 双柏散 (powder), *Dian dao san* 颠倒散 (powder), *Er wei ba du san* 二味拔毒散 (powder), or mashed fresh *ma chi xian* 鲜马齿苋, leaves of *ye ju hua* 野菊花叶, and mashed leaves of *yu zhan hua* 玉簪花叶.[8–10,12]

Broken blisters with small amount of exudate: Topical treatment with *Si huang gao* 四黄膏 (ointment), *Huang lian gao* 黄连膏 (ointment), *Qing dai gao* 青黛膏 (ointment), *Huang ling dan* 黄灵丹 (powder), *Jin huang san* 金黄散 (powder), *Yun nan bai yao* 云南白药; if necrosis appears, alternatively apply *Jiu yi dan* 九一丹 (powder) and *Hai fu san* 海浮散 (powder).[2,8–10,13]

Broken blisters with large amount of exudate: Hydropathic compress with boiled *ku fan* 枯矾, *ma chi xian* 马齿苋, *huang lian* 黄连, *da huang* 大黄, *ku shen* 苦参, *di yu* 地榆, *wu bei zi* 五倍子, and *gan cao* 甘草; or hydropathic compress with cold *Fu fang huang bai ye* 复方黄柏液 (liquid); or apply *zi cao* oil 紫草油 or *qing dai* oil 青黛油 on the infected area.[2,8–10,12]

Large unbroken blisters: Use a three-edged needle or sterilised needle to prick the blisters and clear all liquids to reduce the burning and discomfort.[8,10,12]

Table 2.1   Summary of Chinese Herbal Medicines for Herpes Zoster

Syndrome Differentiation	Treatment Principle	Key Formula
Stagnated heat in Liver meridian 肝经郁热	Subdue pathogenic fire in the Liver, promote Blood circulation and detoxification 清肝泻火, 活血解毒	Long dan xie gan tang 龙胆泻肝汤
Spleen deficiency syndrome with damp retention 脾虚湿蕴	Invigorate Spleen to eliminate dampness, clear heat and detoxify 健脾化湿, 清热解毒	Chu shi wei ling tang 除湿胃苓汤
Qi stagnation and Blood stasis 气滞血瘀	Regulate qi and promote Blood circulation, activate meridians to stop pain 理气活血, 通络止痛	Chai hu shu gan san 柴胡疏肝散 plus Tao hong si wu tang 桃红四物汤; Xue fu zhu yu tang 血府逐瘀汤 plus Jin ling zi san 金铃子散

Dry scabs: Topical treatment with *Bing shi san* 冰石散 (powder), *huang lian gao* 黄连膏 (ointment), or *Shi run shao shang gao* 湿润烧伤膏 (ointment).[9,11]

Acupuncture Therapies

A range of acupuncture therapies have been recommended in key textbooks and guidelines.[8–10,13,14] Recommended interventions include acupuncture (body, ear, and scalp), moxibustion, and magnetic therapy. Many acupuncture points have been recommended in addition to the use of *ashi* points 阿是穴. The selection of points is based on each point's function or location, with points local to the rash being suggested. Treatment details are outlined in Table 2.2.

Analysis of key acupuncture points:[15]

- LI11 *Quchi* 曲池 — clears heat, resolves dampness, cools Blood, regulates nutritive *qi* and Blood, and expels exterior wind;

- PC6 *Neiguan* 内关 — opens the chest, regulates and clears the Triple Energiser, calms the mind, and harmonises the Stomach;
- SP6 *Sanyinjiao* 三阴交 — resolves damp, nourishes Blood and *yin*, cools Blood, stops pain, and strengthens the Spleen;

Table 2.2 Summary of Acupuncture Therapies for Herpes Zoster

Intervention	Acupuncture Points/Body Area
Acupuncture	Main points: LI11 Quchi 曲池, PC6 Neiguan 内关, LI4 Hegu 合谷, GB34 Yanglingquan 阳陵泉, SP6 Sanyinjiao 三阴交, ST36 Zusanli 足三里 Supplementary points: • For lesions around the eyes: EX-HN5 Taiyang 太阳, ST8 Touwei 头维, GB14 Yangbai 阳白 • For lesions on the cheeks: ST2 Sibai 四白, ST7 Xiaguan 下关, BL1 Jingming 睛明 • For lesions on the chin: ST4 Dicang 地仓, ST5 Daying 大迎, ST6 Jiache 颊车 • For lesions under the arms: SI9 Jianzhen 肩贞, HT1 Jiquan 极泉 • For chronic pain: TE6 Zigou 支沟; or with ashi points 阿是穴 around the affected area • For burning pain: EX-B2 Jiaji points 夹脊 on the same body side as the rash, GB34 Yanglingquan 阳陵泉
Electro-acupuncture	Ashi points 阿是穴 around the infected area
Ear acupuncture	CO12 Liver 肝, TF4 Shenmen 神门, AH6a Jiaogan 交感, CO14 Lung 肺, TG2p Shenshangxian 肾上腺
Scalp acupuncture	Sensory area, motor area
Moxibustion	Moxibustion roll: apply to affected area Moxa cone moxibustion: to select acupuncture point, measure the patient's head circumference using a thread. Place the centre of the thread at the front of the patient's neck and place ends on the patient's back, with both ends level. Moxa cones are placed at the level of the thread ends. "Burning rush moxibustion": affected area
Acupuncture-point magnetic therapy	Not specified

- ST36 *Zusanli* 足三里 — tonifies *qi* and Blood, benefits the Stomach and Spleen, expels wind and damp, regulates nutritive and defensive *qi*, and dispels cold.

Acupuncture

Acupuncture points which have the function of clearing heat and dampness, clearing stagnation, and tonifying *qi* and Blood should be selected as main points (see Table 2.2). Supplementary points can be selected according to the location of the rash. Treatment should be administered every second day for 10 days. Reducing manipulation should be used for young, healthy patients, while mild reinforcing-reducing manipulation should be used for aged or weak patients. When selecting EX-B2 *Jiaji* points 夹脊 and GB34 *Yanglingquan* 阳陵泉 for burning pain, use reinforcing-reducing manipulation.[8,9]

Electro-acupuncture

Ashi points 阿是穴 around the affected area can be used with moderate reducing manipulation. After manual stimulation, apply electrical stimulation for 30–40 minutes after the patient feels a sensation of numbness or distension.[14]

Ear Acupuncture

Administer treatment every second day for seven days, with needles retained for 30 minutes each time.[9] See Table 2.2 for acupuncture points.

Scalp Acupuncture

Acupuncture should be applied to the sensory and motor areas on the opposite side to the location of the rash. If the affected area is above the navel, stimulate the lower 3/5 of the sensory and motor areas; if below the navel, stimulate the upper 2/5 of the sensory and motor areas. *Deqi* 得气 should be obtained and needles retained for 30 to 45 minutes. Needles should be stimulated several times during treatment, with treatment administered daily for 10 days.[10]

Moxibustion

Various methods of moxibustion have been recommended in textbooks and guidelines. A moxibustion roll can be applied to the rash location. Light the moxa roll, hold it over the affected area, and slowly move the moxa roll to warm the whole area. This should be applied daily for 20–30 minutes.[13] Moxa cone moxibustion is applied to the back (see Table 2.2), with one moxa cone per day.[13] Burning rush moxibustion uses rushes soaked in sesame oil, and one end of the rush is lit and held over the lesions to warm.[13] Other techniques include garlic moxibustion, cotton stick moxibustion, moxibustion around the eyes, and heat-sensitive moxibustion.[14]

Acupuncture-point Magnetic Therapy

A magnetic disc is applied on the selected acupuncture points. The magnetic disc is retained for three days, after which it is removed for another three days, constituting one course.[13]

Other Chinese Medicine Therapies

In addition to CHM and acupuncture techniques, other CM therapies have been recommended to treat the acute stage of herpes zoster. These include plum-blossom needle therapy and cupping. Plum-blossom needle therapy can be applied to *ashi* points 阿是穴 or along the meridian.[16] The procedure may have minor or no bleeding.[16]

Other Management Strategies

Patients can be encouraged to be involved in their own healthcare as various strategies can be taught as self-management practices. Prevention of herpes zoster may be possible by maintaining a healthy lifestyle, including exercise for physical and emotional wellbeing and ensuring adequate sleep.[13] Good health allows the body to fight disease should it occur.[13] The herpes zoster vaccine may be considered to prevent the development of herpes zoster.[13] If herpes zoster does develop, treatment should be sought quickly and be ongoing during the acute stage.[13] Conventional medicine should be used in the acute stage to reduce the incidence of PHN.[13]

Lifestyle advice which can be provided to patients includes:

- Avoiding exposure to people affected with the varicella zoster virus (chickenpox) or herpes zoster;[13]
- Dressing appropriately for the weather and paying attention to changes in weather to prevent the common cold;[13]
- Maintaining a healthy lifestyle with adequate time for rest and sleep;[13]
- Maintaining a healthy immune system;[13]
- Avoiding excessive mental stimulation and overwork;[13]
- Focusing on mindfulness and emotional wellbeing;[13]
- Ensuring adequate time for recuperation after the acute stage of herpes zoster;[13] and
- Maintaining regular diet and bowel movements.[9]

Diet recommendations include avoiding fatty, oily, sweet, and spicy foods as well as seafood. Diet should be light with adequate amounts of fruits and vegetables.[8,9] Dietary therapy according to CM principles can include the preparation of broth and rice porridge.[13] Rice porridge can be prepared using 30 to 60g of *yi yi ren* 薏苡仁 cooked with rice.[13] This can be used for all herpes zoster syndromes and is especially helpful for cases with dampness heat in the Spleen and Stomach. An alternate recipe uses 100 to 200g of *ma chi xian* 马齿苋 cooked with rice, with a small amount of salt added according to taste preferences.[13] This can be used for syndromes of dampness-heat in the Liver meridian or dampness-heat in the Spleen and Stomach. A broth may also be considered, prepared with 60g of *xi qian gen* 豨莶根 (the root of *xi qian cao* 豨莶草) stewed with a pig hoof 猪蹄 and 100ml of rice wine 黄酒.[13]

References

1. 黄尧洲. 皮肤病中医特色诊疗[M]. 北京: 人民军医出版社; 2008.
2. 中华中医药学会. 中医皮肤科常见病诊疗指南. 北京: 中国中医药出版社; 2012.
3. Shen DH, Wu XF, Wang N. *Manual of Dermatology in Chinese Medicine*. Seattle: Eastland Press Inc; 1995.
4. 禤国维, 陈达灿. 中西医结合皮肤性病学. 北京: 科学出版社; 2008.
5. Xu Y. *Dermatology in Traditional Chinese Medicine*. St Albans, UK: Donica Publishing; 2004.
6. 国家中医药管理局. 中医病证诊断疗效标准. 南京: 南京大学出版社; 1994.
7. World Health Organization. Regional Office for the Western Pacific 2007, WHO International Standard Terminologies on Traditional Medicine in the Western Pacific Region. World Health Organization, Western Pacific Region, Geneva
8. 李曰庆, 何清湖. 中医外科学[M]. 北京: 中国中医药出版社; 2012.
9. 陈德宇. 中西医结合皮肤性病学[M]. 北京: 中国中医药出版社; 2012.
10. 杨志波, 范瑞强, 邓丙戌. 中医皮肤性病学[M]. 北京: 中国中医药出版社; 2010.
11. 刘巧. 中医皮肤病诊疗学[M]. 北京: 人民卫生出版社; 2014.
12. 李元文. 中医皮肤科临证必备[M]. 北京: 人民军医出版社; 2014.
13. 陈达灿, 范瑞强. 皮肤性病科专病中医临床诊治[M]. 北京: 人民卫生出版社; 2013.
14. 范瑞强. 带状疱疹[M]. 北京: 中国中医药出版社; 2012.
15. Deadman P & Al-Khafaji M. (2007). *A Manual of Acupuncture*, 2nd ed. East Sussex, UK: *Journal of Chinese Medicine Publications*.
16. 欧阳卫权. 皮肤病中医外治特色疗法精选[M]. 广州: 广东科技出版社; 2013.

3

Classical Chinese Medicine Literature

OVERVIEW

The classical Chinese medicine literature provides a valuable resource for the prevention and management of disease. This chapter describes the findings of a systematic evaluation of the classical Chinese medicine literature for herpes zoster. A search was conducted on the *Zhong Hua Yi Dian*, one of the largest collections of extant medical works available, and a total of 65 citations describing the treatment of herpes zoster with Chinese medicine were identified. Characteristics of search terms, aetiology and pathogenesis, and clinical management with Chinese herbal medicine and acupuncture techniques are described.

Introduction

Written records of the professional practice of Chinese medicine (CM) date back to the Spring and Autumn (770–476 BC) and Warring states (474–221 BC) periods. In these passages, concepts such as *yin* and *yang* are evident and therapeutic methods included the use of mugwort (*ai* 艾) for moxibustion, herbal decoctions, and acupuncture.[1] Classical CM texts provide a valuable source of information to guide patient management. Clinical cases are described in depth, including detailed explanations of aetiology and pathogenesis, symptoms, and clinical management. Some of this information has contributed to the knowledge of herpes zoster and continues to guide current practice.

Herpes zoster has been described in early classical works. Contemporary texts suggest that descriptions of herpes zoster in classical texts were closely related to symptoms.[2] As such, various terms have been used to describe herpes zoster. In an attempt to standard-ise the terminology, Professor Bingnan Zhao proposed the term *she chuan chuang* 蛇串疮 to be the official name for herpes zoster,[3] and this was accepted and included in contemporary texts. The history of events preceding this proposal remains unclear.

The classical CM literature is vast, but digitalised collections allow for systematic searches and review.[4,5] In order to obtain a sample of the classical and pre-modern CM literature, we conducted electronic searches of the *Zhong Hua Yi Dian* (ZHYD 中华医典) CD-ROM.[6] This collection is the largest currently avail-able and is representative of other large collections of the classical and pre-modern CM literature.[4,5] The findings from the systematic evaluation of the classical literature for herpes zoster are described below.

Search Terms

In order to identify relevant search terms, more than 10 CM works on dermatological and general medicine were hand-searched in 2014. A CM dermatologist was also consulted to identify any additional terms not located through other searches. As many terms have been used to describe herpes zoster historically, a total of 30 search terms were included (see Table 3.1). Many of the search terms describe a red rash

Table 3.1 Terms Used to Identify Classical Literature Citations

Pinyin	Chinese Characters
Bai she chan yao	白蛇缠腰
Chan yao	缠腰
Chan yao chuang	缠腰疮
Chan yao dan	缠腰丹
Chan yao huo dan	缠腰火丹

(*Continued*)

Table 3.1 (*Continued*)

Pinyin	Chinese Characters
Chan yao huo long	缠腰火龙
Chan yao long	缠腰龙
Chuan yao long	串腰龙
Feng chi chuang yi	风赤疮痍
Huo dai chuang	火带疮
Huo dan	火丹
Huo dan chuang	火丹疮
Huo liao chuang	火燎疮
Huo yao dai	火腰带
Huo yao dai du	火腰带毒
Pao zhen	疱疹
Pu xing zhen	匍行疹
She chan chuang	蛇缠疮
She chan dan	蛇缠丹
She chan hu dai	蛇缠虎带
She chuan chuang	蛇串疮
She dan	蛇丹
She dan yu hou tong	蛇丹愈后痛
She ke chuang	蛇窠疮
She pan chuang	蛇盘疮
She xing dan 1	蛇型丹
She xing dan 2	蛇形丹
Sheng she	生蛇
Zeng dai chuang	甑带疮
Zhi zhu chuang	蜘蛛疮

(for example, *huo dan* 火丹, *huo liao chuang* 火燎疮), a rash which affects the waist/belt area (for example, *chan yao* 缠腰, *huo dai chuang* 火带疮, *huo yao dai* 火腰带), or a rash shaped like a snake (for example, *she dan* 蛇丹, *she chuan chuang* 蛇串疮, *she can hu dai* 蛇缠虎带).

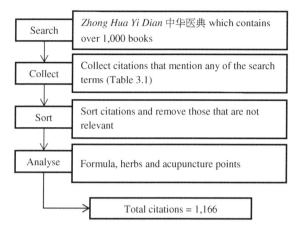

Figure 3.1 Classical literature citations.

Search Procedure and Data Coding

Selected search terms were entered into the search fields of the ZHYD and searches of both the headings and text were conducted (see Fig. 3.1). The search results were downloaded into spreadsheets for data cleaning. A citation was defined as a distinct passage of text referring to one or more of the search terms. Codes were allocated for specific citations, books, and the dynasties in which they were written according to the procedures described in May *et al.*[5] Books written after 1949 were excluded from analysis.

Data Analysis Procedure

The number of hits identified by both heading and text searches were summed to provide the total number of hits for each search term. After removing duplicates, exclusion criteria were applied to remove citations which were judged to be unrelated to herpes zoster. Citations were also excluded if they were unrelated to skin disease, clearly described skin conditions other than herpes zoster, or reported ocular herpes zoster (considered a complication of herpes zoster). Citations which contained no information or insufficient information to judge the likelihood of the reported condition being herpes zoster were also excluded.

Citations were further coded for the likelihood of being herpes zoster based on symptom descriptions. Symptom description terms were grouped according to the distribution of the rash ('belt' 带, 'snake' 蛇, 'encircling' 缠/绕, 'string of beads' 串珠, 'patch' 斑片), the description of pain ('pain' 痛, 'burning pain' 灼痛), the appearance of the rash ('blister' 疱/泡, 'papules' 疹, 'erythema/red spot' 红斑, 'red' 红, 'yellow' 黄, 'white' 白), accompanying symptoms ('itch' 痒), and description of 'heat' 热.

Citations were judged as to whether they were 'possibly' herpes zoster (that is, contained some symptoms but some uncertainty remained) or 'most likely' to be herpes zoster (that is, contained symptoms which are most representative of herpes zoster). Citations that described two of the three symptom categories, namely lesion distribution, lesion appearance, and pain, were judged as 'possibly' herpes zoster citations (see Table 3.2). These citations may or may not have included descriptions of lesion colour, itch, or heat. Citations that described all three symptom categories (lesion distribution, lesion appearance, and pain) were judged to be 'most likely' herpes zoster citations. Again, these citations may or may not have included

Table 3.2   Criteria for Judgment of Herpes Zoster Citations

Symptom Category	Symptom	'Possibly' Herpes Zoster	'Most Likely' Herpes Zoster
Lesion distribution	Belt 带, snake 蛇, encircling 缠/绕, string of beads 串珠, patch 斑片	Described two of these three symptom categories	Described all three symptom categories
Lesion appearance	Blister 疱/泡, papules 疹, erythema/red spot 红斑		
Pain	Pain 痛, burning pain 灼痛		
Lesion colour	Red 红, yellow 黄, white 白	+/-	+/-
Itch	Itch 痒	+/-	+/-
Heat	Heat 热	+/-	+/-

descriptions of lesion colour, itch, or heat. Judgments were made by two researchers independently, in consultation with dermatological experts.

All relevant citations were reviewed to identify the best descriptions of herpes zoster and its aetiology and pathogenesis. Relevant citations that did not provide a description of treatment were excluded from further analysis. The final data set included citations that were considered to potentially refer to herpes zoster ('possibly' and 'most likely' herpes zoster citations), which described treatment with Chinese herbal medicine (CHM), acupuncture and related therapies, or other CM therapies.

For citations that included descriptions of multiple treatments, each treatment was considered as a separate citation for calculation of formulas, herbs, or acupuncture points. Citations that were pharmacopeia-type entries were reviewed for eligibility. Pharmacopeia entries that mentioned any of the terms for herpes zoster (see Table 3.1) but did not include a detailed description of the condition or information about treatment were excluded from further analysis. Pharmacopeia entries that included a description of the condition, with or without reference to other herbs, were included. Single acupuncture points were reviewed in a similar manner.

Included citations were grouped according to the CM intervention for further analysis. Frequency of formulas, herbs, and acupuncture points are presented for two groups:

- 'Possible' herpes zoster, which included citations judged as either possible or most likely to be herpes zoster, and
- 'Most likely' which included only those citations judged as most likely to be herpes zoster.

Search Results

A search of the ZHYD identified 1,166 instances (or hits) of the 30 search terms (see Table 3.3). The search term that produced the

Table 3.3   Hit Frequency by Search Term

Pinyin	Chinese Characters	Hit Frequency n (%)
Huo dan	火丹	853 (73.2)
Chan yao	缠腰	149 (12.8)
Chan yao huo dan	缠腰火丹	89 (7.6)
Sheng she	生蛇	72 (6.2)
Pao zhen	疱疹	33 (2.8)
Zhi zhu chuang	蜘蛛疮	32 (2.7)
She dan	蛇丹	29 (2.5)
Huo dan chuang	火丹疮	26 (2.2)
Chan yao dan	缠腰丹	22 (1.9)
Huo dai chuang	火带疮	20 (1.7)
She chan chuang	蛇缠疮	17 (1.5)
She chuan chuang	蛇串疮	17 (1.5)
She chan dan	蛇缠丹	16 (1.4)
She ke chuang	蛇窠疮	12 (1.0)
Feng chi chuang yi	风赤疮痍	10 (0.9)
Bai she chan yao	白蛇缠腰	7 (0.6)
Chan yao long	缠腰龙	4 (0.3)
Chan yao chuang	缠腰疮	3 (0.3)
Pu xing zhen	匍行疹	3 (0.3)
Huo yao dai	火腰带	2 (0.2)
Huo yao dai du	火腰带毒	2 (0.2)
Zeng dai chuang	甑带疮	2 (0.2)
Huo liao chuang	火燎疮	1 (0.1)
She chan hu dai	蛇缠虎带	1 (0.1)
She pan chuang	蛇盘疮	1 (0.1)

Many passages of text were identified by more than one search term; therefore, the sum for all search terms exceeds the total number of instances found in the literature.

highest number of hits was *huo dan* 火丹 (853 hits, 73.2%). All other search terms were identified in less than 15% of all hits, with several terms returning no results. Many of the terms for herpes zoster described in medical texts and dictionaries were found infrequently in classical CM works. Search terms *chan yao huo long* 缠腰火龙, *chuan yao long* 串腰龙, *she dan yu hou tong* 蛇丹愈后痛, *she xing dan 1* 蛇型丹, and *she xing dan 2* 蛇形丹 did not identify any hits (see Table 3.3).

Citations Related to Herpes Zoster

The citations in which hits were identified were reviewed in further detail. After removal of duplications, citations with no or insufficient information, and those related to other skin conditions, 95 citations were identified that were 'possibly' or 'most likely' to be herpes zoster. Thirty of these were descriptions of the condition which did not include any treatment, and 65 described treatment with either CHM, acupuncture and related therapies, or other approaches. All relevant citations were reviewed to identify passages of text with detailed descriptions of the aetiology and pathogenesis of herpes zoster.

Definitions of Herpes Zoster and Aetiology

Many of the citations contained rich descriptions of herpes zoster, with several describing the aetiology and pathogenesis. The earliest citation comes from *Hua Tuo Shen Fang* 华佗神方 (c. 682) which said that the 'lesion occurs under the waist area, with a length of one or two *cun*. Some skin rash distributes like small rice; some are red colour and hard' (《华佗神方》 c. 682, "生腰下, 长一二寸, 或碎如饭, 或红腰坚硬。").

Other citations suggested that *chan yao huo dan* 缠腰火丹 has two main types, specifically 'dry and damp, and can be differentiated by the lesion colour: red and yellow' (from *Wai Ke Xin Fa Yao Jue* 《外科心法要诀》 c. 1742, "缠腰火丹蛇串名, 干湿红黄似珠形, 肝心脾肺风热湿, 缠腰已遍不能生。若腰肋生之, 系肝火妄动"). The dry type, characterised by red lesions with a 'patchy appearance and small vesicles above the base', is due to heat and wind in the Liver and Heart (from *Yan Fang Xin Bian* 《验方新编》c. 1892, "干者，色红形如云片上起风粟，作痒发热，此心肝二经风火"). The damp type, characterised by yellow lesions with 'white vesicles unequal in size', is caused by the dampness and heat in the Spleen and Lung (from *Tong Yuan Yi Shu — Wai Ke* 《彤园医书-外科》c. 1796, "俗名蛇串疮，有干湿红黄之别。湿者色黄，串起水泡大小不等，溃流黄水，较前多疼，此属脾肺湿热"). Several citations described the aetiology in terms of the location of the rash; for instance, rash located around the waist or chest was due to Liver fire.

The citation described earlier from *Hua Tuo Shen Fang* 华佗神方 (c. 682) is the earliest description of treatment for herpes zoster identified in the ZHYD. The citation describes a topical treatment with the herb *xiong huang* 雄黄: 'Treatment: *xiong huang* 雄黄, combined with vinegar and apply on the rash. This formula works well.' (《华佗神方》c. 682, 以: 雄黄, 研末, 醋调敷, 极效").

One citation included a comprehensive explanation of the aetiology and pathogenesis, characteristics of the condition, and a total of six extensive treatment options. The citation was from *Wai Ke Zheng Zhi Quan Shu* 外科证治全书 (c. 1617) and described herpes zoster as being of either the dry or damp type. The dry type was characterised by red lesions and was associated with heat and wind in the Liver and Gallbladder. The dry type should be treated with *Long dan xie gan tang* 龙胆泻肝汤. The damp type was characterised by yellow lesions and was due to damp-heat in the Liver and Spleen. The damp type could be treated with *Wei ling tang* 胃苓汤, used with *shan zhi zi* 山栀子, *fang feng* 防风, and *shi gao* 石膏. Pricking the lesion to break the skin was also recommended for damp-type herpes zoster (from *Wai Ke Zheng Zhi Quan Shu* 《外科证治全书》 c. 1617, "生腰肋间, 累累如珠形, 有干湿不同, 红黄之异。干者色红赤, 形如云片, 上起风粟, 作痒发热, 属肝胆风热, 宜服龙胆泻肝汤。湿者色黄, 或起白水泡, 大小不等, 作热, 烂流水, 较干者更疼, 属肝脾湿热, 宜服胃苓汤加山栀、防风、石膏, 其小泡用线针穿破。").

Chinese Herbal Medicine

'Possibly' and 'most likely' herpes zoster citations which described multiple CM treatments were split into separate citations for further analysis. The 65 citations which contained treatments were split into 103 separate treatment citations, 94 of which included descriptions of CHM treatment. Several citations were identified by more than one search term. The 94 treatment citations were found in 37 books, with 20 books producing two or more treatment citations. The book which produced the highest number of citations was *Wai Ke Xin Fa Yao Jue* 外科心法要诀 (c. 1742), with 12 CHM treatment citations included.

Frequency of Treatment Citations by Dynasty

The majority of treatment citations were identified in books from the Ming dynasty (c. 1369–1644) and Qing dynasty (c. 1645–1911), with more than two thirds (77.7%) coming from the Qing dynasty (see Table 3.4). The earliest treatment citation was from *Hua Tuo Shen Fang* 华佗神方 (c. 682) and was identified by the search term *chan yao* 缠腰. The most recent citation was from *Ben Cao Jian Yao Fang* 本草简要方 (c. 1938) and was identified by the term *she chan dan* 蛇缠丹.

Table 3.4   Citations by Dynasty

Dynasty	No. of Treatment Citations
Before Tang Dynasty (before 618)	0
Tang and 5 Dynasties (618–960)	1
Song and Jin Dynasties (961–1271)	0
Yuan Dynasty (1272–1368)	1
Ming Dynasty (1369–1644)	18
Qing Dynasty (1645–1911)	73
MinGuo/Republic of China (1912–1949)	1
Total	**94**

The contemporary medical term for herpes zoster is *she chuan chuang* 蛇串疮. Surprisingly, *she chuan chuang* 蛇串疮 was not identified in 'possibly' herpes zoster citations from the most recent MinGuo period. The reasons for this are unclear, but it is possible that this may be due to fewer citations in the MinGuo period overall. The earliest citation of *she chuan chuang* 蛇串疮 was found in *Ben Cao Bei Yao* 本草备要 (c. 1694) and the most recent citation in *Wai Ke Bei Yao* 外科备要 (c. 1904).

Symptoms Described in Treatment Citations

Thirty CHM treatment citations described symptoms of herpes zoster, with symptoms most commonly affecting the waist (22 citations). This finding is consistent with contemporary descriptions of herpes zoster where dermatomes innervated by the thoracic nerves are among the most common presentations.[7] Other locations for the rash included the abdomen, neck, limbs, and skin (generally). Symptoms most commonly described in citations included skin redness 红 (17 citations) and 'encircling' 缠/绕 (16 citations). Other symptom descriptions included 'snake' 蛇 (11 citations), 'string of beads' 串珠 (10 citations), pain 痛 (9 citations), and yellow 黄 (8 citations). While some of these terms can be common to other skin conditions, several terms are unique to contemporary descriptions of herpes zoster, including 'burning pain' 灼痛 and 'belt' 带. These terms may thus be reliable in identifying citations of herpes zoster in the classical CM literature.

Treatment with Chinese Herbal Medicine

The treatments described in 'possibly' herpes zoster citations were analysed. If ingredients were not specified in the included citation, the book where the citation was found was searched to identify other instances of the same formula which listed the ingredients. If identified, these ingredients were used for analysis.

Most Frequent Formulas in 'Possible' Herpes Zoster Citations

Of the 94 treatment citations, 33 described two or more treatments for herpes zoster. Two citations were single herb citations describing *bai shan ni* 白鳝泥 (white eel) and *jian chun luo* 剪春罗 (*Lychnis coronata* Thunb.) for topical use. The remaining citations included 41 named and 51 unnamed formulas. Five named formulas were described in two or more citations (see Table 3.5), although different

Table 3.5   Most Frequent Formulas in 'Possible' Herpes Zoster Citations

Formula Name	Herb Ingredients	No. of Citations
Long dan xie gan tang 龙胆泻肝汤 (oral)	Long dan cao 龙胆草, lian qiao 连翘, sheng di 生地, ze xie 泽泻, che qian zi 车前子, mu tong 木通, huang qin 黄芩, huang lian 黄连, dang gui 当归, zhi zi 栀子, gan cao 甘草, sheng jun 生军 (da huang 大黄)	10
Chai hu qing gan tang/san 柴胡清肝汤/散 (oral)	Chai hu 柴胡, huang qin 黄芩, shan zhi 山栀 (zhi zi 栀子), chuan xiong 川芎, jie geng 桔梗, gan cao 甘草, lian qiao 连翘	6
Bai ye san 柏叶散 (topical)	Ce bai ye 侧柏叶, qiu yin fen 蚯蚓粪, huang bai 黄柏, da huang 大黄, xiong huang 雄黄, chi xiao dou 赤小豆, qing fen 轻粉	4
Chu shi wei ling tang 除湿胃苓汤 (oral)	Wei ling tang 胃苓汤 (cang zhu 苍术, hou pu 厚朴, chen pi 陈皮, zhu ling 猪苓, ze xie 泽泻, fu ling 茯苓, bai zhu 白术, rou gui 肉桂, gan cao 甘草), zhi zi 栀子, hua shi 滑石, fang feng 防风	3
Ru yi jin huang san 如意金黄散 (topical)	Ru yi jin huang san 如意金黄散 (tian hua fen 天花粉, huang bai 黄柏, da huang 大黄, jiang huang 姜黄, bai zhi 白芷, hou pu 厚朴, chen pi 陈皮, gan cao 甘草, cang zhu 苍术, tian nan xing 天南星), xin ji shui 新汲水, dian zhi 靛汁	2

Note: The use of some herbs such as mu tong 木通 may be restricted in some countries under the provisions of CITES. Readers are advised to comply with relevant regulations.

herb ingredient lists were seen. The herb ingredient list from the earliest citation is presented as it is likely that earlier formulas were representative of subsequent formulas.

Two formulas identified in included citations are recommended in key textbooks and clinical practice guidelines (see Chapter 2) — *Long dan xie gan tang* 龙胆泻肝汤 and *Chu shi wei ling tang* 除湿胃苓汤. Two formulas listed base formulas in their ingredient list (*Chu shi wei ling tang* 除湿胃苓汤 and *Ru yi jin huang san* 如意金黄散). Base formula ingredients were not specified in the citation but were instead sourced from other sections of the same book to prepare the ingredient list. The most frequently cited formula was *Long dan xie gan tang* 龙胆泻肝汤, which was included in 10 'possibly' herpes zoster citations.

The majority of formulas were prescribed for topical use (54 citations, 57.4%). Twenty-four (26.1%) formulas were for oral use, one was recommended for both oral and topical use, and 13 did not specify the route of administration. Named formulas were more commonly used orally (21 of 41 citations), with nine citations describing topical application and 11 not specifying the route of administration. For unnamed formulas, topical application was described in 45 citations, oral use in three citations, oral plus topical application in one citation, and two citations did not specify the route of administration.

Most Frequent Herbs in 'Possible' Herpes Zoster Citations

In the 94 'possibly' herpes zoster citations describing treatment with CHM, 165 different ingredients were included. Some ingredients included excipients such as sesame oil 麻油/香油, vinegar 醋, and salt 盐 which were used in preparations to bind the herbs. While these excipients do not have a specific therapeutic action, they are important components of the treatment and as such were included in the analysis. A selection of the most frequently used herbs are described in Table 3.6. The most frequent herb was *gan cao* 甘草 which was used in 26 citations. This is unsurprising as *gan cao* 甘草 is frequently used to harmonize ingredients in a formula. Other herbs

Table 3.6 Most Frequent Herbs in 'Possible' Herpes Zoster Citations

Herb Name	Scientific Name	No. of Citations
Gan cao 甘草	*Glycyrrhiza* spp	26
Xiong huang 雄黄	Arsenic disulfide	25
Shan zhi 山栀/zhi zi; 栀子	*Gardenia jasminoides* Ellis	21
Huang qin 黄芩	*Scutellaria baicalensis* Georgi	19
Lian qiao 连翘	*Forsythia suspensa* (Thunb.) Vahl	18
Ma yao 麻油/Xiang yao 香油	Sesame oil	18
Long dan cao 龙胆草	*Gentiana scabra* Bge.	15
Dang gui 当归	*Angelica sinensis* (Oliv.) Diels	14
Da huang 大黄 (sheng jun 生军)	*Rheum* spp	14
Sheng di 生地	*Rehmannia glutinosa* Libosch.	12
Ze xie 泽泻	*Alisma orientalis* (Sam.) Juzep.	12
Huang lian 黄连	*Coptis* spp	11
Mu tong 木通	*Akebia quinata*	11
Che qian zi 车前子	*Plantago asiatica* L.	9
Fang feng 防风	*Saposhnikovia divaricata* (Turcz.) Schischk.	8
Shi you 柿油/shi qi 柿漆/qing you 清油	Oils	8
Chai hu 柴胡	*Bupleurum chinense* DC	7
Chuan xiong 川芎	*Ligusticum chuangxiong* Hort.	6
Qing fen 轻粉	Mercurous chloride	6

Note: The use of some herbs such as mu tong 木通 may be restricted in some countries under the provisions of CITES. Readers are advised to comply with relevant regulations.

frequently cited in 'possibly' herpes zoster citations include *xiong huang* 雄黄 and *shan zhi* 山栀/*zhi zi*/栀子.

Nine of the most frequently cited herbs in Table 3.6 are included in the formula *Long dan xie gan tang* 龙胆泻肝汤. This may be due to *Long dan xie gan tang* 龙胆泻肝汤 being the most common formula in citations judged as 'possibly' herpes zoster. However, it may also reflect the aetiology and syndromes described in several citations that herpes zoster can be due to Liver fire. Many of the most frequently used herbs have heat clearing actions (*zhi zi* 山栀, *huang qin* 黄芩, *lian qiao* 连翘, *long dan cao* 龙胆草, *sheng di* 生地, *huang lian* 黄连, *da huang* 大黄, *ze xie* 泽泻, and *che qian zi* 车前子).

Two of the most frequently used herbs are typically for topical use (*xiong huang* 雄黄 and *qing fen* 轻粉). As the majority of herbal formulas identified in the search were for topical use, the inclusion of only two topical herbs in the most frequently reported herb list is curious. This may reflect great diversity in herbs used topically (with little overlap in herbal ingredients across citations). Alternatively, this may be due to many of the herbs used in topical formula citations traditionally being used orally.

It is notable that *mu tong* 木通 is included in the most frequently used herb list. *Mu tong* 木通 is described in 11 citations and is included in the ingredient list of all citations which described *Long dang xie gan tang* 龙胆泻肝汤. *Mu tong* 木通 is not included in the ingredient list from the *Guidelines for Diagnosis and Treatment of Common Diseases of Dermatology in Traditional Chinese Medicine* 中医皮肤科常见病诊疗指南.[9] The reason why this herb was omitted in recent guidelines is unclear, but the toxicity of *guan mu tong* 关木通 could be a factor. In clinical guidelines, *tong cao* 通草 is recommended instead of *mu tong* 木通 as it has a similar function without toxicity.

Herbs were further examined according to their route of administration (see Table 3.7). Herbs used orally in 'possibly' herpes zoster citations were similar to those in the overall herb list (see Table 3.6). The most frequently cited herb used topically was *xiong huang* 雄黄. Several of the frequently used topical herbs such as *cu* 醋 (vinegar) and *shi you* 柿油 were used as dissolvents and excipients for making topical preparations.

Table 3.7 Most Frequent Herbs in 'Possible' Herpes Zoster Citations by Route of Administration

Herb Name	Scientific Name	No. of Citations
Oral administration		
Gan cao 甘草	*Glycyrrhiza* spp	17
Shan zhi 山栀/zhi zi; 栀子	*Gardenia jasminoides* Ellis	14
Lian qiao 连翘	*Forsythia suspensa* (Thunb.) Vahl	10
Huang qin 黄芩	*Scutellaria baicalensis* Georgi	10
Dang gui 当归	*Angelica sinensis* (Oliv.) Diels	7
Chai hu 柴胡	*Bupleurum chinense* DC	7
Fang feng 防风	*Saposhnikovia divaricata* (Turcz.) Schischk.	7
Chuan xiong 川芎	*Ligusticum chuangxiong* Hort.	6
Ze xie 泽泻	*Alisma orientalis* (Sam.) Juzep.	6
Sheng di 生地	*Rehmannia glutinosa* Libosch.	6
Topical administration		
Xiong huang 雄黄	Arsenic disulfide	20
Ma you 麻油/Xiang you 香油	Sesame oil	16
Shi you 柿油/Shi qi 柿漆/Qing you 清油	Oils	9
Cu 醋/Mi cu 米醋/Chen cu 陈醋	Vinegars	9
Long dan cao 龙胆草	*Gentiana scabra* Bge.	5
Nuo mi fen 糯米粉	*Oryza sativa* L. var glutinosa	5
Yan 盐	Salt	5
Ce bai ye 侧柏叶	*Platycladus orientalis* (L.) Franco	4

Most Frequent Formulas in 'Most Likely' Herpes Zoster Citations

Thirty-nine CHM treatment citations were judged 'most likely' to be herpes zoster based on symptom descriptions. Several citations described more than one CM treatment, 10 citations included unnamed formulas, and 30 citations included 16 named formulas (several formula names were described in multiple citations). A similar

Table 3.8 Most Frequent Formulas in 'Most Likely' Herpes Zoster Citations

Formula Name	Herb Ingredients	No. of Citations
Long dan xie gan tang 龙胆泻肝汤 (oral)	Long dan cao 龙胆草, lian qiao 连翘, sheng di 生地, ze xie 泽泻, che qian zi 车前子, mu tong 木通, huang qin 黄芩, huang lian 黄连, dang gui 当归, zhi zi 栀子, gan cao 甘草, sheng jun 生军 (da huang 大黄)	5
Chai hu qing gan tang/san 柴胡清肝汤/散 (oral)	Chai hu 柴胡, huang qin 黄芩, shan zhi 山栀 (zhi zi 栀子), chuan xiong 川芎, jie geng 桔梗, gan cao 甘草, lian qiao 连翘	4
Bai ye san 柏叶散 (topical)	Ce bai ye 侧柏叶, qiu yin fen 蚯蚓粪, huang bai 黄柏, da huang 大黄, xiong huang 雄黄, chi xiao dou 赤小豆, qing fen 轻粉	3
Chu shi wei ling tang 除湿胃苓汤 (oral)	Fang feng 防风, cang zhu 苍术, chi ling 赤苓 (fu ling 茯苓), chen pi 陈皮, hou pu 厚朴, shan zhi 山栀, mu tong 木通, ze xie 泽泻, hua shi 滑石, gan cao 甘草, bo he 薄荷, bai zhu 白术, zhu ling 猪苓	2

Note: The use of some herbs such as mu tong 木通 may be restricted in some countries under the provisions of CITES. Readers are advised to comply with relevant regulations.

pattern was seen in 'possibly' herpes zoster citations, with four formulas being described in two or more citations (see Table 3.8). Again, the most frequently reported formula was *Long dan xie gan tang* 龙胆泻肝汤, which was described in five citations.

The numbers of formulas used orally and topically were similar (19 and 17, respectively), while three formulas did not specify the route of administration. Unnamed formulas were more likely to be for topical use (nine citations, compared with one citation for oral use), and named formulas were more likely to be used orally (18 citations, compared with eight for topical use and three not specified).

Most Frequent Herbs in 'Most Likely' Herpes Zoster Citations

In the 39 'most likely' herpes zoster treatment citations, a total of 110 herbal ingredients were described. Again, ingredients considered to be excipients were included in the analysis. A selection of the most frequently used herbs are described in Table 3.9. The herbs included in the list are similar to those in the list for 'possibly' herpes zoster citations, with *gan cao* 甘草 being the most frequently used herb.

Five herbs were included in citations 'most likely' to be herpes zoster which were not in the list for 'possibly' herpes zoster citations:

Table 3.9   Most Frequent Herbs in 'Most Likely' Herpes Zoster Citations

Herb Name	Scientific Name	No. of Citations
Gan cao 甘草	*Glycyrrhiza* spp	18
Shan zhi 山栀/Zhi zi 栀子	*Gardenia jasminoides* Ellis	14
Huang qin 黄芩	*Scutellaria baicalensis* Georgi	12
Lian qiao 连翘	*Forsythia suspensa* (Thunb.) Vahl	10
Dang gui 当归	*Angelica sinensis* (Oliv.) Diels	9
Xiong huang 雄黄	Arsenic disulfide	9
Long dan cao 龙胆草	*Gentiana scabra* Bge.	8
Da huang 大黄 (sheng jun 生军)	*Rheum* spp	8
Fang feng 防风	*Saposhnikovia divaricata* (Turcz.) Schischk.	7
Sheng di 生地	*Rehmannia glutinosa* Libosch.	7
Ze xie 泽泻	*Alisma orientalis* (Sam.) Juzep.	7
Chai hu 柴胡	*Bupleurum chinense* DC	6
Huang lian 黄连	*Coptis* spp	6
Mu tong 木通	*Akebia* spp	6
Chuan xiong 川芎	*Ligusticum chuangxiong* Hort.	5

Note: The use of some herbs such as mu tong 木通 may be restricted in some countries under the provisions of CITES. Readers are advised to comply with relevant regulations.

chen pi 陈皮, *chi xiao dou* 赤小豆, *di long fen* 地龙粪 (*qiu yin fen* 蚯蚓粪), *huang bai* 黄柏, and *jie geng* 桔梗. The inclusion of these herbs may be due to the smaller number of citations in this pool, resulting in herbs with lower frequency being included in the list of most frequently used herbs.

As was seen in the 'possibly' herpes zoster citations, the herbs used orally were similar to the most frequently cited herbs (see Table 3.10). Again, *xiong huang* 雄黄 was the most frequently cited herb used topically. When compared with the 'possibly' herpes zoster citations, a greater number of herbs were seen compared

Table 3.10 Most Frequent Herbs in 'Most Likely' Herpes Zoster Citations by Route of Administration

Herb Name	Scientific Name	No. of Citations
Oral administration		
Gan cao 甘草	*Glycyrrhiza* spp	16
Shan zhi 山栀/Zhi zi 栀子	*Gardenia jasminoides* Ellis	12
Huang qin 黄芩	*Scutellaria baicalensis* Georgi	9
Lian qiao 连翘	*Forsythia suspensa* (Thunb.) Vahl	9
Dang gui 当归	*Angelica sinensis* (Oliv.) Diels	7
Chai hu 柴胡	*Bupleurum chinese* DC	6
Fang feng 防风	*Saposhnikovia divaricata* (Turcz.) Schischk.	6
Sheng di 生地	*Rehmannia glutinosa* Libosch.	6
Ze xie 泽泻	*Alisma orientalis* (Sam.) Juzep.	6
Topical administration		
Xiong huang 雄黄	Arsenic disulfide	5
Ce bai ye 侧柏叶	*Platycladus orientalis* (L.) Franco	4
Ma you 麻油/xiang you 香油/ qing you 清油	Oils	4
Da huang 大黄	*Rheum* spp	3
Shi qi 柿漆	*Diospyros kaki* Thunb	3
Qiu yin fen 蚯蚓粪	*Pheretima aspergillum* (Perrier)	3

(Continued)

Table 3.10   (*Continued*)

Herb Name	Scientific Name	No. of Citations
Chi xiao dou 赤小豆	*Phaseolus* spp	3
Qing fen 轻粉	Mercurous chloride	3
Cu 醋/mi cu 米醋/chen cu 陈醋	Vinegars	3
Huang bo 黄柏	*Phellodendron chinense* Schneid.	3
Long dan cao 龙胆草	*Gentiana scabra* Bge.	3

with excipients for making topical preparations. Actions of these herbs include Blood cooling, purgative, and dampness resolving.

Discussion

CHM has been used as early as c. 682 for the treatment of herpes zoster. While a review of syndromes was not undertaken, several citations described the aetiology and pathogenesis of herpes zoster which align with the concepts of syndrome differentiation described by the contemporary literature (see Chapter 2). There is historical evidence for formulas such as *Long dan xie gan tang* 龙胆泻肝汤 and *Chu shi wei ling tang* 除湿胃苓汤, which are used in contemporary practice and recommended in key textbooks and guidelines. Many of the most frequently described herbs in classical literature are key ingredients of the formula *Long dan xie gan tang* 龙胆泻肝汤, which is likely due to *Long dan xie gan tang* 龙胆泻肝汤 being the most frequently cited herbal formula.

Acupuncture and Other Therapies

Nine treatment citations described treatments other than CHM, with several being identified by two or more search terms. One book, *You Ke Zheng Zhu Zhun Sheng* 幼科证治准绳 (c. 1607), produced two citations. These were the earliest citations of acupuncture and therapies identified, while the most recent citation came from *Wai Ke*

Bei Yao 外科备要 (c. 1904). All citations were from the Ming and Qing dynasties and were found using a variety of terms.

Treatment with Acupuncture and Other Therapies

Interventions in Possible Herpes Zoster Citations

Seven citations judged as 'possibly' herpes zoster described acupuncture and other therapies to manage symptoms. Four citations described the use of acupuncture techniques, three of which used a technique of pricking the lesion with a needle. The remaining citation used a technique of pricking the 'head' or start of the length of the lesion ('snakeheads' 蛇头). Three citations used moxibustion, with moxibustion applied at the beginning and end of the length of the lesion 皮损两头 (1 citation) or using the 'seven *cun* 寸' 七寸处 technique (2 citations). The latter technique probably relates to an ancient saying that the 'seven *cun* 寸' point must be hit to kill a snake as it is the likely location of a snake's heart. As classical descriptions liken herpes zoster to a snake, the 'seven *cun* 寸' point was an important point to treat rash in herpes zoster. Two citations used other techniques for the treatment of herpes zoster and both described prayer 祝由 as a form of treatment delivered by the physician.

Interventions in 'Most Likely' Herpes Zoster Citations

The four citations which used acupuncture treatment for herpes zoster that were included in the 'possibly' herpes zoster pool above were all judged to be 'most likely' herpes zoster. Acupuncture treatment involved pricking the lesions to alleviate symptoms. No other citations describing acupuncture or other therapies were judged as 'most likely' herpes zoster.

Discussion

While acupuncture and other therapies have been described in classical CM texts for the treatment of herpes zoster, their use is less frequent than CHM. The techniques used differ somewhat to those recommended in clinical practice guidelines, although the approach of pricking lesions is described in contemporary dermatology textbooks.[8–10]

Classical Literature in Perspective

Herpes zoster has been described by many terms in CM and they are often related to the description of symptoms.[2] This was certainly the case in this review, with many citations including two or more different terms for herpes zoster. The terms *huo dan* 火丹 and *chan yao* 缠腰 produced the greatest number of hits and may have been the most common terms used to describe herpes zoster in the classical literature.

The official contemporary term for herpes zoster, *she chuan chuang* 蛇串疮, was proposed by Professor Bingna Zhao[3] and was adopted in the 2012 guideline.[11] *She chuan chuang* 蛇串疮 identified seven citations (two were 'possibly' and five were 'most likely' herpes zoster), all of which originated from the Qing dynasty. Compared with other terms for herpes zoster, the historical use of the term *she chuan chuang* 蛇串疮 is relatively short. The earliest included citation identified by *she chuan chuang* 蛇串疮 was from *Ben Cao Bei Yao* 本草备要 (c. 1694). The reasons for why this term was selected to be the official name are unclear. Further, the term *sheng she* 生蛇 is commonly used in southern China[2] but failed to identify any citations describing treatment of 'possibly' or 'most likely' cases of herpes zoster as it might not be a formal medical term.

The earliest citation which described the treatment of possible herpes zoster cases came from *Hua Tuo Shen Fang* 华佗神方 (c. 682). Historical discussions of herpes zoster in CM[2,12] suggest that the earliest discussion of herpes zoster in the classical literature comes from the *Zhu Bing Yuan Hou Lun* 诸病源候论 (c. 610 AD). This citation was not identified in this review as it describes *zeng dai chuang* 甑带疮 as being caused by 'wind-dampness and fighting of Blood and *qi*', which differs slightly from the current understanding of the aetiology of herpes zoster (see Chapter 2) and may reflect a change in understanding of herpes zoster over time.

Aetiology and pathogenesis in included citations was largely consistent with how the contemporary literature understands CM, with one exception — none of the included citations specifically described *qi* stagnation and Blood stasis. Again, this may reflect changes in the understanding of herpes zoster over time. *Qi* stagnation has been described in a passage from the *Lin Zheng Yi De Fang* 临证一得方 (c. 1911).[2] While one citation was identified from *Lin Zheng Yi De Fang* 临证一得方, no description of syndromes was provided. Whether *qi* stagnation and/or Blood stasis were described in relation to herpes zoster in earlier CM works is unclear.

Overall, the number of citations that described the CM management of 'possibly' herpes zoster cases was small. Treatments were consistent with those recommended in clinical practice guidelines,[13] with *Long dan xie gan tang* 龙胆泻肝汤 and *Chu shi wei ling tang* 除湿胃苓汤 both described in the classical literature. CM guidelines also recommend the use of the formula *Chai hu shu gan san* 柴胡疏肝散 with *Tao hong si wu tang* 桃红四物汤, although neither of these formulas were identified in the included citations. Clinical practice guidelines recommend the use of both oral and topical formulations, a finding supported by the classical literature.

Herbs commonly used to treat symptoms were aligned with the aetiology and pathogenesis described in the included citations. Herbs that act by clearing heat and detoxifying, draining dampness releasing the exterior, tonifying, and regulating Blood were among the most frequently used herbs. Acupuncture citations described pricking the lesion with the needle. This technique is not included in clinical practice guidelines but is commonly suggested in CM dermatology textbooks. There is little historical evidence for the use of acupuncture and related techniques in the management of herpes zoster.

References

1. Needham J, Lu GD, Sivin, N. (2000) Science and civilisation in China, Vol 5, Pt VI: Medicine. Cambridge: Cambridge University Press.
2. 范瑞强. 带状疱疹[M]. 北京: 中国中医药出版社; 2012.

3. 赵炳南, 张志礼. 简明中医皮肤病学[M]. 北京: 中国中医药出版社; 2014.

4. May B, Lu C, Xue C. Collections of traditional Chinese medical literature as resources for systematic searches. *J Altern Complement Med*. 2012; **18**(12):1101–7.

5. May BH, Li YB, Lu CJ, Zhang AL, Chang S, Xue CCL. Systematic assessment of the representativeness of published collections of the traditional literature on Chinese Medicine. *J Altern Complement Med*. 2013; **19**:403–9.

6. Hu R. Encyclopedia of Traditional Chinese Medicine. 5th ed. Changsha: Hunan Electronic and Audio-Visual Publishing House; 2000.

7. Gershon AA, Gershon MD, Breuer J, *et al*. Advances in the understanding of the pathogenesis and epidemiology of herpes zoster. *J Clin Virol*. 2010; **48**(Suppl 1):S2–7.

8. 李曰庆, 何清湖. 中医外科学[M]. 北京: 中国中医药出版社; 2012.

9. 杨志波, 范瑞强, 邓丙戌. 中医皮肤性病学[M]. 北京: 中国中医药出版社; 2010.

10. 李元文. 中医皮肤科临证必备[M]. 北京: 人民军医出版社; 2014.

11. 中华中医药学会. *中医皮肤科常见病诊疗指南*. 北京: 中国中医药出版社; 2012.

12. 黄尧洲. 皮肤病中医特色诊疗[M]. 北京: 人民军医出版社; 2008.

13. 国家中医药管理局. *中医病证诊断疗效标准*. 南京: 南京大学出版社; 1994.

4

Methods for Evaluating Clinical Evidence — Herpes Zoster

OVERVIEW

This chapter outlines the methods used to identify and evaluate a range of Chinese medicine (CM) therapies for the treatment of herpes zoster in clinical studies. Comprehensive searches identified studies that were screened against rigorous inclusion criteria. An assessment of the methodological quality of the studies was made using standardised methods. Results from included studies were evaluated to provide an estimate of the treatment effects of a range of CM therapies.

Introduction

Treatment of herpes zoster with Chinese medicine (CM) has been described in the contemporary literature and is supported by historical evidence from the classical CM literature. Several systematic reviews have been conducted which have evaluated the efficacy and safety of CM treatment for herpes zoster (see Chapters 5 and 7). These include reviews of Chinese herbal medicines (CHM) and acupuncture and related therapies.

This chapter describes the methods used to evaluate clinical studies which are presented in subsequent chapters. Studies were evaluated following methods proposed by the Cochrane Handbook of Systematic Reviews.[1] Interventions have been categorised as follows:

1. CHM (Chapter 5);
2. Acupuncture and related therapies (Chapter 7);
3. Combination CM therapies (Chapter 8).

References to clinical studies were obtained and assessed by an expert group (see Appendix 1 for full list of included studies). Randomised controlled trials (RCTs) and controlled clinical trials (CCTs) were evaluated using the same approach and are described in detail. The evidence from non-controlled studies is more difficult to evaluate for efficacy and therefore the approach was taken to describe the characteristics of the study, details of the intervention, and any adverse events. No assessment of efficacy in non-controlled studies was made.

Search Strategy

Searches were conducted in English and Chinese databases following the methods outlined in the Cochrane Handbook of Systematic Reviews.[1] English databases included PubMed, Excerpta Medica Database (Embase), Cumulative Index of Nursing and Allied Health Literature (CINAHL), Cochrane Central Register of Controlled Trials (CENTRAL), and Allied and Complementary Medicine Database (AMED); Chinese databases included China BioMedical Literature (CBM), China National Knowledge Infrastructure (CNKI), Chongqing VIP (CQVIP), and Wanfang. Databases were searched from their inception to February 2015. No restrictions were applied and search terms were mapped to controlled vocabulary (where applicable) as well as keyword searches.

To conduct a comprehensive search of the literature, searches were run according to the study design (reviews, controlled trials, and non-controlled studies). This was done for each of the three intervention types (CHM, acupuncture and related therapies, and other CM therapies) resulting in nine searches in each of the nine databases:

- Reviews of CHM;
- controlled trials of CHM (randomised and non-randomised);
- Non-controlled studies of CHM;
- Reviews of acupuncture and related therapies;
- Controlled trials of acupuncture and related therapies (randomised and non-randomised);

- Non-controlled studies of acupuncture and related therapies;
- Reviews of other CM therapies;
- Controlled trials of other CM therapies (randomised and non-randomised);
- Non-controlled studies of other CM therapies.

Studies of combinations of CM therapies were identified through the above searches. In addition to electronic databases, reference lists of systematic reviews and included studies were searched for additional publications. Clinical trials registers were searched to identify clinical trials which were ongoing or completed, and where required, trial investigators were contacted to obtain data. Trial registers included the Australian New Zealand Clinical Trial Registry (ANZCTR), the Chinese Clinical Trial Registry (ChiCTR), the European Union Clinical Trials Register (EU-CTR), and the US National Institutes of Health registry (ClinicalTrials.gov).

If required, trial investigators were contacted by email or telephone to obtain further information, and if no reply was received, a follow up contact after two weeks was made. Where no response was received after one month, any unknown information was marked as not available.

Inclusion Criteria

- Participants: adult participants (aged ≥ 18 years) with a diagnosis of herpes zoster (acute stage), based either on clinical presentation or laboratory tests (e.g., polymerase chain reaction);
- Interventions: CHM, acupuncture and related therapies, or other CM therapies, alone or in combination with other CM therapies or with pharmacotherapies (see Table 4.1). Studies combining CM therapies with pharmacotherapy were required to use the same pharmacotherapy in both the intervention and comparator groups;
- Comparators: placebos, no treatment, or pharmacotherapies that are recommended in international clinical practice guidelines[2,3]

Table 4.1   Chinese Medicine Interventions Included in Clinical Evidence Evaluation

Chinese herbal medicines (CHM)	Oral CHM, topical CHM
Acupuncture and related therapies	Acupuncture (including surrounding acupuncture and electro-acupuncture), moxibustion, and plum-blossom needle acupuncture

for herpes zoster (antiviral therapy, pain medication, and patient education);
- Outcomes: studies reported at least one of the pre-specified outcome measures in Table 4.2.

Studies were considered eligible if the comparator included at least one guideline-recommended pharmacotherapy.[2,3] Studies were also considered eligible if guideline-recommended pharmacotherapy was used in combination with other treatments, such as acyclovir used with vitamin B1 or B12. Vitamins B1 and B12 are commonly used in China to aid nerve repair, although their efficacy for herpes zoster is unknown.[4,5]

Exclusion Criteria

- Studies of participants with post-herpetic neuralgia (PHN), ophthalmic zoster, herpes zoster oticus (Ramsay Hunt syndrome), zoster encephalitis, zoster sine herpete, visceral herpes zoster, disseminated herpes zoster, or other complications (e.g., bacterial infections, gangrenous zoster);
- Studies examining immunocompromised patients (e.g., HIV infection, cancer, diabetes, pregnant or breastfeeding women);
- Studies which included either children or both adults and children where results were presented in aggregate;
- Studies using herpes zoster vaccine or CM as the comparator.

Outcomes

Included outcomes were determined after consulting the content expert advisory panel (CEAP) which was convened for this monograph.

Table 4.2 Pre-specified Outcomes

Outcome Category	Outcome Measures	Scoring
Pain	1. Pain VAS	1. 0–10 cm or 1–100 mm; lower is better
	2. McGill Pain Questionnaire[6]	2. 0–78 points; lower is better
	3. Time taken for resolution of pain	3. Days or hours; lower is better
Cutaneous Outcomes	1. Time taken for crust formation	1. Days or hours; lower is better
	2. Time taken for cessation of new lesions	2. Days or hours; lower is better
	3. Time taken for resolution of rash	3. Days or hours; lower is better
PHN	1. Incidence of PHN (defined)	1. Number of cases; lower is better
HRQoL	1. SF-36[7]	1. 0–100 points per domain; higher is better
	2. EQ-5D[8]	2. See text
	3. Zoster Brief Pain Inventory[9]	3. See description in text
	4. Zoster Impact Questionnaire[9]	4. See description in text
Effective Rate	1. 30% or greater reduction in lesions, significant reduction in pain	2. Number of cases; higher is better
Adverse Events	Adverse events reported by included studies	

Abbreviations: EQ-5D, EuroQoL 5 Dimensions quality of life questionnaire; HRQoL, health-related quality of life; PHN, post-herpetic neuralgia; SF-36, Medical Outcome Study 36-item Short Form; VAS; visual analogue scale.

Validated assessments of effects and outcomes in herpes zoster research include pain and cutaneous outcomes, measures of health-related quality of life (HRQoL), and clinical effect (effective rate) (Table 4.2). Pain score on a visual analogue scale (VAS) is frequently used to measure zoster-associated pain and is calculated in either centimetres or millimetres. Studies which reported results for the McGill Pain Questionnaire[6] were also included.

The time taken for resolution of pain, crust formation, cessation of new lesions, and resolution of the rash were reported in hours or days. Additional information on the time-point from which measurements were made was also collected to aid analysis. Studies which reported on incidences of PHN were included if the timing of assessment for PHN was described; if not, they were excluded from analysis.

Two generic (Medical Outcome Study 36-item Short Form Health Survey, SF-36; EuroQoL 5 Dimensions, EQ-5D)[7,8] and two disease-specific (Zoster Brief Pain Inventory, ZBPI; Zoster Impact Questionnaire, ZIQ)[9] measures of HRQoL were included. The SF-36[7] is a 36-item questionnaire which assesses health and well-being on eight domains: physical functioning, role functioning due to physical problems, role functioning due to emotional problems, bodily pain, general health perceptions, vitality, social function, and mental health. The SF-36 has been validated in people with herpes zoster and PHN. The EQ-5D[8] includes five questions related to mobility, self-care, usual activities, pain or discomfort, and anxiety or depression. The EQ-5D also includes a 100-point VAS to assess overall health status. Results can be presented in a variety of ways. For the five domains, a higher score indicates a greater level of perceived problems, while for the VAS component, a higher score indicates better health status. No information was identified as to whether the EQ-5D has been validated in people with herpes zoster.

The ZBPI measures both pain intensity and pain interference with daily life activities.[9] Pain intensity is measured on a scale of 0 (no pain) to 10 (worst imaginable pain) at the 'worst', 'least', 'average', and 'now'. Pain intensity domains should be reported separately. Pain interference measures the impact of herpes zoster pain on seven activities of daily living (ADLs): general activity, mood, walking ability, work, relations with others, sleep, and enjoyment of life.[10] Scores for each of the seven pain interference on ADL items can be used to calculate a mean score.

The ZIQ[9] is an extension of the ZBPI designed to assess prodromal pain associated with herpes zoster and includes assessment of the impact of herpes zoster on other ADLs which are not covered in the ZBPI. Prodromal pain is assessed at 'worst' and 'average', and measures severity on a scale from 0 to 10. It includes assessments of the number of days of pain, number of hours on a typical day, and a description of the pain.[11] The impact of herpes zoster on ADLs is assessed through 12 questions about day-to-day behaviours: put on clothing, bathe yourself, eat, groom yourself, travel, do shopping, do housework, prepare meals (cook), get out of the house, participate in leisure activities, concentrate on mental tasks, and be sexually active. Items are scored from 0 (does not interfere) to 10 (completely interferes) and scores of the 12 items are averaged to derive a mean score.

Studies that reported on the effective rate were included if assessment criteria from the *Criteria of Diagnosis and Therapeutic Effect of Diseases and Syndromes in Traditional Chinese Medicine* 中医病证诊断疗效标准 was used,[12] or if a clear and detailed description of assessment criteria was provided that allow for meaningful interpretation of the effective rate. Studies which did not provide a description of criteria for the effective rate were excluded from analysis. The *Criteria of Diagnosis and Therapeutic Effect of Diseases and Syndromes in Traditional Chinese Medicine* 中医病证诊断疗效标准 provides the following criteria for the assessment of effective rate:

- Cure: all lesions resolved, all clinical symptoms resolved, and no PHN;
- Improvement: >30% reduction in skin lesions and significant reduction in pain;
- No improvement: <30% of lesions disappear and pain exists.

For statistical analysis, data for improvement and cure were combined to provide the number of people who achieved a 30% or greater improvement in symptoms. A high number of cases achieving 30% or greater improvement indicates better outcomes. Several studies reported using criteria other than those from the *Criteria of Diagnosis and Therapeutic Effect of Diseases and Syndromes in Traditional Chinese Medicine* 中医病证诊断疗效标准. These were reviewed to identify and judge the criteria used for assessing the effective rate. As none of the other criteria reported by included studies provided a clear and detailed description of assessment criteria which allowed for meaningful interpretation, studies using these criteria were excluded from analysis.

Risk of Bias Assessment

Risk of bias was assessed for RCTs using the Cochrane Collaboration's tool.[1] In clinical trials, bias can be categorised as selection bias, performance bias, detection bias, attrition bias, and reporting bias. Each domain is assessed to determine whether the bias is at low, high, or unclear risk. Low risk of bias indicates that bias is unlikely, high risk indicates plausible risk of bias that seriously weakens confidence in the results, and unclear bias indicates lack of information or uncertainty over potential bias and raises some doubt about the results. Risk of bias assessment was verified by two people and disagreement was resolved by discussion or consultation with a third person.

Risk of bias is categorised using the following six domains:

- Sequence generation: The method used to generate the allocation sequence is given in sufficient detail to allow an assessment of whether it should produce comparable groups. The use of a random number table or computer random generator creates low risk of bias. High risk of bias includes studies that describe a non-random sequence generation such as odd or even date of birth or date of admission.
- Allocation concealment: The method used to conceal the allocation sequence is given in enough detail to determine whether intervention allocations could have been foreseen before or during enrollment. Central randomisation or sealed envelopes create low risk of bias while allocation through open random sequences or date of birth create high risk of bias.

- Blinding of participants and personnel: The measures used to describe if participants and personnel are unaware of the intervention received and information relating to whether the blinding was effective are provided in sufficient detail to enable an assessment of bias risks due to blinding. Studies that ensure blinding of participants and personnel are at low risk of bias. If the study is not blind or incompletely blind it is at high risk of bias.
- Blinding of outcome assessors: The measures used to describe if the outcome assessors are blind from knowledge of which intervention a participant received are given in enough detail to assess bias risks due to blinding. In addition, information relating to whether the blinding was effective is also assessed. Studies that ensure blinding of outcome assessors are at low risk of bias. If the study is not blind or incompletely blind, it is at high risk of bias.
- Incomplete outcome data: The completeness of outcome data for each main outcome, including drop outs and exclusions from the analysis with numbers missing in each group and reasons for drop outs or exclusions, are provided in sufficient detail to assess risk of bias due to missing data. Studies with low risk of bias would include all outcome data or where data are missing, this would be considered unlikely to relate to the true outcome or be balanced between groups. Studies at high risk of bias would have unexplained missing data.
- Selective reporting: The study protocol is available and the pre-specified outcomes are included in the report which enables an assessment of risk of bias due to selective reporting. Studies with a published protocol and include all pre-specified outcomes in their report would be at low risk of bias. Studies that do not include all pre-specified outcomes or have incomplete outcome data reported are at high risk of bias.

Statistical Analyses

Frequency of CM syndromes, CHM formulas and herbs, and acupuncture points reported in included studies are presented using descriptive statistics. CM syndromes reported in two or more studies were presented. The 10 most frequently reported CHM formulas and the 20 most frequently reported herbs are presented if used in at least two studies, although for CHM formulas this was not always possible. The top 10 acupuncture points used in two or more studies are presented, or as available. Where data was limited, reports of single CM syndromes or acupuncture points were provided as a guide for the reader.

Definitions of statistical tests and results are included in the glossary. Dichotomous data are reported as a risk ratio (RR) with 95% confidence intervals (CI) and continuous data are reported as mean difference (MD) or standardised mean difference (SMD) with 95% CI. For dichotomous data, when the RR is greater than one and the upper and lower values of the 95% CI are both greater than one, this indicates we can be 95% certain that there is a difference between the groups and that the true effect lies within these CIs. The same is true for values less than one. In such cases, we say there is a 'significant difference' between the groups. For continuous data, when the MD is greater than zero and both the upper and lower values of the 95% CI are greater than zero, we say there is a 'significant difference' between the groups. The same is true on the negative side of the scale.[1] For all analyses, RR or MD and 95% CI were reported together with a formal test for heterogeneity using the I^2 statistic. An I^2 score greater than 50% may indicate substantial heterogeneity.[1] Sensitivity analyses were undertaken to explore potential sources of heterogeneity based on low risk of bias for one of the risk of bias domains, sequence generation. Where possible and appropriate, planned subgroup analyses included duration of treatment, CM syndromes, CM formula, and comparator type. Available case analysis with a random effects model was used in all analyses. The random effects model was used to take into account the clinical heterogeneity likely to be encountered within and between included studies as well as the variation in treatment effects between included studies.

Assessment Using Grading of Recommendations Assessment, Development, and Evaluation

The Grading of Recommendations Assessment, Development, and Evaluation (GRADE) approach was used.[13] The GRADE approach summarises and rates the quality of evidence in systematic reviews using a structured process for presenting evidence summaries. The results are presented in summary-of-findings tables. The results provide an important overview for herpes zoster outcomes.

A panel of experts was established to evaluate the quality of evidence. The panel included the systematic review team, CM practitioners, integrative medicine experts, research methodologists, and conventional medicine physicians. Experts were asked to rate the clinical importance of key interventions from CHM, acupuncture therapies, and other CM therapies as well as comparators and outcomes. Results were collated and, based on the mean rating scores and subsequent discussion, a consensus on the content for the summary-of-findings tables was achieved.

The quality of evidence for each outcome was rated according to five factors outlined in the GRADE approach. The quality of evidence may be rated down based on:

1. Limitations in study design (risk of bias);
2. Inconsistency of results (unexplained heterogeneity);
3. Indirectness of the evidence (interventions, populations, and outcomes important to the patients with the condition);
4. Imprecision (uncertainty about the results);
5. Publication bias (selective publication of studies).

These five factors are additive and a reduction in more than one factor will reduce the quality of the evidence for that outcome. The GRADE approach also includes three domains that can be rated up, including large magnitude of an effect, dose-response gradient, and effect of plausible residual confounding. However, these three domains are more relevant to observational studies including cohort, case-control, before-after, time series studies, etc. GRADE summaries in this monograph only include RCTs therefore the domains for rating up the quality of evidence were not utilised.

Treatment recommendations can also be assessed using the GRADE approach, but due to the diverse nature of CM practice, treatment recommendations were not included with the summary of findings. Therefore, the reader is able to interpret the evidence with reference to the local practice environment. It should also be noted that the GRADE approach requires judgments about the quality of evidence and some subjective assessment. Nevertheless, the experience of the panel members gives weight to the reliability of these judgments and thus provide transparent representations of the quality of evidence.

The GRADE levels of evidence are grouped into four categories:

1. High quality evidence: Further research is very unlikely to change our confidence in the estimate of the effect;
2. Moderate quality evidence: Further research is likely to have an important impact on our confidence in the estimate of effect and may change the estimate;
3. Low quality evidence: Further research is very likely to have an important impact on our confidence in the estimate of effect and is likely to change the estimate;
4. Very low quality evidence: Any estimate of effect is very uncertain.

References

1. Higgins JPT, Green S, (eds). Cochrane Handbook for Systematic Reviews of Interventions Version 5.1.0 [updated March 2011]. The Cochrane Collaboration, 2011. Available from wwwcochrane-handbookorg2011.
2. Gross G, Schofer H, Wassilew S, *et al.* Herpes zoster guideline of the German Dermatology Society (DDG). *J Clin Virol.* 2003; **26**(3):277–89; discussion 91–3.
3. Dworkin RH, Johnson RW, Breuer J, *et al.* Recommendations for the management of herpes zoster. *Clin Infect Dis.* 2007; **44**(Suppl 1):S1–26.
4. 陈前明, 吴波, 蒋存火. 维生素B12联合伐昔洛韦减少带状疱疹后遗神经痛发生的临床研究, 现代临床医学. 2006; **32**(3):195.
5. 张红星, 黄国付, 杨敏, 中西医结合治疗带状疱疹的临床研究进展, 中国组织工程研究与临床康复. 2007; **11**(29):5810–13.
6. Melzack R. The McGill Pain Questionnaire: Major properties and scoring methods. *Pain.* 1975; **1**:277–99.
7. Ware JJ, Sherbourne C. The MOS 36-item short-form health survey (SF-36). I. Conceptual framework and item selection. *Med Care.* 1992; **30**:473–83.

8. Rabin R, de Charro F. EQ-5D: A measure of health status from the EuroQol Group. *Ann Med.* 2001; **33**:337–43.

9. Coplan P, Schmader K, Nikas A, *et al.* Development of a measure of the burden of pain due to herpes zoster and postherpetic neuralgia for prevention trials: Adaptation of the brief pain inventory. *J Pain.* 2004; **5**(6):344–56.

10. Tsai T, Yao C, Yu H, *et al.* Herpes zoster-associated severity and duration of pain, health-related quality of life, and healthcare utilization in Taiwan: A prospective observational study. *Int J Dermatol.* 2015; **54**(5): 529–36.

11. Benbernou A, Drolet M, Levin M, *et al.* Association between prodromal pain and the severity of acute herpes zoster and utilization of health care resources. *Eur J Pain.* 2011; **15**(10):1100–6.

12. 国家中医药管理局. 中医病证诊断疗效标准. 南京: 南京大学出版社; 1994.

13. Schunemann H, Brozek J, Guyatt G, Oxman A, (eds). *GRADE handbook for grading quality of evidence and strength of recommendations.* Group TGW, editor. The GRADE Working Group: Available from www.guidelinedevelopment.org/handbook; 2013.

5

Clinical Evidence for Chinese Herbal Medicine — Herpes Zoster

OVERVIEW

This chapter provides a review of the clinical study literature and evaluates the evidence using scientific methods. A search conducted using nine English and Chinese databases identified more than 36,600 citations. Studies were screened against rigorous inclusion criteria, resulting in 151 studies being selected for inclusion. There is some evidence that Chinese herbal medicine can alleviate pain and hasten rash healing for people with herpes zoster.

Introduction

Chinese herbal medicine (CHM) has been examined in Chinese and international scientific journals. The evidence for CHM for herpes zoster was evaluated in 100 controlled trials, with a series of meta-analyses conducted to determine efficacy and safety. Details from 51 non-controlled studies are described to provide an overview of the interventions used and the safety of these CHM practices. Included studies are indicated by an 'S' followed by a number (e.g., S1, S2, S3, etc). For the full list of included studies, see Appendix 1.

Previous Systematic Reviews

Searches conducted using the English language databases identified one systematic review of CHM for herpes zoster, while no eligible reviews were identified in the Chinese language databases. Kongkaew and Chaiyakunapruk[1] included four randomised controlled trials

(RCTs) in a review of *Clinacanthus nutans* extract for herpes infections. Two of the studies used *C. nutans* extract to treat herpes zoster and two treated herpes genitalis. Statistical heterogeneity made pooling of results not possible for the herpes zoster trials, and the authors presented results for the higher quality study (based on a Jadad score of ≥ 3). *C. nutans* extract resulted in a greater proportion of patients achieving full lesion crusting at three days compared with a placebo.

Characteristics of Chinese Herbal Medicine Clinical Studies

A search conducted using nine English and Chinese language databases identified 36,621 citations, 5,693 of which required full-text retrieval to determine eligibility for inclusion (see Figure 5.1). After going through rigorous inclusion criteria assessment, 151 clinical studies that evaluated CHM for herpes zoster were included. Ninety-five studies were RCTs (S1–S95), five were controlled clinical trials (CCTs) (S96–S100), and 51 were non-controlled studies (S101–S151). Controlled studies (RCTs and CCTs) were evaluated to assess the efficacy and safety of CHM for herpes zoster while details from non-controlled studies are described.

All studies were conducted in China and published in Chinese. A total of 11,685 people participated in these studies. Treatment was provided for between five (S1, S2) and 42 days (S3). CM syndromes were used either as inclusion criteria or for determining treatment in 27 studies (S4–S17, S101–S113). The most commonly reported syndromes were excess heat in the Liver meridian (11 studies) (S6, S8–S10, S13, S103, S105, S106, S108–S110), *qi* stagnation and Blood stasis (9 studies) (S4, S7, S9, S14, S16, S102–S105), and Liver-Gallbladder dampness-heat (6 studies) (S5, S7, S12, S111–S113).

Many studies evaluated investigator-developed formulas, which resulted in little overlap in formulas observed in two or more studies (see Table 5.1). Further, many studies reported using two or three

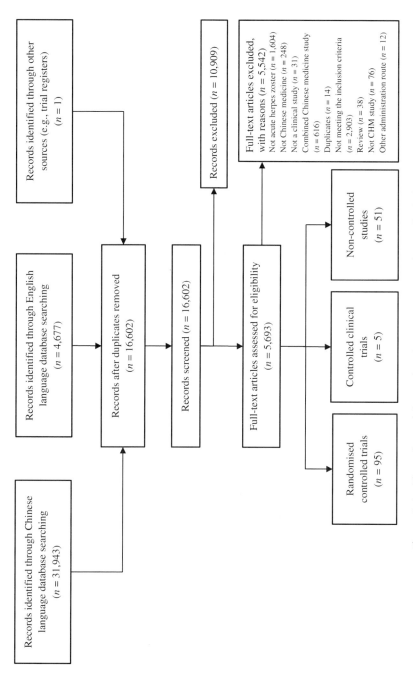

Figure 5.1 Flow chart of the study selection process: Chinese herbal medicine.

Table 5.1 Frequently Reported Formulas in all Chinese Herbal Medicine Clinical Studies

Most Common Formulas	No. of Studies	Ingredients
Long dan xie gan tang (modified) 龙胆泻肝汤	41	Long dan cao 龙胆草, zhi zi 栀子, huang qin 黄芩, mu tong 木通, ze xie 泽泻, che qian zi 车前子, sheng di 生地, dang gui 当归, gan cao 甘草, chai hu 柴胡 (plus modifications)
Chu shi wei ling tang 除湿胃苓汤	8	Fang feng 防风, cang zhu 苍术, bai zhu 白术, chi fu ling 赤茯苓, chen pi 陈皮, hou pu 厚朴, zhu ling 猪苓, shan zhi 山栀, mu tong 木通, ze xie 泽泻, hua shi 滑石, gan cao 甘草, bo he 薄荷, gui zhi 桂枝
Tao hong si wu tang 桃红四物汤	6	Tao ren 桃仁, hong hua 红花, dang gui 当归, shu di huang 熟地黄, shao yao 芍药, chuan xiong 川芎
Liu shen wan 六神丸	4	Zhen zhu fen 珍珠粉, xi niu huang 犀牛黄, she xiang 麝香, xiong huang 雄黄, chan su 蟾酥, bing pian 冰片
Chai hu shu gan san 柴胡疏肝散	4	Chai hu 柴胡, chen pi 陈皮, chuan xiong 川芎, chi shao 赤芍, zhi qiao 枳壳, xiang fu 香附, zhi gan cao 炙甘草
Ji de sheng she yao pian 季德胜蛇药片	3	Qi ye yi zhi hua 七叶一枝花, chan chu pi 蟾蜍皮, wu gong 蜈蚣, di jin cao 地锦草 (S140)
Xiao chai hu tang (modified) 加味小柴胡汤	3	Chai hu 柴胡, huang qin 黄芩, ren shen 人参, ban xia 半夏, gan cao 甘草, sheng jiang 生姜, da zao 大枣 (plus modifications)
Xue fu zhu yu tang 血府逐瘀汤	3	Tao ren 桃仁, hong hua 红花, dang gui 当归, sheng di 生地, zhi ke 枳壳, chi shao 赤芍, chai hu 柴胡, gan cao 甘草, jie geng 桔梗, chuan xiong 川芎, niu xi 牛膝
Er wei ba du san 二味拔毒散	2	Bai fan 白矾, ming xiong huang 明雄黄
Fu fang xiong huang ding/ruan guo 复方雄黄酊	2	Xiong huang 雄黄, bai zhi 白芷, bing pian 冰片 (S133)

(Continued)

Table 5.1 (*Continued*)

Most Common Formulas	No. of Studies	Ingredients
Qing jie hua yu zu fang 清解化瘀组方	2	Hua yu fang 化瘀方, zhi ke 枳壳, jing jie sui 荆芥穗
Wu wei xiao du yin 五味消毒饮	2	Jin yin hua 金银花, ye ju hua 野菊花, pu gong ying 蒲公英, zi hua di ding 紫花地丁, zi bei tian kui zi 紫背天葵子
Xiao yao san 逍遥散	2	Dang gui 当归, gan cao 甘草, fu ling 茯苓, shan yao 芍药, bai zhu 白术, chai hu 柴胡
Xin huang pian 新癀片	2	Jiu jie cha 九节茶, tian qi 田七, niu huang 牛黄, shui niu jiao 水牛角, zhen zhu ceng fen 珍珠层粉 (S78)
Yun nan bai yao jiao nang 云南白药胶囊	2	Not specified

Note: Ingredients are referenced to the *Zhong Yi Fang Ji Da Ci Dian* 中医方剂大辞典 where available, or to an included study if not available.

Note: The use of some herbs such as *mu tong* 木通 may be restricted in some countries under the provisions of CITES. Readers are advised to comply with relevant regulations.

formulas, of which only one was selected according to syndrome differentiation. *Long dan xie gan tang* 龙胆泻肝汤 was the most common formula reported across all clinical studies, evaluated either alone or in combination with other formulas in 41 studies (S2, S4, S5, S7–S9, S12, S14–S16, S18–S25, S26–S32, S96, S101–S103, S105, S106, S109, S111–S119). Other less frequently reported formulas included *Chu shi wei ling tang* 除湿胃苓汤 (8 studies; S4, S7, S15, S27, S101, S103, S105, S119), *Tao hong si wu tang* 桃红四物汤 (6 studies; S7, S15, S101, S103, S105, S119), *Liu shen wan* 六神丸 (4 studies; S22, S33, S120, S121), and *Chai hu shu gan san* 柴胡疏肝散 (4 studies; S27, S34, S104, S119).

A large variety of herbs were reported in included studies, with 174 individual herbs identified (see Table 5.2). As many studies

Table 5.2   Frequently Reported Herbs in all Clinical Studies

Most Common Herbs	Scientific Name	Frequency of Use
Gan cao 甘草	*Glycyrrhiza* spp	80
Huang qin 黄芩	*Scutellaria baicalensis* Georgi	67
Chai hu 柴胡	*Bupleurum* spp	66
Zhi zi 栀子	*Gardenia jasminoides* Ellis	62
Sheng di huang 生地黄	*Rehmannia glutinosa* Libosch.	60
Long dan cao 龙胆草	*Gentiana scabra* Bge.	58
Dang gui 当归	*Angelica sinensis* (Oliv.) Diels	55
Ze xie 泽泻	*Alisma orientalis* (Sam.) Juzep.	48
Yan hu suo 延胡索	*Corydalis yanhusuo* W.T. Wang	46
Ban lan gen 板蓝根	*Isatis indigotica* Fort.	44
Che qian zi 车前子	*Plantago* spp	41
Chi shao 赤芍	*Paeonia* spp	38
Lian qiao 连翘	*Forsythia suspensa* (Thunb.) Vahl	28
Mu tong 木通	*Akebia* spp	28
Jin yin hua 金银花	*Lonicera japonica* Thunb.	27
Mu dan pi 牡丹皮	*Paeonia suffruticosa* Andr.	27
Chuan xiong 川芎	*Ligusticum chuangxiong* Hort.	24
Bing pian 冰片	Borneol	21
Huang lian 黄连	*Coptis* spp	21

Note: The use of some herbs such as *mu tong* 木通 may be restricted in some countries under the provisions of CITES. Readers are advised to comply with relevant regulations.

reported two or more formulas, one herb may have been included multiple times in one study. The frequency count of herbs has not been adjusted to account for this. As such, the number of studies reported hereafter in the herb frequency tables may be greater than the actual number of studies which used the herb (in multiple formulas). The most commonly reported herb was *gan cao* 甘草. Other herbs which were frequently reported included *huang qin* 黄芩, *chai hu* 柴胡, *zhi zi* 栀子, *shu di huang* 熟地黄, and *long dan cao* 龙胆草.

Randomised Controlled Trials of Chinese Herbal Medicine

Ninety-five RCTs were included in this review (S1–S95). One study included three arms, of which two were interventions (S35), and results of the two intervention arms were pooled for analysis. The remaining studies compared CHM with pharmacotherapies in a two-arm parallel design. A total of 8,332 people participated in these RCTs.

The age of participants ranged from 18 (S7, S8, S13, S18, S20, S36–S40) to 90 years (S41, S42), and in the studies that reported the mean age, the median was 54.4 years. There were more males than females included in the studies (4,129 males and 3,735 females). The duration of herpes zoster at the time of study varied widely, ranging from a mean of 1.2 days (S43) up to 27 days (S3). Treatment was provided for between five (S1, S2) and 42 days (S3), and the median duration of treatment was 10 days.

Eleven studies used CM syndrome differentiation as an inclusion criterion or to guide treatment (S5–S13, S16, S17), with several reporting more than one syndrome. The most commonly reported syndromes were excess heat in the Liver meridian (5 studies) (S6, S8–S10, S13), *qi* stagnation and Blood stasis (5 studies) (S4, S7, S9, S14, S16), and Liver-Gallbladder dampness-heat (3 studies) (S5, S7, S12).

CHM was most frequently used in combination with pharmacotherapy (i.e., 'integrative medicine'; IM) (62 studies) and the majority of studies used oral administration of CHM (67 studies). Evaluation of efficacy and safety are reported below according to the route of administration. Fifteen studies did not report a formula name (S6, S41, S44–S56), although all studies listed the herbal ingredients. Seventy formula names were reported in all RCTs and the most commonly reported formula was *Long dan xie gan tang* 龙胆泻肝汤/*Long dan xie gan wan* 龙胆泻肝丸 (S2, S4, S5, S7–S9, S12, S14–S16, S18–S32), which was used in 25 studies (see Table 5.3). In total, 140 different herbs were reported across all studies, with *gan cao* 甘草 as the most frequent (see Table 5.4).

Table 5.3   Frequently Reported Formulas in Randomised Controlled Trials

Most Common Formulas	No. of Studies	Ingredients
Long dan xie gan tang (modified) 龙胆泻肝汤	25	Long dan cao 龙胆草, zhi zi 栀子, huang qin 黄芩, mu tong 木通, ze xie 泽泻, che qian zi 车前子, sheng di 生地, dang gui 当归, gan cao 甘草, chai hu 柴胡 (plus modifications)
Chu shi wei ling tang 除湿胃苓汤	4	Fang feng 防风, cang zhu 苍术, bai zhu 白术, chi fu ling 赤茯苓, chen pi 陈皮, hou pu 厚朴, zhu ling 猪苓, shan zhi 山栀, mu tong 木通, ze xie 泽泻, hua shi 滑石, gan cao 甘草, bo he 薄荷, gui zhi 桂枝
Xiao chai hu tang (modified) 加味小柴胡汤	3	Chai hu 柴胡, huang qin 黄芩, ren shen 人参, ban xia 半夏, gan cao 甘草, sheng jiang 生姜, da zao 大枣 (plus modifications)
Chai hu shu gan san 柴胡疏肝散	2	Chai hu 柴胡, chen pi 陈皮, chuan xiong 川芎, chi shao 赤芍, zhi qiao 枳壳, xiang fu 香附, zhi gan cao 炙甘草
Liu shen wan 六神丸	2	Zhen zhu fen 珍珠粉, xi niu huang 犀牛黄, she xiang 麝香, xiong huang 雄黄, chan su 蟾酥, bing pian 冰片
Qing jie hua yu zu fang 清解化瘀组方	2	Hua yu fang 化瘀方, zhi ke 枳壳, jing jie sui 荆芥穗
Tao hong si wu tang 桃红四物汤	2	Tao ren 桃仁, hong hua 红花, dang gui 当归, shu di huang 熟地黄, shao yao 芍药, chuan xiong 川芎
Wu wei xiao du yin 五味消毒饮	2	Jin yin hua 金银花, ye ju hua 野菊花, pu gong ying 蒲公英, zi hua di ding 紫花地丁, zi bei tian kui zi 紫背天葵子
Xin huang pian 新癀片	2	Jiu jie cha 九节茶, tian qi 田七, niu huang 牛黄, shui niu jiao 水牛角, zhen zhu ceng fen 珍珠层粉 (S78)

Note: Ingredients are referenced to the *Zhong Yi Fang Ji Da Ci Dian* 中医方剂大辞典 where available, or to the included study if not available.

Note: The use of some herbs such as *mu tong* 木通 may be restricted in some countries under the provisions of CITES. Readers are advised to comply with relevant regulations.

Table 5.4   Frequently Reported Herbs in Randomised Controlled Trials

Most Common Herbs	Scientific Name	Frequency of Use
Gan cao 甘草	*Glycyrrhiza* spp	46
Huang qin 黄芩	*Scutellaria baicalensis* Georgi	42
Chai hu 柴胡	*Bupleurum* spp	39
Long dan cao 龙胆草	*Gentiana scabra* Bge.	38
Dang gui 当归	*Angelica sinensis* (Oliv.) Diels	36
Zhi zi 栀子	*Gardenia jasminoides* Ellis	36
Sheng di huang 生地黄	*Rehmannia glutinosa* Libosch.	35
Ze xie 泽泻	*Alisma orientalis* (Sam.) Juzep.	31
Ban lan gen 板蓝根	*Isatis indigotica* Fort.	29
Yan hu suo 延胡索	*Corydalis yanhusuo* W.T. Wang	25
Che qian zi 车前子	*Plantago* spp	24
Chi shao 赤芍	*Paeonia* spp	21
Mu tong 木通	*Akebia* spp	19
Lian qiao 连翘	*Forsythia suspensa* (Thunb.) Vahl	16
Jin yin hua 金银花	*Lonicera japonica* Thunb.	16
Mu dan pi 牡丹皮	*Paeonia suffruticosa* Andr.	15
Chuan xiong 川芎	*Ligusticum chuangxiong* Hort.	15
Zi cao 紫草	*Arnebia* spp	14
Bing pian 冰片	Borneol	14
Fu ling 茯苓	*Poria cocos* (Schw.) Wolf	13

Note: The use of some herbs such as *mu tong* 木通 may be restricted in some countries under the provisions of CITES. Readers are advised to comply with relevant regulations.

Risk of Bias

The methodological quality of included studies was low to moderate (see Table 5.5). Fourteen studies used appropriate methods to allocate participants to groups, including random number lists (S10, S12, S14, S34, S43, S47, S57–S59), computer-generated randomisation schedules (S60, S61), block randomisation (S20), or drawing lots (S62, S63). These studies were thus judged as having low risk of bias in terms of group allocation. The majority (70.5%) were judged as having unclear bias risk for sequence generation. There was

Table 5.5   Risk of Bias of Randomised Controlled Trials: Chinese Herbal Medicine

Risk of Bias Domain	Low Risk n (%)	Unclear Risk n (%)	High Risk n (%)
Sequence generation	14 (14.7)	67 (70.5)	14 (14.7)
Allocation concealment	1 (1.1)	94 (98.9)	0 (0)
Blinding of participants	0 (0)	5 (5.3)	90 (94.7)
Blinding of personnel	0 (0)	5 (5.3)	90 (94.7)
Blinding of outcome assessor	0 (0)	95 (100)	0 (0)
Incomplete outcome data	93 (97.9)	2 (2.1)	0 (0)
Selective outcome reporting	0 (0)	95 (100)	0 (0)

insufficient information to judge potential bias risks arising from allocation concealment in all but one study which used opaque, sealed envelopes to conceal group allocation (S57).

Five studies mentioned blinding (either single or double) but did not provide sufficient detail (S11, S17, S48, S53, S64) and thus were judged as having unclear bias risk for blinding of participants, personnel, and outcome assessors. The remaining studies lacked adequate blinding of participants and personnel, and also provided insufficient detail on blinding of outcome assessment, and thus were judged as having high risk of bias in terms of blinding. In terms of completeness of data, two studies were judged as having unclear bias risk as they had missing data that was not explained and did not account for the missing data in their analysis of results (S20, S65). On the other hand, over 97% of studies had data available for all people randomised and were judged as having low bias risk. None of the studies had a published trial protocol or trial registration and therefore all were judged as having unclear risk of bias for selective outcome reporting.

Oral Chinese Herbal Medicine

In total, 66 RCTs evaluated oral CHM for herpes zoster. Twenty-one studies compared oral CHM with pharmacotherapies (S7, S8, S15,

S17–S21, S28, S31, S32, S36, S38, S57, S66–S72) and meta-analysis was possible for most outcomes. Forty-five RCTs evaluated oral CHM as IM (S2–S6, S9–S14, S23–S27, S30, S34, S39, S42, S44, S45, S50, S53, S55, S58–S62, S73–S84) and meta-analyses were possible for all oral CHM outcomes. The most commonly reported outcome was adverse events (38 studies) followed by time taken for crust formation (37 studies).

Pain Score

Oral Chinese Herbal Medicine Alone

Four studies reported pain score on a visual analogue scale (VAS) at the end of treatment (S7, S8, S57, S72), but one study reported data in a way that did not permit re-analysis and was excluded (S7). Oral CHM was more beneficial compared with pharmacotherapy in reducing the pain score at the end of treatment (mean difference, MD, −0.60 cm, [−1.12, −0.07], $I^2 = 62\%$) (see Table 5.6). Statistical heterogeneity was explored through subgroup analysis. Heterogeneity was reduced to acceptable levels when studies that provided oral CHM

Table 5.6   Oral Chinese Herbal Medicine *vs.* Pharmacotherapy: Pain Score (Visual Analogue Scale)

Outcome	No. of Studies (Participants)	Effect Size MD [95% CI] I^2	Included Studies
Pain score (cm)	3 (189)	−0.60 [−1.12, −0.07]* 62%	S8, S57, S72
Subgroup: *antivirals alone*	2 (133)	−0.73 [−1.52, 0.07] 68%	S8, S57
Subgroup: *treatment duration 7–10 days*	2 (121)	−0.34 [−0.72, 0.05] 0%	S57, S72
Subgroup: *guideline-recommended dose of antivirals*	2 (133)	−0.73 [−1.52, 0.07] 68%	S8, S57

*Statistically significant.
Abbreviations: CI, confidence interval; MD, mean difference.

for between seven and 10 days were grouped for analysis, although there was no benefit shown over pharmacotherapy.

Oral Chinese Herbal Medicine as Integrative Medicine

Nine studies which used oral CHM as IM reported pain score as the outcome (S6, S10, S16, S30, S42, S60, S61, S63, S74). One study reported pain only at follow-up (and not at the end of treatment) and is reported separately (S74). Meta-analysis of eight studies found that people treated with oral CHM as IM had a pain score on the VAS that was 1.18cm lower than those who received pharmacotherapy ([–1.74, –0.63], I^2 = 89%) (see Table 5.7). Statistical heterogeneity was explored through planned subgroup analysis.

Table 5.7 Oral Chinese Herbal Medicine as Integrative Medicine *vs.* Pharmacotherapy: Pain Score (Visual Analogue Scale)

Outcome	No. of Studies (Participants)	Effect Size MD [95% CI] I^2	Included Studies
Pain score (cm)	8 (521)	–1.18 [–1.74, –0.63]* 89%	S6, S10, S16, S30, S42, S60, S61, S63
Subgroup: *antivirals plus other treatments*	4 (274)	–1.61 [–1.95, –1.26]* 37%	S6, S30, S42, S60
Subgroup: *treatment duration 7–10 days*	3 (165)	–0.97 [–2.08, –0.66]* 93%	S10, S60, S61
Subgroup: *treatment duration >10 days*	5 (156)	–1.32 [–1.77, –0.87]* 63%	S6, S16, S30, S42, S63
Subgroup: *Low RoB sequence generation*	4 (217)	–0.94 [–1.75, –0.13]* 90%	S10, S60, S61, S63

*Statistically significant.
Abbreviations: CI, confidence interval; MD, mean difference; RoB, risk of bias.

When compared with antivirals used in combination with other treatments, oral CHM as IM reduced the pain score on the VAS by 1.61 cm ([−1.95, −1.26], I^2 = 37%) with lower levels of statistical heterogeneity. Other subgroup analyses also produced results which favoured oral CHM as IM; however, statistical heterogeneity remained. The greatest effect size was seen when oral CHM as IM was compared with antivirals plus other treatments.

One study reported pain assessment at one month follow-up (S74) and indicated that oral CHM as IM reduced the pain score on the VAS by 2.36 cm ([−2.85, −1.87]) compared with acyclovir, vitamin B1, and vitamin B12.

Time Taken for Resolution of Pain

Oral Chinese Herbal Medicine Alone

Ten studies reported on the time taken for resolution of pain (S15, S20, S21, S28, S32, S36, S69–S72) (see Table 5.8). Time was

Table 5.8 Oral Chinese Herbal Medicine *vs.* Pharmacotherapy: Time Taken for Resolution of Pain

Outcome	No. of Studies (Participants)	Effect Size MD [95% CI] I^2	Included Studies
Time from treatment start to resolution of pain (days)	4 (446)	−2.64 [−3.74, −1.53]* 81%	S15, S20, S21, S28
Subgroup: *antivirals alone*	2 (274)	−1.93 [−3.08, −0.79]* 75%	S15, S20
Subgroup: *antivirals plus pain management plus other treatments*	2 (172)	−3.40 [−4.24, −2.56]* 0%	S21, S28
Subgroup: *treatment duration 7–10 days*	2 (184)	−2.96 [−3.67, −2.26]* 0%	S20, S21
Subgroup: *Long dan xie gan tang* 龙胆泻肝汤	3 (320)	−3.07 [−3.72, −2.43]* 0%	S20, S21, S28

*Statistically significant.
Abbreviations: CI, confidence interval; MD, mean difference.

measured from either the start of treatment (S15, S20, S21, S28, S71) or an unspecified time-point (S32, S36, S69, S70, S72). Studies that did not specify the time-point from which measurement was made were not included in analyses. Four studies that evaluated time from the start of treatment to pain resolution found that oral CHM decreased the time taken for pain to resolve by 2.64 days ([–3.74, –1.53], $I^2 = 81\%$) (Table 5.8). Statistical heterogeneity was eliminated whilst retaining the treatment effect in subgroups according to comparators of antivirals plus pain management plus other treatments (MD –3.40 days [–4.24, –2.56], $I^2 = 0\%$), the use of formula *Long dan xie gan tang* 龙胆泻肝汤 (MD –3.07 days [–3.72, –2.43, $I^2 = 0\%$), and treatment duration of seven to 10 days (MD –2.96 days [–3.67, –2.26]), $I^2 = 0\%$). Statistical heterogeneity remained in studies which used antivirals alone as the comparator (MD –1.93 days [–3.08, –0.79], $I^2 = 75\%$).

One study reported the time from start of treatment to resolution of pain in hours (S71) and indicated that oral CHM reduced the time taken for resolution of pain by 573.2 hours ([–644.31, –502.09]) compared with acyclovir and moroxydine. This equates to a reduction of 23.9 days, which is unusually high. The reliability of this data is uncertain and should be interpreted with great caution.

Oral Chinese Herbal Medicine as Integrative Medicine

Seventeen studies reported on the time taken for resolution of pain. One study reported data in a way that did not allow for re-analysis and was excluded (S34). Nine studies reported the time from the start of treatment (S6, S12, S23, S74, S75, S78, S79, S82, S83) while seven studies did not specify the time-point from which measurement was made (S2, S9, S26, S53, S62, S84, S85) (see Table 5.9). Therefore, these seven studies were excluded from further analysis. Oral CHM as IM reduced the time from the start of treatment to resolution of pain by 2.43 days ([–3.16, –1.70], $I^2 = 90\%$). Statistical heterogeneity was explored through planned subgroup analyses.

Table 5.9 Oral Chinese Herbal Medicine as Integrative Medicine vs. Pharmacotherapy: Time Taken for Resolution of Pain

Outcome	No. of Studies (Participants)	Effect Size MD [95% CI] I^2	Included Studies
Time from treatment start to resolution of pain (days)	9 (865)	−2.43 [−3.16, −1.70]* 90%	S6, S12, S23, S74, S75, S78, S79, S82, S83
Subgroup: *antivirals alone*	4 (439)	−1.98 [−2.42, −1.54]* 0%	S12, S75, S78, S83
Subgroup: *antivirals plus other treatments*	4 (366)	−2.45 [−3.72, −1.19]* 96%	S6, S74, S79, S82
Subgroup: *treatment duration 7–10 days*	7 (719)	−1.98 [−2.58, −1.37]* 80%	S12, S23, S74, S75, S78, S79, S83
Subgroup: *treatment duration > 10 days*	2 (146)	−3.59 [−4.07, −3.10]* 0%	S6, S82
Subgroup: *guideline-recommended doses*	4 (410)	−2.52 [−4.35, −0.70]* 95%	S6, S12, S23, S79

*Statistically significant.

Abbreviations: CI, confidence interval; MD, mean difference.

Statistical heterogeneity was eliminated when studies using antiviral therapies alone in both the treatment and comparator groups were pooled (MD −1.98 days [−2.42, −1.54], I^2 = 0%) and when studies with treatment durations of more than 10 days were pooled (MD −3.59 days [−4.07, −3.10], I^2 = 0%). Other subgroup analyses produced considerable statistical heterogeneity.

Time Taken for Crust Formation

Oral Chinese Herbal Medicine Alone

Twelve studies reported on the time taken for the formation of crusts (S7, S15, S20, S21, S28, S32, S36, S57, S69–S72) (see Table 5.11). Time was measured from the start of treatment (S15, S20, S21, S28, S71) or an unspecified time-point (S7, S32, S36, S57, S69, S70, S72). Studies which did not specify the time-point from measurement were not analysed. Oral CHM reduced the time from the start of treatment to crust formation by 1.70 days compared with pharmacotherapy (4 studies, 446 participants; [–2.10, –1.29]), and there was low statistical heterogeneity ($I^2 = 10\%$) (S15, S20, S21, S28).

One study which reported the time from treatment start to crust formation in hours indicated that oral CHM was beneficial (MD –85.00 hours [–117.88, –52.12]) (S71). This equates to a reduction in time by approximately 3.5 days, which is greater than the result seen for studies that were pooled for meta-analysis (see above).

Oral Chinese Herbal Medicine as Integrative Medicine

Time taken for crust formation was reported in 25 studies. Time was measured from the onset of the rash in one study (S61) and the start of treatment in ten studies (S6, S12, S23, S44, S74, S75, S78, S79, S82, S83), but was not specified in 14 studies (S2, S9, S11, S13, S26, S42, S53, S55, S58, S62, S63, S76, S84, S85). Studies which did not specify the time-point from which measurement was made were excluded from analysis. The time from start of treatment to crust formation was 2.28 days less in participants who received oral CHM as IM compared with pharmacotherapy ([–2.86, –1.71], $I^2 = 88\%$) (see Table 5.10). Statistical heterogeneity was explored through planned subgroup analysis but failed to reduce heterogeneity to acceptable levels. As such, the certainty of this finding remains unclear.

One study reported the time from onset of the rash to crust formation (S61). The time taken for crust formation occurred 1.47 days faster in participants who received oral CHM as IM compared with famciclovir and diclofenac alone ([–2.78, –0.16]).

Time Taken for Cessation of New Lesions

Oral Chinese Herbal Medicine Alone

Ten studies reported the time taken for new lesions to stop forming (S7, S15, S20, S28, S32, S36, S57, S70–S72) (Table 5.11). Some

Table 5.10 Oral Chinese Herbal Medicine as Integrative Medicine *vs.* Pharmacotherapy: Time Taken for Crust Formation

Outcome	No. of Studies (Participants)	Effect Size MD [95% CI] I^2	Included Studies
Time from start of treatment to crust formation (days)	10 (945)	−2.28 [−2.86, −1.71]* 88%	S6, S12, S23, S44, S74, S75, S78, S79, S82, S83
Subgroup: *antivirals alone*	4 (439)	−2.54 [−3.05, −2.03]* 53%	S12, S75, S78, S83
Subgroup: *antivirals plus other treatments*	4 (366)	−1.90 [−3.16, −0.63]* 95%	S6, S74, S79, S82
Subgroup: *antivirals plus pain management plus other treatments*	2 (140)	−2.40 [−3.74, −1.05]* 80%	S23, S44
Subgroup: *guideline-recommended doses*	4 (410)	−2.38 [−3.34, −1.42]* 93%	S6, S12, S23, S79
Subgroup: *Long dan xie gan tang/ wan* 龙胆泻肝汤/丸	2 (238)	−2.52 [−3.43, −1.61]* 79%	S12, S23
Subgroup: *treatment duration 7–10 days*	8 (799)	−2.12 [−2.72, −1.52]* 86%	S12, S23, S44, S74, S75, S78, S79, S83
Subgroup: *treatment duration > 10 days*	2 (146)	−2.89 [−3.96, −1.81]* 81%	S6, S82

*Statistically significant.

Abbreviations: CI, confidence interval; MD, mean difference.

studies recorded the time-point that treatment started (S15, S20, S28, S71) while some did not specify the starting time-point (S7, S32, S36, S57, S70, S72). Studies which did not specify the time-point from which measurement was made were not analysed. No benefit was seen for oral CHM over pharmacotherapy when time taken for cessation of new lesions was measured from the start of treatment, and this was accompanied by considerable heterogeneity (MD −1.16

Table 5.11   Oral Chinese Herbal Medicine *vs.* Pharmacotherapy: Time Taken for Cessation of New Lesions

Outcome	No. of Studies (Participants)	Effect Size MD [95% CI] I²	Included Studies
Time from treatment start to cessation of new lesions (days)	3 (410)	−1.16 [−2.53, 0.22] 96%	S15, S20, S28
Subgroup: *antivirals alone*	2 (274)	−0.24 [−0.71, 0.23] 66%	S15, S20
Subgroup: *Long dan xie gan tang* 龙胆泻肝汤	2 (274)	−0.24 [−0.71, 0.23] 66%	S15, S20

Abbreviations: CI, confidence interval; MD, mean difference.

days [−2.53, 0.22], I² = 96%) (see Table 5.11). Subgroup analysis was conducted according to comparator and formula type, which included the same studies. Statistical heterogeneity was reduced, although not to acceptable levels.

One study found that oral CHM reduced the time from the start of treatment to cessation of lesions by 209.6 hours compared with acyclovir, vitamin B1, and vitamin B12 ([−237.59, −181.61]) (S71). This was equivalent to a reduction of 8.73 days, which was much greater than that seen in meta-analyses. The certainty of these results remains unclear.

Oral Chinese Herbal Medicine as Integrative Medicine

Time taken for new lesions to cease forming was reported in 23 studies. One study reported the time from rash onset to cessation of new lesions (S61), 10 studies reported the time from treatment start to cessation of new lesions (S6, S12, S23, S44, S74, S75, S78, S79, S82, S83), and 12 studies reported the time taken for cessation of new lesions from an unspecified time-point (S2, S9, S11, S13, S26, S42, S53, S58, S62, S63, S76, S85). Studies which did not specify the starting time-point for measurement were not analysed. Studies which reported the time from start of treatment to cessation of new lesions

Table 5.12   Oral Chinese Herbal Medicine as Integrative Medicine *vs.* Pharmacotherapy: Time Taken for Cessation of New Lesions

Outcome	No. of Studies (Participants)	Effect Size MD [95% CI] I^2	Included Studies
Time from treatment start to cessation of new lesions (days)	10 (945)	−1.80 [−2.33, −1.27]* 94%	S6, S12, S23, S44, S74, S75, S78, S79, S82, S83
Subgroup: *antivirals alone*	4 (439)	−2.32 [−3.30, −1.35]* 94%	S12, S75, S78, S83
Subgroup: *antivirals plus other treatments*	4 (366)	−1.26 [−2.03, −0.49]* 94%	S6, S74, S79, S82
Subgroup: *antivirals plus pain management plus other treatments*	2 (140)	−1.88 [−2.48, −1.28]* 56%	S23, S44
Subgroup: *guideline-recommended doses*	4 (410)	−1.58 [−2.41, −0.74]* 95%	S6, S12, S23, S79
Subgroup: *Long dan xie gan tang* 龙胆泻肝汤	2 (238)	−1.68 [−2.61, −0.75]* 89%	S12, S23
Subgroup: *treatment duration 7–10 days*	8 (799)	−1.82 [−2.41, −1.23]* 94%	S12, S23, S44, S74, S75, S78, S79, S83
Subgroup: *treatment duration > 10 days*	2 (146)	−1.71 [−3.28, −0.14]* 93%	S6, S82

*Statistically significant.

Abbreviations: CI, confidence interval; MD, mean difference.

showed a reduction in the time taken for new lesions to stop forming by 1.80 days ([−2.33, −1.27], I^2 = 94%) (see Table 5.12). Subgroup analyses were performed to identify potential sources of statistical heterogeneity. As none of the subgroup analyses reduced statistical heterogeneity to acceptable levels, the certainty of these findings remains unclear.

The time from rash onset to cessation of new lesions was reported in one study (S61). Oral CHM as IM therapy reduced the time taken for lesions to stop forming by 1.70 days ([−2.52, −0.88]) compared with famciclovir and diclofenac.

Time Taken for Resolution of Rash

Oral Chinese Herbal Medicine Alone

Time taken for rash resolution was reported in six studies (S7, S20, S21, S28, S32, S71). Time was either measured from the start of treatment (S20, S21, S28, S71) or not specified (S7, S32). The two studies which did not specify the time-point for measurement were excluded from analysis. Oral CHM reduced the time from treatment start to resolution of the rash by 4.11 days compared with pharmacotherapy (3 studies, 320 participants; [−5.07, −3.15]), and no statistical heterogeneity was detected ($I^2 = 0\%$) (S20, S21, S28). One study which reported the time taken for rash resolution in hours (S71) found that oral CHM reduced the time from the start of treatment to resolution of the rash by 470.4 hours compared with acyclovir, vitamins B1 and B12, and moroxydine ([−537.24, −403.56]). This is equivalent to 19.6 days, which seems to be an unusually fast resolution of the rash. The findings of this study should be viewed in light of the usual healing time for herpes zoster.

Oral Chinese Herbal Medicine as Integrative Medicine

Thirteen studies reported information for the time taken for the rash to resolve. Two studies reported the time from the onset of the rash to resolution (S26, S61), five reported the time from the start of treatment to rash resolution (S6, S12, S34, S44, S79), and six did not specify the time-point from which measurements were made (S11, S13, S55, S58, S62, S63). These six studies were excluded from further analysis. Of the five studies that reported the time from the start of treatment to resolution of the rash, one study was excluded from analysis because it reported data in a way that did not permit re-analysis (S34).

Table 5.13   Oral Chinese Herbal Medicine as Integrative Medicine *vs.* Pharmaco-therapy: Time Taken for Resolution of Rash

Outcome	No. of Studies (Participants)	Effect Size MD [95% CI] I^2	Included Studies
Time from onset to resolution of rash (days)	2 (155)	−4.35 [−9.49, 0.79] 86%	S26, S61
Time from start of treatment to resolution of rash (days)	4 (430)	−3.43 [−5.58, −1.28]* 95%	S6, S12, S44, S79
Subgroup: *antivirals plus other treatments*	2 (172)	−1.98 [−3.42, −0.54]* 81%	S6, S79
Subgroup: *guideline-recommended doses*	3 (350)	−3.30 [−6.09, −0.51]* 97%	S6, S12, S79
Subgroup: *treatment duration 7–10 days*	3 (358)	−3.64 [−6.58, −0.71]* 97%	S12, S44, S79

*Statistically significant.

Abbreviations: CI, confidence interval; MD, mean difference.

In studies which measured time from onset of the rash, there was no statistical difference between groups (MD −4.35 days [−9.49, 0.79], I^2 = 86%) (see Table 5.13). While statistical heterogeneity was detected, this could not be explored through subgroup analysis due to the small number of included studies. The time from start of treatment to rash resolution was 3.43 days less in those who received oral CHM as IM compared with pharmacotherapy ([−5.58, −1.28], I^2 = 95%) (see Table 5.13). Subgroup analyses were possible according to comparators and duration of treatment, and while all subgroup analyses showed that oral CHM as IM was beneficial, statistical heterogeneity was not reduced to acceptable levels. Therefore, the reliability of these findings is uncertain.

Incidence of Post-herpetic Neuralgia

Oral Chinese Herbal Medicine Alone

The incidence of PHN was reported in seven studies (S7, S8, S17, S38, S57, S72). One study provided a definition which was unlikely

Table 5.14 Oral Chinese Herbal Medicine *vs.* Pharmacotherapy: Incidence of Post-herpetic Neuralgia

Outcome	No. of Studies (Participants)	Effect Size RR [95% CI] I^2	Included Studies
PHN: 3 months from resolution of rash	2 (246)	0.13 [0.03, 0.47]* 0%	S17, S38
PHN: 1 month from rash onset	2 (121)	0.28 [0.05, 1.77] 0%	S57, S72

*Statistically significant.
Abbreviations: CI, confidence interval; PHN, post-herpetic neuralgia; RR, risk ratio.

to be representative of PHN and was excluded from analysis (S20). Two studies assessed PHN three months after resolution of the rash (S17, S38) and two studies assessed PHN one month from the onset of the rash (S57, S72). Meta-analyses were performed for these various time-points (see Table 5.14). Oral CHM reduced the incidence of PHN measured three months from the resolution of rash (risk ratio RR 0.13 [0.03, 0.47], $I^2 = 0\%$), while no benefit was seen when PHN was assessed one month after rash onset (RR 0.28 [0.05, 1.77], $I^2 = 0\%$). This finding may reflect potential issues with the timing of PHN assessment. At one month from resolution of the rash, the pain experienced by patients may be residual pain from the acute rash or sub-acute herpetic neuralgia rather than PHN. The former finding (three months from resolution of the rash) more accurately captures incidence of PHN according to current consensus.[2]

Two studies reported PHN at time-points other than those above (S7, S8). When measured at one month from resolution of the rash, oral CHM did not reduce the incidence of PHN (RR 0.48 [0.09, 2.45]) (S7). Oral CHM also showed no benefit when PHN was assessed one month after the end of treatment (the treatment duration was 21 days) (RR 0.30 [0.09, 1.00], p = 0.05) (S8).

Oral Chinese Herbal Medicine as Integrative Medicine

Seventeen studies measured the incidence of PHN. Three studies assessed PHN three or more months after resolution of the rash

(S3, S10, S27), seven assessed PHN one month to six weeks after resolution of the rash (S4, S53, S60, S62, S63, S74, S83), four assessed PHN four weeks to 40 days after treatment began (S5, S11, S12, S73), two assessed PHN one month after treatment ended (S23, S75), and one assessed PHN three weeks after resolution of the rash (S14). One study that described measuring the incidence of PHN did not report the number of cases and was excluded from analysis (S27).

Irrespective of the time at which PHN was assessed, oral CHM as IM reduced the chance of PHN occurring compared with pharmacotherapy alone (see Table 5.15), and there was no statistical heterogeneity. When the most accepted definition of PHN (three months or more after resolution of the rash) was used the chance of developing PHN with oral CHM as IM was 0.17 that of the pharmacotherapy group ([0.05, 0.63], $I^2 = 0\%$). There is some evidence that oral CHM used in combination with pharmacotherapy can reduce the incidence of PHN, although the number of studies using a robust definition was small.

One study which studied the incidence of PHN three weeks after rash resolution found fewer cases of PHN among participants who received oral CHM as IM (RR 0.22 [0.07, 0.72]) (S14).

Table 5.15 Oral Chinese Herbal Medicine as Integrative Medicine *vs.* Pharmacotherapy: Incidence of Post-herpetic Neuralgia

Outcome	No. of Studies (Participants)	Effect Size RR [95% CI] I^2	Included Studies
PHN: ≥ 3 months from resolution of rash	2 (156)	0.17 [0.05, 0.63]* 0%	S3, S10
PHN: 1 month/6 weeks from rash onset	7 (527)	0.13 [0.05, 0.33]* 0%	S4, S53, S60, S62, S63, S74, S83
PHN: 4 weeks-40 days after start of treatment	4 (493)	0.24 [0.14, 0.40]* 0%	S5, S11, S12, S73
PHN: 1 month after treatment finished	2 (149)	0.18 [0.04, 0.78]* 0%	S23, S75

*Statistically significant.
Abbreviations: CI, confidence interval; RR, risk ratio.

Table 5.16   Oral Chinese Herbal Medicine *vs.* Pharmacotherapy: Effective Rate

Outcome	No. of Studies (Participants)	Effect Size RR [95% CI] I^2	Included Studies
Effective rate	3 (470)	1.15 [0.73, 1.83] 98%	S18, S19, S38
Subgroup: *antiviral plus pain management plus other treatments*	2 (250)	1.09 [0.79, 1.58] 96%	S19, S38
Subgroup: *treatment duration 7–10 days*	2 (320)	1.25 [1.13, 1.38]* 0%	S18, S19

*Statistically significant.
Abbreviations: CI, confidence interval; RR, risk ratio.

Effective Rate

Oral Chinese Herbal Medicine Alone

Ten studies reported on a defined effective rate (S8, S17–S19, S38, S57, S66, S68, S69, S72). The criteria for effective rate could not be verified in five studies (S8, S57, S66, S69, S72) and two studies referred to the 1994 guideline but used different criteria (S17, S68). These data were excluded from analysis. Three studies reported the effective rate of treatment according to the 1994 guideline (S18, S19, S38) (see Table 5.16). Oral CHM did not significantly increase the chance of achieving a 30% reduction in lesions and significant pain relief (RR 1.15 [0.73, 1.83], I^2 = 98%). Subgroup analysis suggested that studies with shorter treatment durations (seven to 10 days) may produce more reliable results (I^2 = 0%) and showed statistically that oral CHM was beneficial.

Oral Chinese Herbal Medicine as Integrative Medicine

Eighteen studies provided definitions of the effective rate measure employed (S2, S3, S10, S12, S14, S25, S30, S34, S53, S58, S59, S62, S75, S77, S80, S81, S83). One study cited effective rate criteria which could not be verified (S75) and five studies cited the 1994 guideline but also used additional criteria which were not from the guideline (S12, S30, S34, S58, S81). These studies were not analysed.

Twelve studies reported the effective rate according to the selected CM guideline (S2, S3, S10, S14, S25, S53, S59, S62, S77, S80, S83, S84). Oral CHM as IM increased the chance of achieving a 30% or greater reduction in lesions and significant pain relief compared with pharmacotherapy alone (RR 1.16 [1.09, 1.23], I^2 = 54%) (see Table 5.17). Statistical heterogeneity was slightly above accepted

Table 5.17 **Oral Chinese Herbal Medicine as Integrative Medicine *vs.* Pharmacotherapy: Effective Rate**

Outcome	No. of Studies (Participants)	Effect Size RR [95% CI] I^2	Included Studies
Effective rate	12 (1,118)	1.16 [1.09, 1.23]* 54%	S2, S3, S10, S14, S25, S53, S59, S62, S77, S80, S83, S84
Subgroup: *antivirals alone*	3 (278)	1.12 [0.98, 1.28] 60%	S10, S59, S62
Subgroup: *antivirals plus other treatments*	6 (598)	1.16 [1.06, 1.28]* 64%	S14, S53, S59, S77, S80, S84
Subgroup: *antivirals plus pain management plus other treatments*	2 (164)	1.21 [1.08, 1.35]* 0%	S2, S25
Subgroup: *guideline-recommended doses of antiviral therapies*	2 (318)	1.26 [1.14, 1.38]* 0%	S59, S77
Subgroup: *Long dan xie gan tang* 龙胆泻肝汤	2 (164)	1.56 [0.86, 2.86] 71%	S2, S25
Subgroup: *treatment duration 7–10 days*	6 (638)	1.19 [1.07, 1.32]* 64%	S10, S59, S62, S77, S80, S83
Subgroup: *Low RoB sequence generation*	4 (331)	1.15 [1.03, 1.28]* 60%	S10, S14, S59, S62

*Statistically significant.

Abbreviations: CI, confidence interval; RoB, risk of bias; RR, risk ratio.

levels (I^2 = 54%) and potential causes of heterogeneity were explored through subgroup analyses.

Statistical heterogeneity was reduced while maintaining the treatment effect for subgroups antiviral therapies plus pain management and other treatments (RR 1.21 [1.08, 1.35], I^2 = 0%), as well as in studies which used advocated doses of guideline-recommended antiviral therapies (RR 1.26 [1.14, 1.38], I^2 = 0%). For all other subgroup analyses, statistical heterogeneity remained high.

Frequently Reported Orally Used Herbs in Meta-analyses Showing Favourable Effects

Analysis was conducted to identify the most frequently reported herbs which may be contributing to the positive effects seen in the main meta-analyses. Subgroup analyses were not included in the calculations. Outcomes were grouped into four categories:

(1) Pain outcomes: pain score and time taken for resolution of pain;
(2) Cutaneous outcomes: time taken for crust formation, time taken for cessation of new lesions, and time taken for resolution of rash;
(3) Incidence of PHN; and
(4) Effective rate.

Studies that reported two or more outcomes in the same outcome category were counted only once in analysis. No calculation of herb lists were made if meta-analyses were not conducted. Similarly, if there was no overlap in herbs across studies (i.e., each herb has a frequency of one), the results are not presented. Herbs are presented if they are reported in at least two or more studies, and the final selection presents the highest frequency herbs. Relevant meta-analyses and studies included in each outcome category calculation are noted in each table.

The most frequently used herbs in positive meta-analyses were identified when oral CHM was used alone (see Table 5.18) or as IM (see Table 5.19). When oral CHM alone produced benefits compared with pharmacotherapy, the herbs which may be contributing to the effect are similar to the most frequently used herbs in all clinical studies. Many of these herbs act by clearing heat, resolving dampness,

Table 5.18 Frequently Reported Herbs in Meta-Analyses Showing Favourable Effect: Oral Chinese Herbal Medicine *vs.* Pharmacotherapy

Herb	Scientific Name	Frequency of Use
Pain outcomes: 2 meta-analyses, 7 RCTs (Tables 5.6, 5.8)		
Gan cao 甘草	*Glycyrrhiza* spp	8*
Ban lan gen 板蓝根	*Isatis indigotica* Fort.	7
Huang qin 黄芩	*Scutellaria baicalensis* Georgi	7
Zhi zi 栀子	*Gardenia jasminoides* Ellis	7
Chai hu 柴胡	*Bupleurum* spp	5
Long dan cao 龙胆草	*Gentiana scabra* Bge.	5
Sheng di huang 生地黄	*Rehmannia glutinosa* Libosch.	5
Ze xie 泽泻	*Alisma orientalis* (Sam.) Juzep.	5
Che qian zi 车前子	*Plantago* spp	4
Dang gui 当归	*Angelica sinensis* (Oliv.) Diels	4
Cutaneous outcomes: 2 meta-analyses, 4 RCTs (see Time to crust formation; Time to resolution of rash)		
Lian qiao 连翘	*Forsythia suspensa* (Thunb.) Vahl	2
Mu dan pi 牡丹皮	*Paeonia suffruticosa* Andr.	2
Ze xie 泽泻	*Alisma orientalis* (Sam.) Juzep.	2
Zi cao 紫草	*Arnebia* spp	2

*The frequency of use for some herbs may be greater than the actual number of studies which used the herb, for example, in studies where multiple formulas were reported.

Note: The use of some herbs may be restricted in some countries. Readers are advised to Comply with relevant regulations.

and tonifying and cooling the Blood, which are key treatment principles in herpes zoster. Only one herb, *ze xie* 泽泻, was common to both outcome categories (pain and cutaneous outcomes). The lack of overlap may be a result of the small number of studies that contributed to the positive effects seen with oral CHM for cutaneous outcomes.

Where oral CHM as IM produced favourable results compared with pharmacotherapy, three herbs which may have contributed to the observed effects were common to all outcome categories (see Table 5.19). These were *gan cao* 甘草, *Sheng di huang* 生地黄, and

Table 5.19 Frequently Reported Herbs in Meta-Analyses Showing Favourable Effect: Oral Chinese Herbal Medicine as Integrative Medicine *vs.* Pharmacotherapy

Herb	Scientific Name	Frequency of Use
Pain outcomes: 2 meta-analyses, 16 RCTs (Tables 5.7, 5.9)		
Yan hu suo 延胡索	*Corydalis yanhusuo* W.T. Wang	8
Chai hu 柴胡	*Bupleurum* spp	7
Sheng di huang 生地黄	*Rehmannia glutinosa* Libosch.	6
Gan cao 甘草	*Glycyrrhiza* spp	6
Chi shao 赤芍	*Paeonia* spp	5
Cutaneous outcomes: 3 meta-analyses, 10 RCTs (see Tables 5.10, 5.12, 5.13)		
Yan hu suo 延胡索	*Corydalis yanhusuo* W.T. Wang	3
Chai hu 柴胡	*Bupleurum* spp	2
Chi shao 赤芍	*Paeonia* spp	2
Gan cao 甘草	*Glycyrrhiza* spp	2
Hong hua 红花	*Carthamus tinctorius* L.	2
Huang qin 黄芩	*Scutellaria baicalensis* Georgi	2
Jin yin hua 金银花	*Lonicera japonica* Thunb.	2
Lian qiao 连翘	*Forsythia suspensa* (Thunb.) Vahl	2
Niu huang 牛黄	*Bos taurus domesticus* Gmelin	2
Sheng di huang 生地黄	*Rehmannia glutinosa* Libosch.	2
Shui niu jiao 水牛角	*Bubalus bubalis* Linnaeus	2
Yu jin (guang) 郁金	*Curcuma* spp	2
Zhen zhu 珍珠	Pearl	2
Incidence of PHN: 1 meta-analysis, 15 RCTs (see Table 5.15)		
Gan cao 甘草	*Glycyrrhiza* spp	6
Huang qin 黄芩	*Scutellaria baicalensis* Georgi	6
Chai hu 柴胡	*Bupleurum* spp	4
Che qian zi 车前子	*Plantago* spp	4
Chi shao 赤芍	*Paeonia* spp	4
Fu ling 茯苓	*Poria cocos* (Schw.) Wolf	4
Long dan cao 龙胆草	*Gentiana scabra* Bge.	4
Sheng di huang 生地黄	*Rehmannia glutinosa* Libosch.	4
Ze xie 泽泻	*Alisma orientalis* (Sam.) Juzep.	4

(Continued)

Table 5.19   (*Continued*)

Herb	Scientific Name	Frequency of Use
Effective rate: 1 meta-analysis, 12 RCTs (see Table 5.17)		
Chai hu 柴胡	*Bupleurum* spp	8
Huang qin 黄芩	*Scutellaria baicalensis* Georgi	8
Gan cao 甘草	*Glycyrrhiza* spp	7
Chuan xiong 川芎	*Ligusticum chuangxiong* Hort.	6
Long dan cao 龙胆草	*Gentiana scabra* Bge.	6
Dang gui 当归	*Angelica sinensis* (Oliv.) Diels	5
Ze xie 泽泻	*Alisma orientalis* (Sam.) Juzep.	5
Zhi zi 栀子	*Gardenia jasminoides* Ellis	5
Huang qi 黄芪	*Astragalus* spp	4
Shu di huang 熟地黄	*Rehmannia glutinosa* Libosch.	4

chai hu 柴胡. It was not surprising that *gan cao* 甘草 was seen in the herb lists for all outcomes as it is frequently used as a harmonizing herb. *Chai hu* 柴胡 facilitates release of the exterior which may aid the healing process, and the other important action of *chai hu* 柴胡 is to spread Liver *qi*, which would benefit patients with *qi* stagnation. *Shu di huang* 熟地黄 clears heat and tonifies and nourishes Blood.

An interesting finding was the low herb frequency for cutaneous outcomes. When used as IM, the number of studies was larger than for oral CHM alone, which makes it reasonable to expect less herb diversity in a larger pool. This was not found to be the case. While the reasons for this remain unclear, one plausible explanation could be that there is a greater diversity in formulas and herbs used to target skin symptoms compared with treating pain.

Safety of Oral Chinese Herbal Medicine for Herpes Zoster

Oral Chinese Herbal Medicine Alone

Twelve studies (621 participants in the intervention groups and 596 in the comparator groups) provided information on adverse events

(S7, S8, S18, S20, S31, S36, S38, S57, S66, S67, S69, S72), with four studies stating that no adverse events were experienced (S36, S38, S69, S72). Adverse events in people who received oral CHM included five cases of diarrhoea, four cases of nausea, and three cases of mild stomach discomfort and loss of appetite. Adverse events in the comparator group included 11 cases of nausea, five cases of headache, three cases of mild drowsiness, three cases of stomach discomfort, two cases of dizziness, two cases of mild dizziness and fatigue, and one case of dizziness and nausea.

Oral Chinese Herbal Medicine as Integrative Medicine

Twenty-six studies (1,276 participants in the intervention groups and 1,084 in the comparator groups) reported details about adverse events (S5, S6, S10, S11, S12, S13, S23, S24, S35, S39, S44, S50, S60, S61, S63, S73, S74, S76–S80, S82–S85). Twelve studies reported that no adverse events occurred (S6, S10, S11, S35, S50, S61, S73, S76, S82–S85). In participants who received oral CHM as IM, adverse events included 10 cases of mild abdominal pain and diarrhoea, eight cases of dizziness, eight cases of nausea, six cases of diarrhoea, three cases of gastrointestinal discomfort, and one case each of rash, pain at site of intramuscular injection, increased frequency of bowel movement, and headache. Adverse events in the comparator groups included 10 cases of dizziness, eight cases of nausea, five cases of gastrointestinal discomfort, five cases of headache, two cases of a transient increase in alanine transaminase and aspartate transaminase, and one case each of diarrhoea, pain at site of intramuscular injection, sore throat, and back pain.

Topical Chinese Herbal Medicine

Nineteen studies evaluated topical CHM for the treatment of herpes zoster. Six studies compared topical CHM with pharmacotherapy (S1, S41, S46–S48, S86). Due to diversity in reported outcomes, meta-analysis was possible for two outcomes: time taken for crust formation and effective rate. Thirteen studies used topical CHM as IM

(S35, S37, S43, S49, S51, S52, S54, S87–S92). The outcome most frequently reported was time taken for crust formation in 11 studies (S37, S41, S43, S46, S47, S49, S51, S54, S87, S88, S92). Meta-analyses were possible for cutaneous outcomes and effective rate.

Pain Score

Topical Chinese Herbal Medicine Alone

One study reported the pain score on the VAS at the end of treatment (S47). Topical CHM reduced the pain score at the end of treatment by 1.64 cm ([–2.52, –0.76]) compared with valacyclovir, carbamazepine, vitamin B1, mecobalamin (a form of vitamin B12), penciclovir cream, and health education.

Topical Chinese Herbal Medicine as Integrative Medicine

One study which used topical CHM in combination with pharmacotherapy reported the VAS pain score at the end of treatment (S49). Topical CHM as IM reduced the pain score by 0.93 cm compared with acyclovir, indomethacin, and acyclovir eye drops ([–1.12, –0.74]).

Time Taken for Resolution of Pain

Topical Chinese Herbal Medicine Alone

Two studies reported the time taken until pain was resolved (S41, S46), with time recorded from the start of treatment in one (S46) and the other reporting an unspecified time-point; the latter study was excluded from analysis. When measured from the start of treatment, topical CHM reduced the time taken for resolution of pain by 4.40 days ([–4.88, –3.92]) compared with acyclovir (S46).

Topical Chinese Herbal Medicine as Integrative Medicine

Seven studies reported the time until resolution of pain (S35, S43, S49, S51, S54, S88, S92). One study reported the time from the start of treatment to pain resolution (S35). This study was a three-arm study with two treatment arms, which were considered sufficiently similar to be merged for analysis. All other studies did not specify the time-point from which measurement was made and were excluded from analysis. Topical CHM as IM resulted in a faster time taken for the resolution of pain compared with acyclovir (MD –6.76 days [–7.42, –6.10]).

Time Taken for Crust Formation

Topical Chinese Herbal Medicine Alone

Three studies reported on the time taken for crusts to form (S41, S46, S47). Two studies did not specify the time-point from which measurement was made (S41, S47) and were thus not analysed. One study reported the time from start of treatment to crust formation (S46). Compared with acyclovir, topical CHM reduced the time taken for crust formation by 3.00 days ([–3.45, –2.55]).

Topical Chinese Herbal Medicine as Integrative Medicine

Nine studies reported the time taken for the formation of crusts (S35, S37, S43, S49, S51, S54, S87, S88, S92). Data for one study were not presented in a way which permitted re-analysis (S37). Further, six studies which did not specify the time-point from which measurement was made were also excluded from analysis (S43, S51, S54, S87, S88, S92). When measured from the start of treatment, topical CHM as IM decreased the time taken for crust formation by 1.65 days (2 studies, 230 participants; [–2.08, –1.22], $I^2 = 0\%$) (S35, S49).

Time Taken for Cessation of New Lesions

Topical Chinese Herbal Medicine Alone

Three studies reported the time taken for cessation of new lesions (S41, S46, S47), with time measured from the start of treatment for one study (S46). This study found that topical CHM reduced the time taken from treatment start to cessation of new lesions by 2.90 days

([–3.25, –2.55]) compared with acyclovir. Two studies did not specify the time-point from which measurement was made and were excluded from analysis (S41, S47).

Topical Chinese Herbal Medicine as Integrative Medicine

Six studies reported the time taken until no new lesions formed (S35, S43, S49, S51, S88, S92). Time measurements were made from the start of treatment (S35, S49) or from an unspecified time-point (S43, S51, S88, S92). Studies which did not specify the time-point from which measurement was made were excluded from analysis. The time from treatment start to cessation of new lesions when topical CHM was used as IM was 1.61 days less that pharmacotherapy (2 studies, 230 participants; [–2.27, –0.96], I^2 = 81%) (S35, S49). Statistical heterogeneity could not be examined due to the small number of studies included in the meta-analysis.

Time Taken for Resolution of Rash

Topical Chinese Herbal Medicine Alone

Two studies reported on the time taken for the rash to resolve (S41, S46). One study did not specify the time-point from which measurement was made and was excluded from analysis (S41). One study reported the time from start of treatment to rash resolution and found that topical CHM reduced the time by 4.30 days ([–4.72, –3.88]) compared with acyclovir (S46).

Topical Chinese Herbal Medicine as Integrative Medicine

Four studies reported on the time taken for resolution of the rash (S35, S54, S87, S88). Three studies which did not specify the time-point from which measurement was made were excluded from analysis (S54, S87, S88). One study reported the time from the start of treatment to resolution of the rash (S35). In this study, topical CHM as IM reduced the time taken for resolution of the rash by 5.58 days ([–6.58, –4.58]).

Incidence of Post-herpetic Neuralgia

Topical Chinese Herbal Medicine Alone

One study assessed the incidence of PHN one month after resolution of the rash (S47). The chance of developing PHN with topical CHM was 0.18 that of valacyclovir, carbamazepine, vitamin B1, mecobalamin (a form of vitamin B12), penciclovir cream, and health education ([0.04, 0.76]).

Topical Chinese Herbal Medicine as Integrative Medicine

None of the included studies of topical CHM as IM reported on this outcome.

Effective Rate

Topical Chinese Herbal Medicine Alone

Four studies reported outcomes according to a defined effective rate (S1, S46, S47, S86). All studies referred to the 1994 guideline; however, one study reported an effective rate that was not in accordance with the 1994 guideline (S46) and was excluded from analysis. In studies reporting the effective rate according to the 1994 guideline, the chance of achieving a 30% or greater reduction in lesions and significant pain relief with topical CHM was 1.10 that of pharmacotherapy (3 studies, 192 participants; [1.02, 1.18], $I^2 = 0\%$) (S1, S47, S86).

Topical Chinese Herbal Medicine as Integrative Medicine

Seven studies reported outcomes according to a defined effective rate (S49, S51, S87–S90, S92). Four studies cited references which did not include detailed effective rate criteria and were excluded from analysis (S51, S87, S89, S92). Another study was excluded from analysis as it referred to the 1994 guideline but did not report the effective rate in accordance with the guideline (S88). Two studies evaluated the effective rate of topical CHM as IM according to the

1994 guideline (S49, S90). The number of people achieving a 30% reduction in lesions and significant pain relief was not different between those who received topical CHM as IM and those who received pharmacotherapy (2 studies, 160 participants; RR 1.00 [0.85, 1.17], $I^2 = 69\%$). Planned subgroup analyses to investigate possible reasons for statistical heterogeneity could not be performed due to the small number of included studies.

Frequently Reported Topically Used Herbs in Meta-analyses Showing Favourable Effects

The process for determining the herbs which may contribute to positive effects has been outlined above (see *Frequently Reported Orally Used Herbs in Meta-analyses Showing Favourable Effects*). Topical CHM alone resulted in a greater number of people achieving a clinical benefit (based on the effective rate). One herb was present in two of the three studies included in that meta-analysis — *bing pian* 冰片. This herb acts by clearing heat and draining fire. While this herb was common to two studies, whether this herb contributed to the positive result seen remains uncertain due to the low frequency and small number of studies included in the meta-analysis.

When used as IM, topical CHM was found to be superior to pharmacotherapy for cutaneous outcomes (time taken for crust formation) and effective rate. No overlap in herbs was seen for either meta-analysis, which is likely due to each meta-analysis including only two studies. From the available data, it is unclear whether one particular herb (or more) contributed to the effect size or whether the result is due to a synergistic action of the various herbs.

Safety of Topical Chinese Herbal Medicine for Herpes Zoster

Topical Chinese Herbal Medicine Alone

Two studies (86 participants in intervention groups and 71 in comparator groups) reported information about adverse events (S47, S48), with one study reporting that no adverse events were observed (S47) and the other reporting that abdominal fullness, nausea, and loss of appetite occcurred in an unspecified number of cases (S48).

Topical Chinese Herbal Medicine as Integrative Medicine

Five studies (220 participants in intervention groups and 198 in comparator groups) reported on adverse events (S49, S52, S54, S87, S91), with four studies reporting that no adverse events occurred during the trial (S49, S54, S87, S91). In one study (S52), an unspecified number of cases of people who received topical CHM as IM reported feeling cold.

Oral plus Topical Chinese Herbal Medicine

Ten studies evaluated the combination of oral and topical CHM for herpes zoster. Six studies used oral plus topical CHM alone for herpes zoster (S29, S40, S56, S64, S65, S93). Meta-analysis was possible for both pain and cutaneous outcomes. Four studies used oral plus topical CHM as IM (S22, S33, S94, S95). The most frequently reported outcome was time taken for crust formation.

Pain Score

Oral plus Topical Chinese Herbal Medicine Alone

Two studies reported the pain score on the VAS at the end of treatment (S29, S64). The combination of oral and topical CHM did not produce a difference in the pain score at the end of treatment compared with pharmacotherapy (2 studies, 226 participants; MD 0.30 cm [−2.88, 3.47]), $I^2 = 98\%$).

Oral plus Topical Chinese Herbal Medicine as Integrative Medicine

One study reported the pain score using a 0–4 point scale (S95). No explanation was provided on how the pain score was calculated and the results presented were outside of the 0–4 range. This study was excluded from analysis.

Time Taken for Resolution of Pain

Oral plus Topical Chinese Herbal Medicine Alone

Two studies reported on the time taken for the resolution of pain (S40, S64). One study which did not specify the time-point from which measurement was made was excluded from analysis (S64). When measured from the start of treatment, oral plus topical CHM reduced the time taken for pain resolution by 4.30 days compared with oral and topical acyclovir and vitamin B1 ([−6.25, −2.35]) (S40).

Oral plus Topical Chinese Herbal Medicine as Integrative Medicine

One study which compared oral plus topical CHM as IM with acyclovir and vitamin B12 reported on the time taken for pain to resolve (S33). However, data were reported in such a way that re-analysis was not possible. The evidence for oral plus topical CHM as IM in reducing the time taken for resolution of pain is unclear.

Time Taken for Crust Formation

Oral plus Topical Chinese Herbal Medicine Alone

Four studies reported on the time taken for crust formation (S40, S64, S65, S93). One study did not specify the time-point from which measurement was made and was excluded from analysis (S64). Three studies were pooled for analysis (S40, S65, S93). Oral plus topical CHM reduced the time from the start of treatment to crust formation by 1.66 days compared with pharmacotherapy (3 studies, 225 participants; [−2.16, −1.15], $I^2 = 31\%$).

Oral plus Topical Chinese Herbal Medicine as Integrative Medicine

Two studies reported the time taken to achieve crust formation (S33, S94). One study reported the results in a way that did not permit re-analysis (S33), while the other study did not specify the time-point from which measurement was made (S94). Thus, both were excluded from analysis and the evidence for oral plus topical CHM as IM in hastening crust formation remains unclear.

Time Taken for Cessation of New Lesions

Oral plus Topical Chinese Herbal Medicine Alone

Four studies reported the time taken for no new lesions to develop (S40, S64, S65, S93). One study which did not specify the time-point from which measurement was made was excluded from analysis (S64). Meta-analysis was possible for the other three studies (S40, S65, S93) (see Table 5.20). The time from the start of treatment to cessation of new lesions was 1.09 days less in those who received oral plus topical CHM compared with pharmacotherapy ([−2.09, −0.10], $I^2 = 84\%$). Statistical heterogeneity was explored through subgroup analysis. When studies which provided oral plus topical CHM for 7–10 days were pooled, statistical heterogeneity was eliminated whilst benefit remained (MD −1.55 days [−2.02, −1.07], $I^2 = 0\%$).

Oral plus Topical Chinese Herbal Medicine as Integrative Medicine

One study reported the time taken for cessation of new lesions from an unspecified time-point (S94) and thus this study had to be excluded

Table 5.20   Oral plus Topical Chinese Herbal Medicine *vs.* Pharmacotherapy: Time Taken for Cessation of New Lesions

Outcome	No. of Studies (Participants)	Effect Size MD [95% CI] I^2	Included Studies
Time from treatment start to cessation of new lesions (days)	3 (225)	−1.09 [−2.09, −0.10]* 84%	S40, S65, S93
Subgroup: *antivirals plus other treatments*	2 (147)	−0.93 [−2.59, 0.74] 89%	S40, S93
Subgroup: *treatment duration 7–10 days*	2 (142)	−1.55 [−2.02, −1.07]* 0%	S65, S93

*Statistically significant.

Abbreviations: CI, confidence interval; MD, mean difference.

from analysis. The evidence for oral plus topical CHM as IM in reducing the time taken to cease the further forming of lesions remains unclear.

Time Taken for Resolution of Rash

Oral plus Topical Chinese Herbal Medicine Alone

One study reported the time taken for resolution of rash from the start of treatment (S40). Oral plus topical CHM reduced the time taken for the rash to resolve by 3.00 days compared with oral and topical acyclovir and vitamin B1 ([−3.73, −2.27]).

Oral plus Topical Chinese Herbal Medicine as Integrative Medicine

One study which evaluated oral plus topical CHM as IM reported the time taken for the rash to resolve (S94). The study did not report the time-point from which measurement was made and was not subject to re-analysis. The evidence for oral plus topical CHM in reducing the time taken for rash resolution remains unclear.

Incidence of Post-herpetic Neuralgia

Oral plus Topical Chinese Herbal Medicine Alone

The incidence of PHN one month after resolution of the rash was reported in one study (S64). The chance of developing PHN with oral plus topical CHM was not statistically different from that of acyclovir, vitamin B1, and mecobalamin (a form of vitamin B12) (RR 0.10 [0.01, 1.85]).

Oral plus Topical Chinese Herbal Medicine as Integrative Medicine

The incidence of PHN six months after the resolution of rash was lower with oral plus topical CHM as IM compared to oral and topical acyclovir, carbamazepine, indomethacin, and vitamins B1 and B12 (RR 0.25 [0.09, 0.66]) (S95). The incidence of PHN was also lower in those who received oral and topical CHM as IM when measured 30 days after treatment started (RR 0.35 [0.13, 0.89]) (S22).

Effective Rate

Oral plus Topical Chinese Herbal Medicine Alone

Three studies reported outcomes in terms of a defined effective rate (S56, S64, S65). However, the criteria for one study was not described in detail (S56) and the data were excluded from further analysis. Two studies reported on the effective rate with oral plus topical CHM in accordance with the selected CM clinical practice guideline (S64, S65). No benefit was seen for oral plus topical CHM compared with pharmacotherapy in reducing lesions and pain (2 studies, 208 participants; RR 1.01 [0.98, 1.04]).

Oral plus Topical Chinese Herbal Medicine as Integrative Medicine

None of the included studies using oral plus topical CHM as IM reported outcomes in terms of effective rate.

Safety of Oral plus Topical Chinese Herbal Medicine for Herpes Zoster

Oral plus Topical Chinese Herbal Medicine Alone

Three studies (121 participants in the intervention groups and 106 in comparator groups) reported on the safety of oral plus topical CHM for herpes zoster (S40, S65, S93), with two studies reporting that no adverse events occurred (S40, S65). In one study, no adverse events were reported in participants who received oral plus topical CHM (S93) while adverse events in the control group included two cases of increased pustules in the rash.

Oral plus Topical Chinese Herbal Medicine as Integrative Medicine

One study (50 participants in the intervention group and 45 in the comparator group) reported the occurrence of adverse events (S22). Two cases of dizziness were seen with oral and topical CHM as IM and four cases each of dizziness and gastrointestinal discomfort were reported with acyclovir, cimetidine, polyinosinic acid, and vitamin B12.

Chinese Herbal Medicine Compared with Guideline-recommended Doses of Antiviral Therapy

Eighteen studies used guideline-recommended doses of antiviral therapies (see Chapters 1 and 4). Studies used various routes of administration of CHM, including oral CHM alone (S8, S18, S57, S68), oral CHM as IM (S6, S11, S12, S23, S45, S58, S59, S61, S77, S79), topical CHM as IM (S87, S88, S91), and oral plus topical CHM as IM (S94). While many studies presented findings in terms of both pain and cutaneous outcomes, several did not specify the time-point from which measurement was made for 'time taken' outcomes (e.g., time taken for resolution of pain, time taken for resolution of rash, etc). These data were excluded from further analysis. Therefore, evidence is available for oral CHM alone (S8, S18, S57, S68) and oral CHM as IM (S6, S11, S12, S23, S45, S58, S59, S61, S77, S79).

Oral CHM was not statistically different from pharmacotherapy in reducing the pain score on the VAS at the end of treatment (2 studies, 133 participants; MD −0.73 cm [−1.52, 0.07], $I^2 = 68\%$) (S8, S57). Results from single studies showed no difference between oral CHM and pharmacotherapy in the incidence of PHN one month from the onset of rash (RR 0.48 [0.05, 5.09]) (S57) or one month after the end of treatment (RR 0.30 [0.09, 1.00], p = 0.05) (S8). Oral CHM was superior to pharmacotherapy in increasing the chance of achieving a 30% or greater reduction in lesions and significant pain relief (RR 1.29 [1.13, 1.48]) (S18).

In studies which used oral CHM as IM, several meta-analyses were possible (see Table 5.21). Compared with guideline-recommended doses of antiviral therapies, oral CHM as IM:

- Decreased the time from the start of treatment to no pain by 2.52 days ([−4.35, −0.70], $I^2 = 95\%$);

Table 5.21   Oral Chinese Herbal Medicine as Integrative Medicine *vs.* Guideline-recommended Doses of Antiviral Therapies

Outcome	No. of Studies (Participants)	Effect Size MD/RR [95% CI] I^2	Included Studies
Pain score (cm)	2 (129)	MD −0.93 [−2.60, 0.74]	S6, S61
Time from treatment start to resolution of pain (days)	4 (410)	MD −2.52 [−4.35, −0.70]* 95%	S6, S12, S23, S79
Time from treatment start to crust formation (days)	4 (410)	MD −2.38 [−3.34, −1.42]* 93%	S6, S12, S23, S79
Time from treatment start to cessation of new lesions (days)	4 (410)	MD −1.58 [−2.41, −0.74]* 95%	S6, S12, S23, S79
Time from treatment start to resolution of the rash (days)	3 (350)	MD −3.30 [−6.09, −0.51]* 97%	S6, S12, S79
PHN: 30 to 40 days after start of treatment	2 (262)	RR 0.22 [0.08, 0.64]* 0%	S11, S12
Effective rate	2 (318)	RR 1.26 [1.14, 1.38]* 0%	S59, S77

*Statistically significant.
Abbreviations: CI, confidence interval; MD, mean difference; PHN, post-herpetic neuralgia; RR, risk ratio.

- Decreased the time from the start of treatment to crust formation by 2.38 days ([−3.34, −1.42], I^2 = 93%);
- Decreased the time from the start of treatment to cessation of new lesions by 1.58 days ([−2.41, −0.74], I^2 = 95%);
- Decreased the time from the start of treatment to resolution of the rash by 3.30 days ([−6.09, −0.51], I^2 = 97%);
- Decreased the incidence of PHN measured between four weeks and 40 days after the start of treatment (RR 0.22 [0.08, 0.64], I^2 = 0%), and;

- Increased the chance of achieving a 30% or greater reduction in lesions and significant pain relief (RR 1.26 [1.14, 1.38], $I^2 = 0\%$).

The findings for incidence of PHN and effective rate had little statistical heterogeneity and may be more reliable than other outcomes, although the number of studies in both analyses was small. From the meta-analyses, no benefit was seen in reducing the pain score on the VAS at the end of treatment (MD –0.93 cm [–2.60, 0.74], $I^2 = 96\%$).

Oral CHM as IM was also compared with guideline-recommended doses of antiviral therapy in several studies which were unable to be pooled for analysis. Results from single studies showed that CHM as IM was superior to antiviral therapy in reducing the time taken from onset of the rash to crust formation (MD –1.47 days [–2.78, –0.16]) (S61) as well as time taken from onset of the rash to cessation of new lesion formation (MD –1.70 days [–2.52, –0.88]) (S61). Oral CHM as IM was statistically not superior to guideline-recommended doses of antiviral therapy in terms of reducing the time elapsed from onset to resolution of the rash (MD –1.54 days [–4.90, 1.82]) (S61) or reducing the incidence of PHN one month after the end of treatment (RR 0.17 [0.02, 1.30]) (S23).

Assessment Using Grading of Recommendations

Summary-of-findings tables using Grading of Recommendations Assessment, Development, and Evaluation (GRADE) were prepared to present the quality of the evidence for the main comparisons. Interventions, comparators, and outcomes to be included were selected based on a consensus process as described in Chapter 4. At the conclusion of the rating process, it was determined that summary-of-findings tables should be prepared for CHM overall as well as for *Long dan xie gan tang* 龙胆泻肝汤.

For CHM overall, two tables were prepared for the main routes of administration, specifically oral and topical CHM, and both included studies where CHM was used in IM, which is more reflective of practice. When studies which evaluated *Long dan xie gan tang* 龙胆泻肝汤 were reviewed, it was found that none of the studies reported on the outcomes selected by the panel and/or used comparators that are of interest to this review. As a result, the summary-of-findings table for *Long dan xie gan tang* 龙胆泻肝汤 was not prepared, and further evaluation of this intervention compared with the preferred treatment of antivirals plus pain management therapies is needed. Summary-of-findings tables are presented below for oral and topical CHM as IM.

Oral Chinese Herbal Medicine as Integrative Medicine vs. Antivirals plus Pain Management Therapies

Four studies compared oral CHM as IM with antivirals plus pain management therapies (S3, S16, S45, S50), three of which reported on outcomes selected for inclusion in the summary-of-findings table (S3, S16, S50) (see Table 5.22).

- Evidence for oral CHM as IM *vs.* antivirals plus pain management therapies was judged to be of 'very low' or 'low' quality. None of the studies reported on outcomes in terms of time taken for resolution of pain and time taken for resolution of rash. No benefit was seen in one study which reported pain severity (VAS) at the end of treatment and there was no statistical difference between groups in the incidence of PHN.

Topical Chinese Herbal Medicine as Integrative Medicine vs. Antivirals plus Pain Management Therapies

Two studies evaluated topical CHM as IM compared with antivirals and pain management treatments alone (S49, S51) (see Table 5.23). Both studies reported on at least one outcome selected for inclusion in the summary-of-findings table. Neither study reported on the time taken for rash to resolve or PHN incidence.

Table 5.22   GRADE: Oral Chinese Herbal Medicine as Integrative Medicine *vs.* Antivirals plus Pain Management Therapies

Outcomes (Treatment Duration)	No of Participants (Studies)	Quality of the Evidence (GRADE)	Relative Effect (95% CI)	Anticipated Absolute Effects	
				Risk with Antiviral plus Pain	Risk Difference with Oral CHM as IM
Pain severity (VAS) (12 days)	60 (1 RCT)	⊕⊕◯◯ LOW[1,2]	—	The mean pain severity was **2.78 cm**	MD **0.57 cm** lower (1.44 lower to 0.3 higher)
				Study population	
Incidence of PHN (3 months) (range 7 to 42 days)	78 (1 RCT)	⊕◯◯◯ VERY LOW[2,3]	RR 0.08 (0.00 to 1.32)	15 per 100	14 fewer per 100 (15 fewer to 5 more)
Adverse events (3 weeks)	52 (1 RCT)	No adverse events reported			

The risk in the intervention group (and its 95% confidence interval) is based on the assumed risk in the comparison group and the relative effect of the intervention (and its 95% CI).

Abbreviations: CI, confidence interval; GRADE, Grading of Recommendations Assessment, Development, and Evaluation; MD, mean difference; RR, risk ratio; PHN, post-herpetic neuralgia; RCT, randomised controlled trial; VAS, visual analogue scale.

1. High risk of bias due to lack of blinding
2. Uncertainty in results due to small sample size
3. High risk of bias due to lack of blinding, inadequate sequence generation, and allocation concealment

Study References

Pain severity (VAS): S16
Incidence of PHN (3 months): S3
Adverse events: S50

Table 5.23   GRADE: Topical Chinese Herbal Medicine as Integrative Medicine *vs.* Antivirals plus Pain Management Therapies

Outcomes (Treatment Duration)	No of Participants (studies)	Quality of the Evidence (GRADE)	Relative Effect (95% CI)	Anticipated Absolute Effects	
				Risk with Antiviral plus Pain	Risk Difference with Topical CHM as IM
Pain severity (VAS) cm (10 days)	80 (1 RCT)	⊕⊕◯◯ LOW[1,2]	—	The mean pain severity was **2.15 cm**	MD **0.93 cm** lower (1.12 lower to 0.74 lower)
Time taken for resolution of pain (days) (mean 10 days)	161 (2 RCTs)	⊕◯◯◯ VERY LOW[1,2,3]	—	The mean time taken for resolution of pain was **7.04 days**	MD **2.63 days** fewer (5.98 fewer to 0.72 more)
Adverse events (mean 10 days)	80 (1 RCT)	No adverse events were reported			

The risk in the intervention group (and its 95% confidence interval) is based on the assumed risk in the comparison group and the relative effect of the intervention (and its 95% CI).

Abbreviations: CI, confidence interval; GRADE, Grading of Recommendations Assessment, Development, and Evaluation; MD, mean difference; RR, risk ratio; PHN, post-herpetic neuralgia; RCT, randomised controlled trial; VAS, visual analogue scale.

1. High risk of bias due to lack of blinding
2. Uncertainty in results due to small sample size
3. No overlap in confidence intervals

Study References

Pain severity (VAS) cm: S49
Time taken for resolution of pain (days): S49, S51
Adverse events: S49

- Evidence for topical CHM as IM *vs.* antivirals plus pain management therapies was judged to be of 'very low' or 'low' quality. Topical CHM as IM resulted in pain severity that was 0.93 cm lower than antivirals plus pain management on the VAS at the end of treatment. No difference was observed between groups in the time taken for resolution of pain.

Randomised Controlled Trial Evidence from Individual Formulas

Several formulas were used in multiple RCTs, thereby allowing meta-analyses to be conducted. The evidence from meta-analyses is presented where the study used only the formula of interest (i.e., not in combination with other formulas). *Long dan xie gan tang* 龙胆泻肝汤 was used as the sole formula in 16 studies (S2, S5, S8, S12, S18–S21, S23–S26, S28, S30–S32) (see Table 5.24). In these studies where *Long dan xie gan tang* 龙胆泻肝汤 was the sole treatment in the intervention group, the time taken from start of treatment to:

- Resolution of pain was 3.07 days less than pharmacotherapy ([–3.72, –2.43], $I^2 = 0\%$);
- Crust formation was 1.91 days less than pharmacotherapy ([–2.54, –1.28], $I^2 = 12\%$);
- Resolution of the rash was 4.11 days less than pharmacotherapy ([–5.07, –3.15], $I^2 = 0\%$).

The chance of achieving a 30% or greater reduction in symptoms and significant pain relief was greater with *Long dan xie gan tang* 龙胆泻肝汤 compared with pharmacotherapy (RR 1.25 [1.13, 1.38], $I^2 = 0\%$). No difference was seen between *Long dan xie gan tang* 龙胆泻肝汤 and pharmacotherapy in terms of the time taken for cessation of new lesion formation (MD –1.78 days [–4.33, 0.77], $I^2 = 97\%$).

Table 5.24   Long Dan Xie Gan Tang 龙胆泻肝汤 *vs.* Pharmacotherapy

Outcome	No. of Studies (Participants)	Effect Size MD/RR [95% CI] I^2	Included Studies
Time from treatment start to resolution of pain	3 (320)	MD –3.07 [–3.72, –2.43]* 0%	S20, S21, S28
Time from treatment start to crust formation	3 (320)	MD –1.91 [–2.54, –1.28]* 12%	S20, S21, S28
Time from treatment start to cessation of new lesions	2 (284)	MD –1.78 [–4.33, 0.77] 97%	S20, S28
Time from treatment start to resolution of rash	3 (320)	MD –4.11 [–5.07, –3.15]* 0%	S20, S21, S28
Effective rate	2 (320)	RR 1.25 [1.13, 1.38]* 0%	S18, S19

*Statistically significant.

Abbreviations: CI, confidence interval; MD, mean difference; RR, risk ratio.

When used as IM, *Long dan xie gan tang/wan* 龙胆泻肝汤/丸 also reduced the time taken from start of treatment to:

- Resolution of pain by 2.99 days ([–3.98, –2.01], I^2 = 11%);
- Crust formation by 2.52 days ([–3.43, –1.61], I^2 = 79%), and;
- Cessation of new lesions by 1.68 days ([–2.61, –0.75], I^2 = 89%) (see Table 5.25).

Meta-analysis was also possible in two studies which used *Xiao chai hu tang* (modified) 加味小柴胡汤 as IM. The chance of achieving a 30% or greater reduction in symptoms and significant pain relief was 1.78 that of pharmacotherapy alone (2 studies, 114 participants; [1.31, 2.42, I^2 = 0%) (S59, S80). There is some evidence to support the use of these formulas in reducing the pain caused by herpes zoster and helping with rash healing.

Table 5.25   Long Dan Xie Gan Tang/Wan 龙胆泻肝汤/丸 as Integrative Medicine *vs.* Pharmacotherapy

Outcome	No. of Studies (Participants)	Effect Size MD/RR [95% CI] I²	Included Studies
Time from treatment start to resolution of pain	2 (238)	MD −2.99 [−3.98, −2.01]* 11%	S12, S23
Time from treatment start to crust formation	2 (238)	MD −2.52 [−3.43, −1.61]* 79%	S12, S23
Time from treatment start to cessation of new lesions	2 (238)	MD −1.68 [−2.61, −0.75]* 89%	S12, S23
Effective rate	2 (164)	RR 1.56 [0.86, 2.86] 71%	S2, S25

*Statistically significant.

Abbreviations: CI, confidence interval; MD, mean difference; RR, risk ratio.

Randomised Controlled Trial Evidence for Formulas Commonly Used in Clinical Practice

Many studies used formulas recommended in key textbooks and clinical practice guidelines (see Chapter 2). These include *Long dan xie gan tang* 龙胆泻肝汤, *Xin huang pian* 新癀片, *San huang* powder 三黄散, and topical *qing dai* powder 青黛散. An attempt was made to evaluate the clinical evidence of several formulas recommended in Chapter 2. However, many were used in combination with other formulas, therefore making it impossible to evaluate the effects of these formulas alone. Evidence from RCTs for *Long dan xie gan tang* 龙胆泻肝汤 has been presented above.

Xin huang pian 新癀片 was used as IM in two studies (S60, S78). As a form of IM therapy compared with oral and topical acyclovir, *Xin huang pian* 新癀片 shortened the time from start of treatment to no pain by 3.14 days ([−4.69, −1.59]), time taken for crust formation by 2.49 days ([−3.18, −1.80]), and time taken for cessation of new lesions by 2.70 days ([−3.09, −2.31]) (S78). When combined with valacyclovir and helium-neon laser treatment, *Xin huang pian* 新癀片 reduced pain scores on the VAS at the end of treatment by 1.70 cm ([−2.26, −1.14]) (S60). The study also reported on the incidence of PHN, with no cases seen in either group.

Controlled Clinical Trials of Chinese Herbal Medicine

Five CCTs of CHM for herpes zoster were eligible for inclusion (S96–S100). A total of 832 participants were included. One study was a three-arm trial with two intervention groups (S100), while all others used a two-arm, parallel design. Two studies used CHM alone (S96, S97) and three used CHM as IM (S98–S100). All studies were conducted in China, with two conducted in both inpatient and outpatient departments (S96, S97), two in outpatient departments only (S99, S100), and one that did not specify the trial setting (S98).

There was some variation across studies in the duration of the condition, with four studies reporting conditions that lasted 12 days or less (S97–S100) and one reporting durations between one and 23 days (S96). Studies included more males than females (440 vs. 392, respectively) and while age ranged from 18 (S98, S99) to 75 years (S98), the majority of participants were middle-aged (the median of the mean age was 51.9 years). Treatment duration ranged from seven (S96, S100) to 14 days (S96), or continued until loss of crusts was achieved (S99). Three studies followed up participants after treatment finished, at 7 days (S100), 15 days (S99), or three months (S97).

None of the studies reported using CM syndrome differentiation for inclusion of participants or for treatment. Two studies used oral CHM (S97, S98) and three used oral plus topical CHM (S96, S99, S100). Named oral formulas included *Long dan xie gan tang* 龙胆泻肝汤 (S96), *Jie du tong luo huo xue tang* 解毒通络活血汤 (S98), *Mie tong xiao pao tang* 灭痛消疱汤 (S99), and compound glycyrrhizin 复方甘草酸苷片 tablets (S100). There were no overlaps in formulas. Forty-five different herbs were used, with the most common being *gan cao* 甘草/compound glycyrrhizin 复方甘草酸苷片, *ban lan gen* 板蓝根, *che qian zi* 车前子, *zhi zi* 栀子, *long dan cao* 龙胆草, and *yan hu suo* 延胡索 (see Table 5.26).

All studies included antiviral therapy, with two using antiviral therapy alone (S99, S100), two using antiviral therapy in combination with analgesics and vitamins (S96, S98), and one using antiviral therapy with vitamins (S97). Two studies used antiviral therapy at a

Table 5.26 Frequently Reported Herbs in Controlled Clinical Trials

Most Common Herbs	Scientific Name	Frequency of Use
Gan cao 甘草/ compound glycyrrhizin 复方甘草酸苷片	*Glycyrrhiza* spp	4
Ban lan gen 板蓝根	*Isatis indigotica* Fort.	3
Che qian zi 车前子	*Plantago* spp	3
Jiao zhi zi 焦栀子	*Gardenia jasminoides* Ellis	3
Jin long dan cao 金龙胆草	*Conyza blinii* Lévl.	3
Yan hu suo 延胡索	*Corydalis yanhusuo* W.T. Wang	3
Bai zhi 白芷	*Angelica dahurica* spp	2
Chai hu 柴胡	*Bupleurum* spp	2
Da huang 大黄	*Rheum* spp	2
Fu ling 茯苓	*Poria cocos* (Schw.) Wolf	2
Huang bai 黄柏	*Phellodendron chinense* Schneid.	2
Huang qin 黄芩	*Scutellaria baicalensis* Georgi	2
Jiang huang 姜黄	*Curcuma longa* L.	2
Ku shen 苦参	*Sophora flavescens* Ait.	2
Mu dan pi 牡丹皮	*Paeonia suffruticosa* Andr.	2
Pu gong ying 蒲公英	*Taraxacum* spp	2
Sheng di huang 生地黄	*Rehmannia glutinosa* Libosch.	2
Ze xie 泽泻	*Alisma orientalis* (Sam.) Juzep.	2

Note: The use of some herbs may be restricted in some countries. Readers are advised to comply with relevant regulations. The frequency of use for some herbs may be greater than the actual number of studies which used the herb, i.e., where multiple formulas were reported.

dosage that is recommended in clinical practice guidelines (S99, S100). One study used helium-neon laser irradiation as a co-intervention in both groups (S99). One study that documented the time taken for the resolution of rash reported the mean time but not the standard deviation, and thus re-analysis was not possible (S97).

Two studies comparing the combination of oral and topical CHM plus famciclovir with famciclovir alone reported on the same outcomes (time taken for crust formation, time taken for cessation of new lesions, and time taken for resolution of rash) (S99, S100). One study measured the time from the start of treatment (S100) while the other did not indicate a specific time-point and was excluded from analysis. The analysed study (S100) was a three-arm trial study and the two intervention arms both included CHM, and data for these arms were merged for analysis.

The combination of oral plus topical CHM with famciclovir reduced the time taken for crust formation (MD −1.15 days [−2.14, −0.16], S100) and the time taken for resolution of the rash (MD −1.93 days [−2.92, −0.94], S100) compared with famciclovir alone. No benefit over famciclovir was seen with oral plus topical CHM as IM in reducing the time taken for cessation of new lesions (MD 0.46 days [−0.99, 0.07], S100).

Results from other studies showed that oral plus topical CHM used alone increased the number of people achieving a 30% or greater improvement in pain and lesions compared with acyclovir, indomethacin, polyinosinic acid (an immunostimulant), and vitamins C and B1 (RR 1.11 [1.01, 1.23]) (S96). Oral plus topical CHM as IM reduced the time taken from start of treatment to resolution of pain by 1.31 days ([−2.41, −0.21]) (S100), but no benefit was seen on the incidence of PHN seven days after cessation of treatment (RR 0.53 [0.28, 1.00], $p = 0.05$) (S100). This finding was not surprising as PHN is usually diagnosed at least one month after the resolution of the rash but treatment was provided for only seven days.

Three studies (252 participants in the intervention groups and 248 in the comparator groups) reported outcomes for adverse events (S98, S99, S100), with one reporting no adverse events occurring (S98). Thirty-seven adverse events were reported in the CHM groups and 20 adverse events were reported with pharmacotherapy. Adverse events in the treatment groups included 12 cases of nausea, seven cases of gastrointestinal discomfort, six cases of diarrhoea, three cases of erythema associated with laser irradiation, two cases of dizziness, and one case each of malaise and skin rash. In the pharmacotherapy group, the most common adverse event was nausea (9 cases) followed by gastrointestinal discomfort (2 cases), diarrhoea (2 cases), and one case each of skin rash and dizziness.

Non-controlled Studies of Chinese Herbal Medicine

Fifty-one non-controlled studies evaluated CHM (S101–S151). A total of 2,521 adults were involved in these studies which were all conducted in China. Seven studies were case reports (S106–S108, S112, S113, S122, S123) and the remaining were case series. Sample sizes ranged from one in case reports up to 146 (S124), and the median sample size was 40.

Thirteen studies reported using CM syndrome differentiation either for inclusion or to guide treatment (S101–S113). The most frequently reported syndrome was excess heat in the Liver meridian (6 studies) (S103, S105, S106, S108–S110). Other syndromes reported in two or more studies included the pattern/syndrome of *qi* stagnation and Blood stasis (4 studies) (S102–S105), Liver-Gallbladder dampness-heat (3 studies) (S111–S113), and Spleen deficiency with dampness (3 studies) (S101, S103, S110).

CHM was used alone in 31 studies (S101, S104–S113, S115, S116, S121–S138) and in combination with pharmacotherapy in 20 studies (S102, S103, S114, S117–S120, S139, S140–S151). Forty studies used oral CHM either alone (S101–S104, S106, S108–S114, S117, S118, S123–S126, S131, S134, S135, S137, S138, S141–S143, S145–S148,) or in combination with topical CHM (S105, S107, S115, S116, S119, S121, S122, S136, S150). Twelve studies used topical CHM alone (S120, S127–S130, S132, S133, S139, S140, S144, S149, S151).

The most frequently reported formula was *Long dan xie gan tang* 龙胆泻肝汤 (15 studies) (see Table 5.27). Several other formulas were used in two or more studies, with both *Chu shi wei ling tang* 除湿胃苓汤 and *Tao hong si wu tang* 桃红四物汤 used in four studies each. The most commonly reported herbs were *gan cao* 甘草, *zhi zi* 栀子, *chai hu* 柴胡, *huang qin* 黄芩, and *di huang* 地黄 (see Table 5.28).

Eleven studies (620 participants) reported the occurrence of adverse events (S101, S105, S120, S127, S134, S141, S142, S145, S146, S150, S151). Adverse events occurred in three studies (S142, S146, S151) and included five cases of mild epigastric discomfort (S142) and one case of dizziness and nausea (S146) with oral CHM,

Table 5.27 Frequently Reported Formulas in Non-controlled Studies

Most Common Formulas	No. of Studies	Ingredients
Long dan xie gan tang 龙胆泻肝汤	15	Long dan cao 龙胆草, zhi zi 栀子, huang qin 黄芩, mu tong 木通, ze xie 泽泻, che qian zi 车前子, sheng di 生地, dang gui 当归, gan cao 甘草, chai hu 柴胡
Chu shi wei ling tang 除湿胃苓汤	4	Fang feng 防风, cang zhu 苍术, bai zhu 白术, chi fu ling 赤茯苓, chen pi 陈皮, hou pu 厚朴, zhu ling 猪苓, shan zhi 山栀, mu tong 木通, ze xie 泽泻, hua shi 滑石, gan cao 甘草, bo he 薄荷, gui zhi 桂枝
Tao hong si wu tang 桃红四物汤	4	Tao ren 桃仁, hong hua 红花, dang gui 当归, shu di huang 熟地黄, shao yao 芍药, chuan xiong 川芎
Xue fu zhu yu tang 血府逐瘀汤	3	Tao ren 桃仁, hong hua 红花, dang gui 当归, sheng di 生地, zhi ke 枳壳, chi shao 赤芍, chai hu 柴胡, gan cao 甘草, jie geng 桔梗, chuan xiong 川芎, niu xi 牛膝
Chai hu shu gan san 柴胡疏肝散	2	Chai hu 柴胡, chen pi 陈皮, chuan xiong 川芎, chi shao 赤芍, zhi qiao 枳壳, xiang fu 香附, zhi gan cao 炙甘草
Er wei ba du san 二味拔毒散	2	Bai fan 白矾, ming xiong huang 明雄黄
Fu fang xiong huang ding 复方雄黄酊	2	Xiong huang 雄黄, bai zhi 白芷, bing pian 冰片 (S133)
Ji de sheng she yao pian 季德胜蛇药片	2	Qi ye yi zhi hua 七叶一枝花, chan chu pi 蟾蜍皮, wu gong 蜈蚣, di jin cao 地锦草 (S140)
Liu shen wan 六神丸	2	Zhen zhu fen 珍珠粉, xi niu huang 犀牛黄, she xiang 麝香, xiong huang 雄黄, chan su 蟾酥, bing pian 冰片
Yun nan bai yao jiao nang 云南白药胶囊	2	Not specified

Note: Ingredients are referenced to the *Zhong Yi Fang Ji Da Ci Dian* 中医方剂大辞典 where available, or to an included study if not available.

Note: The use of some herbs such as *mu tong* 木通 may be restricted in some countries under the provisions of CITES. Readers are advised to comply with relevant regulations.

Table 5.28   Frequently Reported Herbs in Non-controlled Studies

Most Common Herbs	Scientific Name	Frequency of Use
Gan cao 甘草	*Glycyrrhiza* spp	30
Zhi zi 栀子	*Gardenia jasminoides* Ellis	26
Chai hu 柴胡	*Bupleurum* spp	25
Huang qin 黄芩	*Scutellaria baicalensis* Georgi	23
Sheng di huang 生地黄	*Rehmannia glutinosa* Libosch.	22
Long dan cao 龙胆草	*Gentiana scabra* Bge.	20
Yan hu suo 延胡索	*Corydalis yanhusuo* W.T. Wang	18
Dang gui 当归	*Angelica sinensis* (Oliv.) Diels	18
Chi shao 赤芍	*Paeonia* spp	16
Ze xie 泽泻	*Alisma orientalis* (Sam.) Juzep.	15
Che qian zi 车前子	*Plantago* spp	14
Lian qiao 连翘	*Forsythia suspensa* (Thunb.) Vahl	12
Ban lan gen 板蓝根	*Isatis indigotica* Fort.	12
Jin yin hua 金银花	*Lonicera japonica* Thunb.	11
Mu dan pi 牡丹皮	*Paeonia suffruticosa* Andr.	10
Huang lian 黄连	*Coptis* spp	9
Da huang 大黄	*Rheum* spp	9
Chuan xiong 川芎	*Ligusticum chuangxiong* Hort.	9
Mu tong 木通	*Akebia* spp	9

Note: The use of some herbs such as *mu tong* 木通 may be restricted in some countries under the provisions of CITES. Readers are advised to comply with relevant regulations. The frequency of use for some herbs may be greater than the actual number of studies which used the herb, i.e., where multiple formulas were reported.

and three cases of erythema, burning, and peeling at the skin lesion in a study using topical CHM (S151).

Summary of Clinical Evidence for Chinese Herbal Medicine

This evaluation of the clinical evidence found that CHM formulas and routes of administration vary and there was a diverse range of outcomes reported. Oral CHM was the most frequently investigated

CHM and was used in the majority of studies. Treatment durations were short which corresponded with the transient nature of herpes zoster. Syndromes used as inclusion criteria and for selection of treatment were broadly consistent with those in key CM textbooks and clinical practice guidelines described in Chapter 2. The most frequently reported syndromes included excess heat in the Liver meridian, Liver-Gallbladder dampness-heat, and *qi* stagnation and Blood stasis. The formula *Long dan xie gan tang* 龙胆泻肝汤 was evaluated most frequently across all clinical studies and is consistent with CM syndromes reported.

Some promising clinical evidence was seen with oral CHM, topical CHM, and the combination of oral and topical CHM. Oral CHM may reduce the incidence of PHN, an important finding considering the burden associated with PHN and that acyclovir (one of the most commonly used antiviral therapies) has been shown to be ineffective in inhibiting the incidence of PHN.[3] Promising evidence was seen with the formula *Long dan xie gan tang* 龙胆泻肝汤 alone for all cutaneous outcomes and for effective rate. In addition, *Long dan xie gan tang* 龙胆泻肝汤 worked well as IM for improving all cutaneous outcomes and shortening the time taken for the resolution of pain. The clinical evidence also showed that modified *Xiao chai hu tang* 加味小柴胡汤 can improve the effective rate and *Xin huang pian* 新癀片 as IM can alleviate pain and improve cutaneous outcomes.

While benefits were seen for pain and cutaneous outcomes, the importance of these findings remains uncertain if the clinical changes are only modest. Many pain studies suggest that a 50% reduction in pain is clinically important. Differences seen between groups in pain scores from the VAS were typically in the range of one to two centimetres. Whether these indicate a clinically important reduction in pain is dependent on baseline pain scores, which were not analysed as part of this review. Findings for pain outcomes should be interpreted in light of this.

Herbs that may have contributed to the positive effects observed include *bing pian* 冰片 for topical use and *chai hu* 柴胡, *gan cao* 甘草, *shu di huang* 熟地黄, and *long dan cao* 龙胆草 for oral use. Practitioners may consider these herbs when preparing prescriptions for patients with herpes zoster. Few side effects were reported, with CHM considered to be safe for treating herpes zoster based on included studies.

Much of the most promising evidence discussed in this chapter came from analyses where time taken for cutaneous outcomes was measured from the start of treatment. The duration that participants have been afflicted with herpes zoster upon beginning their trials varied in RCTs from one to 27 days, making the time from start of treatment a less reliable indicator of treatment effect. Current conventions in clinical practice and clinical trials dictate that antiviral therapy should be initiated within 72 hours of rash onset,[4] although this is dependent on patients presenting for treatment. Only four of the 103 RCTs reported the duration of herpes zoster as three or fewer days for included participants which further limits the interpretation of the findings. Clinical trials should be designed with careful consideration of guideline recommendations to ensure that treatment effects can be evaluated appropriately.

Many studies did not report the time-point from which measurement was made and the data had to be excluded from analysis. As herpes zoster is a self-limiting condition of relatively short duration, the time-point from which measurements are made is important in the interpretation of results. Consistent reporting of these details in future studies is imperative to ensure that accurate interpretations of potential benefits are possible.

Many studies used antiviral therapies at doses less than those recommended in clinical practice guidelines. A Chinese clinical practice guideline draft published in 2013[5] recommended doses for oral acyclovir (400 mg three times daily) and oral valacyclovir (300 mg twice daily) that are below those recommended in international guidelines (800 mg five times daily and 1000 mg three times daily, respectively). Many of the studies included in this review pre-date this draft guideline and yet were still conducted after the publication of two key international guidelines.[4,6] Why the guideline-recommended doses of antiviral therapy differ is unclear. Regardless, this has an influence on the interpretation of results as the comparator may have a sub-threshold clinical effect.

Many studies also combined guideline-recommended treatments with other treatments for which the evidence is unclear, or for which there is no evidence of benefit. For example, many studies used oral and topical acyclovir, but clinical practice guidelines recommend against the use of topical acyclovir as it has not been demonstrated to be beneficial.[5] Many studies also combined antiviral therapies with vitamins B1 or B12 (or forms of B12). Vitamins B1 and B12 are commonly used in China to aid nerve repair[7,8] but have not been evaluated for efficacy in herpes zoster treatment.

The best available evidence comes from the few studies which used guideline-recommended doses of antiviral therapy, with benefits shown for oral CHM as IM in reducing the time taken for resolution of pain, crust formation, cessation of new lesions, and resolution of rash, inhibiting the incidence of PHN between four weeks to 40 days after start of treatment, and effective rate. Finally, none of the included studies reported on the pre-specified measures of health-related quality of life. Herpes zoster is known to be a significant health burden, so future clinical trials should include measures to assess its impact on quality of life.

References

1. Kongkaew CC, N. Efficacy of Clinacanthus nutans extracts in patients with herpes infection: Systematic review and meta-analysis of randomised clinical trials. *Complement Ther Med.* 2011; **19**(1):47–53.
2. Dubinsky RM, Kabbani H, El-Chami Z, Boutwell C, Ali H. Practice parameter: Treatment of postherpetic neuralgia: An evidence-based report of the Quality Standards Subcommittee of the American Academy of Neurology. *Neurology.* 2004; **63**(6):959–65.
3. Chen N, Li Q, Yang J, Zhou M, Zhou D, He L. Antiviral treatment for preventing postherpetic neuralgia. Cochrane Database of Systematic Reviews. 2014(2).
4. Dworkin RH, Johnson RW, Breuer J, *et al.* Recommendations for the management of herpes zoster. *Clin Infect Dis.* 2007; **44** (Suppl 1):S1–26.
5. 周冬梅, 陈维文. 蛇串疮中医诊疗指南 (2014 年修订版) [J]. 中医杂志. 2015; **13**:1163–1168.

6. Gross G, Schofer H, Wassilew S, *et al*. Herpes zoster guideline of the German Dermatology Society (DDG). *J Clin Virol.* 2003; **26**(3):277–89; discussion 91-3.

7. 陈前明, 吴波, 蒋存火. 口服及肌注维生素 B12 和维生素 B1 对治疗带状疱疹疼痛的疗效比较. 现代临床医学, 2006; **32**(3), 195.

8. 张红星, 黄国付, 杨敏. 中西医结合治疗带状疱疹的临床研究进展. 中国组织工程研究与临床康复. 2007; **11**(29), 5810–5813.

6

Pharmacological Actions of Frequently Used Herbs — Herpes Zoster

OVERVIEW

Many of the herbs frequently used in clinical trials have been evaluated in experimental research. Eleven of the most frequently used herbs in randomised controlled trials included in the previous chapter were reviewed to examine their pharmacological actions. Experimental research has shown that herbs may exert their actions through antiviral and anti-inflammatory mechanisms, which are important in the treatment of herpes zoster.

Introduction

Formulas and herbs mediate physiological effects through their phytochemicals. Clinical studies provide some insight into whether Chinese herbal medicine (CHM) is effective and safe while experimental studies suggest possible mechanisms that underlie the actions and effects of CHM. Mechanisms relevant to herpes zoster have been described in Chapter 1. A selection of the most frequently reported herbs in randomised controlled trials included in Chapter 5 were examined in further detail to identify possible mechanisms of action. This section describes the evidence from experimental studies.

Methods

This chapter provides a general overview of the experimental evidence relating to the pharmacology of herbs and their constituent compounds for herpes zoster. The constituent compounds were identified by searching herbal monographs, high-quality reviews of CHM, herbal medicine encyclopedia,[1] materia medica,[2] and/or PubMed. To identify preclinical publications, a literature search of PubMed was undertaken. Studies were screened for relevance in terms of the mechanisms of action underlying herpes zoster. When reviewing and reporting results, scientific methods were considered as well as the impact of the research citations and the journals in which the articles were published. Relevant data were extracted and a summary of the findings is reported here. The search strategy included the terms for each herb and their constituent compounds *in vitro* and *in vivo*.

Experimental Studies on *Gan Cao* 甘草

Gan cao 甘草 (*Glycyrrhiza uralensis* Fisch., *Glycyrrhiza inflata* Bat., *Glycyrrhiza glabra* L.) contains triterpene saponins, flavonoids, and coumarin derivatives.[2] The effects of *Gan cao* and its compounds have been extensively researched in a variety of skin conditions, and its effects on herpes zoster symptoms have also been examined. Both antiviral and analgesic properties have been demonstrated in animal models and cell lines.

Aikawa *et al.*[3] found that administration of *gan cao* decreased human leukocyte antigen-antigen D-related (HLA-DR+) expression in CD8+ T cells from the peripheral blood of patients with acute stage herpes zoster, and this was correlated with pain reduction. The authors postulate that reduction in HLA-DR+ expression may reflect *gan cao*'s anti-inflammatory actions. The findings from this study suggest antiviral activity, as cytolytic CD8+ T cells contribute to controlling the replication of varicella zoster virus (VZV) during the acute stage of herpes zoster.[4]

Glycyrrhizin (GL), a key compound of *gan cao*, suppressed VZV replication when VZV-infected human embryonic fibroblast (HEF) cells were both pre-treated and post-treated with GL.[5] Suppression was greater in the post-treated cells. Inhibition of viral spreading was also seen when GL was added 16 hours post-infection. The action of GL may proceed through the inhibition of the penetration, uncoating, or release of VZV particles.

One study examined the antiviral activity of GL in Vero cell-cultured VZV from vesicular aspirates in children with chickenpox.[6] The antiviral activity of GL (mean log virus titre) was lower than that of acyclovir and interferon, which may be due to the use of *gan cao* powder extract rather than the pure form of GL. GL may have properties that prevent the VZV from becoming latent in the dorsal or cranial root ganglia by inducing cell death. In BALB/c mice, apoptotic cell death was induced in mature splenic and thymic lymphocytes *in vitro.*[7]

Gan cao may also exhibit analgesic effects. In an inflamed rat model, a compound of glycyrrhetinic acid (GA), olean-11,13(18)-dien-3β,30-*O*-dihemiphthalate (compound 5), suppressed flinching behaviour induced by capsaicin in a dose-dependent manner.[8] Compound 5 also suppressed flinching pain behaviours in the late phase of the formalin test and inhibited tachykinin-induced increases in the number of Chinese hamster ovary (CHO)-K1-expressing tachykinin receptors (a neurotransmitter of pain perception).

Experimental Studies on *Huang Qin* 黄芩

Many compounds have been identified in *huang qin* 黄芩 (*Scutellaria baicalensis* Georgi), including flavonoids, flavone glycosides, and chalcones.[2] Experimental evidence suggests that *huang qin* has anti-inflammatory and immunomodulatory effects. Baicalin, a flavonoid, inhibited interleukin (IL)-6 activity (an inflammatory cytokine), induced dose-dependent increases in Foxp3[+] expression in CD4[+]CD25[−] murine T cells, and led to increased differentiation of T cells and T cell regulation.[9] T cell regulation has been identified as a key mechanism in immune system homeostasis.

Another compound, baicalein, has been shown to attenuate nitric oxide (NO) production (generated from phagocytes as part of the immune response) and apoptosis in lipopolysaccharide (LPS)-activated mouse microglial cells.[10] In the same study, inhibition of LPS-induced nuclear factor-κB (NF-κB) activity in mouse microglial BV-2 cells was also observed. Two flavonoids, baicalein and wogonin, concentration-dependently inhibited LPS-induced NO production in murine RAW 264.7 macrophage cells. The effect was short-lived and was only seen when baicalein and wogonin were added to RAW 264.7 cells shortly after LPS stimulation.[10] The effects were stronger with wogonin than baicalein. Both compounds inhibited inducible nitric oxide synthase (iNOS).[11]

Experimental Studies on *Chai Hu* 柴胡

Chai hu 柴胡 (*Bupleurum chinense* DC., *Bupleurum scorzonerifolium* Willd.) contains two key groups of compounds: triterpene saponines and volatile oils.[2] D-limonene is a compound common to many herbs, including *chai hu*. Much of the research for *chai hu* has focused on D-limonene and immunomodulatory effects have been demonstrated. D-limonene and metabolites, limonene-1–2-diol and perillic acid (which are the main circulating metabolites in humans), inhibited production of interferon-gamma (IFN-γ), IL-2, IL-4, IL-13, and tumour necrosis factor-α (TNF-α) by CD3$^+$CD4$^+$ T cells, and also inhibited the production of IFN-γ, IL-2 and TNF-α by CD3$^+$CD8$^+$ T cells.[12]

Similar results were seen in LPS-stimulated murine macrophage RAW 264.7 cells, where D-limonene dose-dependently decreased expression of IL-1β, IL-6, and TNF-α.[13] In the same study, D-limonene also inhibited NO and prostaglandin E2 (PGE$_2$) production and also dose-dependently decreased expression of iNOS and cyclooxygenase (COX)-2 proteins.

Perillic acid suppressed IL-2 and IL-10 production in human mitogen-activated T cells and peripheral blood mononuclear cells (PBMC) and also dose-dependently decreased levels of phosphorylated mitogen-activated protein kinases.[14] Limonene also had an immunomodulatory effect in BALB/c mice.[15] Limonene and perillic acid increased white blood cell count, bone marrow cell count, plaque forming cells in the spleen, and circulating antibody count in BALB/c mice.

Experimental Studies on *Long Dan Cao* 龙胆草

Long dan cao 龙胆草 (*Gentiana scabra* Bge.) is commonly used in the treatment of herpes zoster. However, there is little research that examines its biological mechanism of action on this condition. Major constituents of *long dan cao* are secoiridoid glycosides,[2] which have been researched in experimental studies. The secoiridoid and iridoid glycosides are likely contributors to the anti-inflammatory effect seen with *long dan cao*. Many secoiridoid glycoside compounds have shown effects on LPS-induced murine macrophage RAW 264 cells.[16] Compounds have showed inhibition of IL-6, NO, and IL-6 production, which are mediators in the immune response.[16] Weak inhibition was seen in a TNF-α bioassay.

Iridoid and secoiridoid glycosides were examined for their anti-inflammatory activity in LPS-stimulated bone marrow-derived dendritic cells (BMDCs) from wild mice.[17] Compounds were shown to significantly inhibit IL-6 and IL-12 p40 activity, as well as TNF-α.

Experimental Studies on *Sheng Di Huang* 生地黄

Sheng di huang 生地黄 (*Rehmannia glutinosa* Libosch) contains four major groups of chemical constituents: iridoids and iridoid glycosides, sugars, organic acids, and amino acids.[2] Despite being one of the most commonly reported herbs in clinical studies of CHM, there is little experimental evidence of the biological actions of *sheng di huang*. Findings from one study suggest that *sheng di huang* has actions that are immunomodulatory. *Rehmannia glutinosa* polysaccharides (RGP) enhanced cellular and humoral immune activity through increasing B and T lymphocyte proliferation in mice spleens.[18] The effects of RGP were increased when RGP was applied concurrently with LPS to B cells, and with phytohemagglutinin (PHA) applied to T cells, suggesting that RGP has a synergistic effect with other mitogens. In the same study, RGP also upregulated IL-2 and IFN-γ in T cells.

Experimental Studies on *Zhi Zi* 栀子

Zhi zi 栀子 (*Gardenia jasminoides* Ellis) has been well researched for its role in inflammation. Several compounds of *zhi zi* have shown anti-inflammatory and immunomodulatory effects which may explain their actions in the acute stage of herpes zoster. Two constituents, genipin and geniposide, have been the focus of many experimental studies. Genipin, an iridoid compound, inhibited LPS-induced NO release, reduced LPS-induced production of TNF-α, IL-1β, PGE_2, and intracellular reactive oxygen species, and reduced activation of NF-κB in rat brain microglial cells.[19] In the same study, genipin reduced microglial activation in a mouse model of neuropathic pain. Genipin concentration-dependently reduced NO release and iNOS expression while inhibiting NF-κB activation in LPS-stimulated RAW 264.7 cells.[20]

Koo *et al.*[20] also found that topical application of genipin inhibited croton oil-induced ear oedema in mice. Similar effects were seen in a later study, with genipin inhibiting carrageenan-induced rat paw oedema to a greater extent than geniposide, another compound of *zhi zi.*[21] The authors suggest that genipin's effects on acute inflammation is due to the inhibition of COX-2 expression. In the same study, genipin produced similar reductions as dexamethasone in the volume of exudate and nitrite levels in the carrageenan-induced air pouch model of acute inflammation. The mechanism of genipin in acute inflammation appeared to be through suppression of NO production and COX-2 expression.

While Koo *et al.*[21] found geniposide to be less potent than genipin, geniposide also inhibited NO, PGE_2, TNF-α, and IL-6 expression in LPS-stimulated RAW 264.7 murine macrophage cells and peritoneal macrophages.[22] Geniposide also downregulated messenger RNA (mRNA) levels as well as iNOS and COX-2 expression compared with LPS. Six compounds of *zhi zi* were found to inhibit IL-2 in human T cells: geniposide, genipin gentiobioside, 6α-hydroxygeniposide, 6β-hydroxygeniposide, ixoroside, and shanzhiside.[23]

Experimental Studies on *Dang Gui* 当归

Dang gui 当归 (*Angelica sinensis* (Oliv.) Diels) contains many volatile oils in addition to amino acids, sugars, and sterols.[2] Actions appear to be both anti-inflammatory and immunomodulatory. Four hydrosoluble fractions of *dang gui* (*Angelica* polysaccharide (APS),

Angelica oligosaccharide, *Angelica* sucrose, and *Angelica* total amino acid) were examined for effects on cell proliferation in macrophages in female ICR mice.[24] Dose-dependent increases in proliferation were seen with all fractions, with the greatest increase seen with the APS fraction. Phagocytic and lysosomal activity was greater at higher concentrations with all four fractions compared with LPS, and an increase in the production of hydrogen peroxide was seen.

The effects of APS were investigated by Yang *et al.*[25] APS promoted cell proliferation in total spleen cell population, macrophage-depleted cell population, peritoneal macrophages, and macrophage/B cell-depleted cell population from BALB/c mice. Dose-dependent increases in IL-2 and IFN-γ production were seen in total spleen cells, where IL-2 increases were time-dependent and IFN-γ peaked at 12 hours and remained high after exposure to APS.

In chickens vaccinated with Newcastle disease, three selenizised polysaccharides of *dang gui* promoted lymphocyte proliferation and increased serum antibody titer, IFN-γ, and IL-6.[26] An acidic APS dose-dependently increased lysosomal enzyme activity in murine peritoneal macrophages *in vitro* and increased both lysosomal activity and NO production *in vivo*, mediated by expression of iNOS.[27] Increased TNF-α released from macrophages was also reported.

In addition to polysaccharides, other components of *dang gui* have shown potential benefits. N-butylidenephthalide increased the endocytic action of LPS-stimulated murine dendritic cells (DCs; specifically DC2.4 cell), decreased IL-6 and TNF-α production, inhibited major histocompatibility complex (MHC) class II, CD86, and CD40 expression, and decreased the antigen-presenting action of DCs.[28] Ligustilide inhibited LPS-induced production of NO, PGE_2, and TNF-α in murine RAW 264.7 cells, and also induced the expression of iNOS and its mRNA, suggesting ligustilide modulates NO production via transcription.[29] Furthermore, pre-treatment of cells with ligustilide prior to LPS stimulation significantly suppressed NF-κB p65 expression and reduced the nuclear level of c-Jun (indicative of transcription of activator protein 1). Ligustilide appears to exert its effects through inhibiting NF-κB and activator protein 1 pathways.

Experimental Studies on *Ze Xie* 泽泻

Despite being commonly included in clinical studies, few experimental studies have examined the possible biological mechanisms of *ze xie* 泽泻 (*Alisma orientalis* (Sam.) Juzep.). Constituents of *ze xie* which have been studied suggest that *ze xie* exhibits immunomodulatory and anti-inflammatory effects. Two compounds from *ze xie*, alismol and alisol B monoacetate, dose-dependently inhibited NO production in LPS- and IFN-γ stimulated RAW 264.7 cells. These compounds also decreased iNOS mRNA levels.[30]

A constituent of *ze xie*, alisol B-23 monoacetate, was found to induce cell apoptosis and reduce the mitochondrial cell membrane potential in A7r5 rat aortic smooth muscle cells and human CEM lymphocytes.[31] Some sequiterpenes and triterpenes of *ze xie* inhibited NO production in LPS-stimulated murine macrophages, and alismol and alisol F also suppressed induction of iNOS.[32]

Experimental Studies on *Ban Lan Gen* 板蓝根

Several groups of compounds have been identified in *ban lan gen* 板蓝根 (*Isatis indigotica* Fort.), including alkaloids, amino acids, and glycosides.[2] Findings from experimental studies suggest that *ban lan gen* can enhance cellular and humoral immunity. Several compounds from *ban lan gen* protected Vero cells from infection with herpes simplex virus type 1 (HSV-1).[33] Methanolic extracts of *ban lan gen* dose-dependently inhibited production of NO and PGE_2 in LPS-activated RAW 264.7 murine macrophage cells, reduced expression of iNOS and to a lesser extent COX-2 proteins, and reduced inflammation in 12-O-Tetradecanolyphorbol 13-acetate induced ear edema in mice.[34] Production of pro-inflammatory cytokines TNF-α and IL-6 was also inhibited in LPS-activated RAW 264.7 cells. Inhibition of the degradation of Iκ-B, a protein that inactivates the NF-κB transcription factor, occurred 30 minutes after exposure.

Another study of *ban lan gen* extract confirmed that it suppresses NO production, although the extent of the effect differed with varying *in vitro* conditions.[35] Polysaccharides from *ban lan gen* were found to increase phagocytosis in BALB/c mice after being intraperitoneally injected with chicken red blood cell solution and subsequently enhanced the production of serum hemolysin (which leads to lysis of red blood cells by destroying the cell membrane).[36] Further, lymphocyte proliferation and expression of IL-2 and IFN-γ increased dose-dependently.

Experimental Studies on *Che Qian Zi* 车前子

Che qian zi 车前子 (*Plantago asiatica* L., *Plantago depressa* Willd.) contains iridoid and phenylpropane glycosides, organic acids, and other constituents such as β-sitosterol.[2] *Che qian zi* appears to have antiviral and immunomodulatory actions which may be relevant to herpes zoster. Hot water extract of *che qian zi* was shown to have weak antiviral activity against the herpes simplex type 2 (HSV-2) virus.[37] The study also found that *che qian zi* increased PBMC proliferation at low doses, but inhibited proliferation at high doses (≥50 μg/mL). Inhibition of IFN-γ also varied according to dose.

Seed extract of *che qian zi* increased the surface expression of MHC class II molecules from CD11c+ DCs, enhanced the ability of mitomycin C-treated DCs to induce proliferation in allogenic T cells, and promoted the antigen presenting capacity of DCs.[38] Plantagoside, identified from the seed extract of *Plantago asiatica* L., was identified as having inhibitory actions on jack bean α-mannosidase activity and was subject to further investigation.[39] Plantagoside dose-dependently decreased the antigen-forming ability against sheep red blood cells in spleen cells from BALB/c mice and suppressed T cell proliferation from concanavalin A, but not T cell proliferation due to PHA or LPS.

Experimental Studies on *Yan Hu Suo* 延胡索

Yan hu suo 延胡索 (*Corydalis yanhusuo* W.T. Wang) contains many identified alkaloids.[2] Constituents of *yan hu suo* have demonstrated both anti-inflammatory and analgesic mechanisms.

Dehydrocorydaline decreased cell viability in RAW 246.7 cells when incubated alone or with LPS. A decrease in cell viability was also seen in primary macrophages.[40] In the same study, dehydrocorydaline inhibited elevation in mitochondrial membrane potential when used alone, inhibited the increase in IL-1β and IL-6 production in LPS-stimulated RAW 264.7 macrophages *in vitro*, and inhibited IL-6 levels *in vivo*.

Another constituent, dehydrocorybulbine, dose-dependently induced antinociception in an acute pain model in CD1 mice and demonstrated weak activity at the μ opioid receptor which was not antagonised by nalaxone.[41] Further, dehydrocorybulbine reduced the time that mice spent licking the injured paw following the formalin test, indicating acute analgesia. Pre-treatment with berberine, another alkaloid of *yan hu suo*, dose-dependently promoted IL-12 production in splenic macrophages and DCs while increasing the production of IL-12 when subsequently stimulated with either LPS or heat-killed *Listeria* monocytogenes.[42] Increases in mRNA levels of IL-12 were also seen, suggesting that changes occur at the transcription level.

The analgesic actions of DL-tetrahydropalmatine were dose-dependently demonstrated through reductions in acetic acid-induced writhing in mice, and corresponding increases in plasma concentrations were also seen.[43] Tetrahydropalmatine dose-dependently inhibited LPS-induced IL-8 production in human monocytic cell line THP-1, inhibited extracellular signal-regulated kinase, and blocked the phosphorylation of mitogen-activated protein kinase.[44]

Experimental Studies on Herbal Formulas

Identifying experimental studies of herbal formulas is more challenging compared with that of individual herbs. In experimental studies of individual herbs, the action of the herb is clearly identifiable. In experimental studies of herbal formulas, the actions are harder to attribute and are instead broadly attributed to the synergistic actions of all included herbs. One such study evaluated the actions of *Long dan xie gan tang* 龙胆泻肝汤 in mice.[45] *Long dan xie gan tang* promoted macrophage phagocytosis within three to six hours and enhanced lymphocyte transformation in a dose-dependent manner.

Summary of Pharmacological Actions of the Frequently Used Herbs

Evidence from experimental studies suggest that key herbs used for herpes zoster inhibit production of NO and iNOS and also reduce the production of pro-inflammatory cytokines. For many herbs commonly evaluated in clinical trials, there is evidence of analgesic, anti-inflammatory, and immunomodulatory actions.

References

1. Zhou J, Xie G, Yan X. Encyclopedia of Traditional Chinese Medicine: Molecular structures, pharmacological activities, natural sources and applications. Berlin: Springer; 2011.
2. Bensky D, Clavey S, Stoger E. *Chinese herbal medicine Materia Medica*. 3rd ed. Seattle, US: Eastland Press, Inc; 2004.
3. Aikawa Y, Yoshiike T, Ogawa H. Effect of glycyrrhizin on pain and HLA-DR antigen expression on CD8-positive cells in peripheral blood of herpes zoster patients in comparison with other antiviral agents. *Skin Pharmacol.* 1990; **3**(4):268–71.
4. Steain M, Sutherland JP, Rodriguez M, *et al.* Analysis of T cell responses during active varicella-zoster virus reactivation in human ganglia. *J Virol.* 2014; **88**(5):2704–16.
5. Baba M, Shigeta S. Antiviral activity of glycyrrhizin against varicella-zoster virus *in vitro. Antiviral Res.* 1987; **7**(2):99–107.
6. Shebl RI, Amin MA, Emad-Eldin A, *et al.* Antiviral activity of liquorice powder extract against varicella zoster virus isolated from Egyptian patients. *Chang Gung Med J.* 2012; **35**(3):231–9.
7. Oh C, Kim Y, Eun J, *et al.* Induction of T lymphocyte apoptosis by treatment with glycyrrhizin. *Am J Chin Med.* 1999; **27**(2):217–26.
8. Akasaka Y, Sakai A, Takasu K, *et al.* Suppressive effects of glycyrrhetinic acid derivatives on tachykinin receptor activation and hyperalgesia. *J Pharmacol Sci.* 2011; **117**(3):180–8.

9. Yang J, Yang X, Li M. Baicalin, a natural compound, promotes regulatory T cell differentiation. *BMC Complement Altern Med.* 2012; **12**:64.

10. Suk K, Lee H, Kang SS, Cho GJ, Choi WS. Flavonoid baicalein attenuates activation-induced cell death of brain microglia. *J Pharmacol Exp Ther.* 2003; **305**(2):638–45.

11. Wakabayashi I. Inhibitory effects of baicalein and wogonin on lipopolysaccharide-induced nitric oxide production in macrophages. *Pharmacol Toxicol.* 1999; **84**(6):288–91.

12. Lappas CM, Lappas NT. D-Limonene modulates T lymphocyte activity and viability. *Cell Immunol.* 2012; **279**(1):30–41.

13. Yoon WJ, Lee NH, Hyun CG. Limonene suppresses lipopolysaccharide-induced production of nitric oxide, prostaglandin E2, and pro-inflammatory cytokines in RAW 264.7 macrophages. *J Oleo Sci.* 2010; **59**(8):415–21.

14. Schulz S, Reinhold D, Schmidt H, Ansorge S, Hollt V. Perillic acid inhibits Ras/MAP kinase-driven IL-2 production in human T lymphocytes. *Biochem Biophys Res Commun.* 1997; **241**(3):720–5.

15. Raphael TJ, Kuttan G. Immunomodulatory activity of naturally occurring monoterpenes carvone, limonene, and perillic acid. *Immunopharmacol Immunotoxicol.* 2003; **25**(2):285–94.

16. He YM, Zhu S, Ge YW, *et al.* The anti-inflammatory secoiridoid glycosides from gentianae scabrae radix: The root and rhizome of Gentiana scabra. *J Nat Med.* 2015; **69**(3):303–12.

17. Li W, Zhou W, Kim S, *et al.* Three new secoiridoid glycosides from the rhizomes and roots of Gentiana scabra and their anti-inflammatory activities. *Nat Prod Res.* 2015; **29**(20):1920–7.

18. Huang Y, Jiang C, Hu Y, *et al.* Immunoenhancement effect of rehmannia glutinosa polysaccharide on lymphocyte proliferation and dendritic cell. *Carbohydr Polym.* 2013; **96**(2):516–21.

19. Nam KN, Choi YS, Jung HJ, *et al.* Genipin inhibits the inflammatory response of rat brain microglial cells. *Int Immunopharmacol.* 2010; **10**(4):493–9.

20. Koo HJ, Song YS, Kim HJ, *et al.* Antiinflammatory effects of genipin, an active principle of gardenia. *Eur J Pharmacol.* 2004; **495**(2–3):201–8.

21. Koo HJ, Lim KH, Jung HJ, Park EH. Anti-inflammatory evaluation of gardenia extract, geniposide and genipin. *J Ethnopharmacol.* 2006; **103**(3):496–500.

22. Shi Q, Cao J, Fang L, *et al.* Geniposide suppresses LPS-induced nitric oxide, PGE2 and inflammatory cytokine by downregulating NF-κB,

MAPK and AP-1 signaling pathways in macrophages. *Int Immunopharmacol.* 2014; **20**(2):298–306.

23. Chang WL, Wang HY, Shi LS, Lai JH, Lin HC. Immunosuppressive iridoids from the fruits of Gardenia jasminoides. *J Nat Prod.* 2005; **68**(11):1683–5.

24. Chen Y, Duan JA, Qian D, *et al.* Assessment and comparison of immunoregulatory activity of four hydrosoluble fractions of Angelica sinensisin vitro on the peritoneal macrophages in ICR mice. *Int Immunopharmacol.* 2010; **10**(4):422–30.

25. Yang T, Jia M, Meng J, Wu H, Mei Q. Immunomodulatory activity of polysaccharide isolated from Angelica sinensis. *Int J Biol Macromol.* 2006; **39**(4–5):179–84.

26. Qin T, Chen J, Wang D, *et al.* Selenylation modification can enhance immune-enhancing activity of Chinese angelica polysaccharide. *Carbohydr Polym.* 2013; **95**(1):183–7.

27. Yang X, Zhao Y, Wang H, Mei Q. Macrophage activation by an acidic polysaccharide isolated from Angelica sinensis (Oliv.) Diels. *J Biochem Mol Biol.* 2007; **40**(5):636–43.

28. Fu RH, Hran HJ, Chu CL, *et al.* Lipopolysaccharide-stimulated activation of murine DC2.4 cells is attenuated by n-butylidenephthalide through suppression of the NF-κB pathway. *Biotechnol Lett.* 2011; **33**(5):903–10.

29. Su YW, Chiou WF, Chao SH, *et al.* Ligustilide prevents LPS-induced iNOS expression in RAW 264.7 macrophages by preventing ROS production and down-regulating the MAPK, NF-κB and AP-1 signaling pathways. *Int Immunopharmacol.* 2011; **11**(9):1166–72.

30. Kim NY, Kang TH, Pae HO, *et al. In vitro* inducible nitric oxide synthesis inhibitors from Alismatis Rhizoma. *Biol Pharm Bull.* 1999; **22**(10):1147–9.

31. Chen HW, Hsu MJ, Chien CT, Huang HC. Effect of alisol B acetate, a plant triterpene, on apoptosis in vascular smooth muscle cells and lymphocytes. *Eur J Pharmacol.* 2001; **419**(2–3):127–38.

32. Matsuda H, Kageura T, Toguchida I, *et al.* Effects of sesquiterpenes and triterpenes from the rhizome of Alisma orientale on nitric oxide production in lipopolysaccharide-activated macrophages: Absolute stereostructures of alismaketones-B 23-acetate and -C 23-acetate. *Bioorg Med Chem Lett.* 1999; **9**(21):3081–6.

33. He LW, Liu HQ, Chen YQ, *et al.* Total synthesis and anti-viral activities of an extract of Radix isatidis. *Molecules.* 2014; **19**(12):20906–12.

34. Shin EK, Kim DH, Lim H, Shin HK, Kim JK. The anti-inflammatory effects of a methanolic extract from Radix Isatidis in murine macrophages and mice. *Inflammation.* 2010; **33**(2):110–8.

35. Xiao P, Huang H, Chen J, Li X. *In vitro* antioxidant and anti-inflammatory activities of Radix Isatidis extract and bioaccessibility of six bioactive compounds after simulated gastro-intestinal digestion. *J Ethnopharmacol.* 2014; **157**:55–61.

36. Zhao YL, Wang JB, Shan LM, *et al.* Effect of Radix isatidis polysaccharides on immunological function and expression of immune related cytokines in mice. *Chin J Integr Med.* 2008; **14**(3):207–11.

37. Chiang LC, Chiang W, Chang MY, Lin CC. *In vitro* cytotoxic, antiviral and immunomodulatory effects of Plantago major and Plantago asiatica. *Am J Chin Med.* 2003; **31**(2):225–34.

38. Huang DF, Xie MY, Yin JY, *et al.* Immunomodulatory activity of the seeds of Plantago asiatica L. *J Ethnopharmacol.* 2009; **124**(3):493–8.

39. Yamada H, Nagai T, Takemoto N, *et al.* Plantagoside, a novel alpha-mannosidase inhibitor isolated from the seeds of Plantago asiatica, suppresses immune response. *Biochem Biophys Res Commun.* 1989; **165**(3):1292–8.

40. Ishiguro K, Ando T, Maeda O, Watanabe O, Goto H. Dehydrocorydaline inhibits elevated mitochondrial membrane potential in lipopolysaccharide-stimulated macrophages. *Int Immunopharmacol.* 2011; **11**(9):1362–7.

41. Zhang Y, Wang C, Wang L, *et al.* A novel analgesic isolated from a traditional Chinese medicine. *Curr Biol.* 2014; **24**(2):117–23.

42. Kim TS, Kang BY, Cho D, Kim SH. Induction of interleukin-12 production in mouse macrophages by berberine, a benzodioxoloquinolizine alkaloid, deviates CD4+ T cells from a Th2 to a Th1 response. *Immunology.* 2003; **109**(3):407–14.

43. Liao ZG, Liang XL, Zhu JY, *et al.* Correlation between synergistic action of Radix Angelica dahurica extracts on analgesic effects of Corydalis alkaloid and plasma concentration of dl-THP. *J Ethnopharmacol.* 2010; **129**(1):115–20.

44. Oh YC, Choi JG, Lee YS, *et al.* Tetrahydropalmatine inhibits pro-inflammatory mediators in lipopolysaccharide-stimulated THP-1 cells. *J Med Food.* 2010; **13**(5):1125–32.

45. Shen LL, Wu HS, Wang XY. The efficacy of long-dan-xie-gan-tang in the treatment of herpes zoster: A clinical trial and animal experimental data. *J Tongji Med Univ.* 1986; **6**(2):109–11.

7

Clinical Evidence for Acupuncture and Related Therapies — Herpes Zoster

OVERVIEW

Acupuncture therapies for herpes zoster have been evaluated by many clinical studies published in both Chinese and international journals. This chapter provides an assessment of the evidence for acupuncture therapies from clinical studies. A comprehensive search of nine English and Chinese language databases identified more than 36,600 citations. Screening against rigorous inclusion criteria resulted in the selection of 47 clinical studies for further evaluation. Acupuncture, moxibustion, and plum-blossom needle therapy were found to reduce pain and hasten rash healing, and these therapies were also well-tolerated.

Introduction

Acupuncture is part of a family of techniques that stimulate acupuncture points to correct imbalances of energy and restore health to the body. Methods of stimulating acupuncture points include:

- Acupuncture: insertion of an acupuncture needle into acupuncture points. This includes manual acupuncture (manual stimulation of acupuncture needles), surrounding acupuncture (insertion of needles around a lesion or rash site), and electro-acupuncture (stimulation of the inserted needle by an electrical device);
- Moxibustion: burning of herbs (usually artemesia vulgaris) close to or on the skin to induce a warming sensation;

- Plum-blossom needle therapy: application of a plum-blossom needle which contains a bundle of short embedded needles, usually tapped lightly on the skin.

Previous Systematic Reviews

No systematic reviews of acupuncture therapies were identified in the English language databases. One systematic review authored by Zheng and Xu[1] was identified from the Chinese literature. The authors included five RCTs using moxibustion alone or with acupuncture as interventions. The comparators were acyclovir that was either orally ingested or injected. The intervention groups produced greater improvement in curative rate relative to the comparators. The authors noted that there were methodological flaws in the included studies, such as insufficient information on randomisation, failure to describe allocation concealment, and lack of blinding.

Characteristics of Clinical Studies of Acupuncture and Related Therapies

Over 36,600 citations were identified in English and Chinese databases, and 5,693 full articles were reviewed for eligibility (see Figure 7.1). A total of 47 clinical studies which evaluated acupuncture therapies for herpes zoster were eligible for inclusion. Of these, 27 were randomised controlled trials (RCTs) (S152–S178), four were controlled clinical trials (CCTs) (S179–S182), and 16 were non-controlled studies (S183–S198). All studies were conducted in China and published in Chinese. Evidence from RCTs and CCTs were evaluated to establish the efficacy and safety of acupuncture therapies for herpes zoster. Details from non-controlled studies are described.

In total, 3,498 people with acute stage herpes zoster participated in these studies. Treatment duration ranged from five (S152) to 28 days (S153). Chinese medicine (CM) syndromes were used for selecting study participants or for treatment, with three studies reporting syndromes (S154, S183, S184). There were no overlaps in

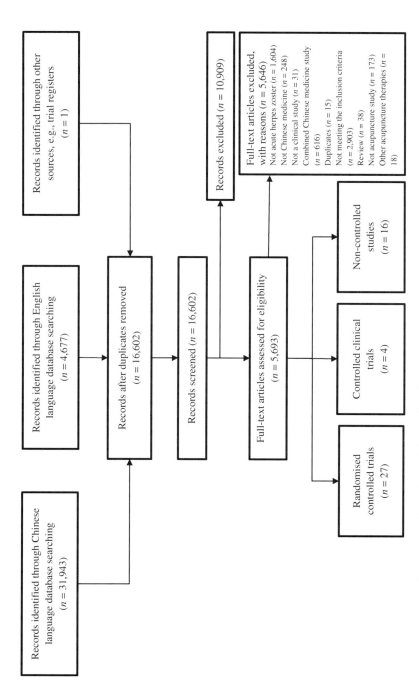

Figure 7.1   Flow chart of the study selection process: Acupuncture and related therapies.

syndromes reported and these included the pattern/syndrome of *qi* stagnation and Blood stasis (S154), Spleen deficiency with dampness encumbrance (S154), Liver-Gallbladder fire (S183), and dampness-heat (S184).

Interventions used in clinical studies included acupuncture (including manual acupuncture, surrounding acupuncture, and electro-acupuncture), plum-blossom needle therapy, and moxibustion. Many studies used various combinations of these interventions, and one three-arm RCT compared two combinations with a control group (S155). Not surprisingly, the most common intervention was acupuncture, which was evaluated alone or in combination with other acupuncture therapies in 33 studies.

A total of 47 acupuncture points or treatment approaches were reported. The most common approaches were to treat the rash area (used in 36 studies), use EX-B2 *Huatuojiaji* points 夹脊穴 (20 studies), and GB34 *Yanglingquan* 阳陵泉 (13 studies). Other commonly reported approaches included using *ashi* points 阿是穴 (12 studies), LR3 *Taichong* 太冲 (11 studies), ST36 *Zusanli* 足三里 (11 studies), TE6 *Zhigou* 支沟 (10 studies), LI4 *Hegu* 合谷 (nine studies), LI11 *Quchi* 曲池 (7 studies), and TE5 *Waiguan* 外关 (6 studies).

Randomised Controlled Trials of Acupuncture and Related Therapies

Twenty-seven RCTs which used acupuncture therapies to treat herpes zoster were included. Five studies included three or more arms (S155–S159) while all other studies used a two-arm parallel group design. In three-arm trials, only the relevant arm was included in the analysis (for example, if one arm included Chinese herbal medicine plus acupuncture therapies, this arm was excluded from this section).

Participant age ranged from 18 (S157–S162) to 82 years (S152, S159). In studies that reported the mean age of participants, the median of the mean was 50 years. The number of males and females was similar (1,006 males, 957 females). The duration of treatment ranged from five (S152) to 28 days (S153) with a median of 10 days.

CM syndromes were used as an inclusion criterion or for treatment selection in one study (S154). Syndromes included Spleen deficiency with dampness encumbrance and *qi* stagnation and Blood stasis (S154).

Interventions included variations of acupuncture such as manual acupuncture, surrounding acupuncture, and electro-acupuncture. Plum-blossom needle therapy and moxibustion were also evaluated in RCTs. Thirteen studies used combinations of acupuncture therapies (S154, S155, S158, S160, S163–S171). The most common intervention was acupuncture, used in 19 studies (S153–S160, S162–S165, S167–S173), and the most common combination was acupuncture plus moxibustion, used in nine studies (S154, S155, S158, S160, S163, S165, S167–S169). Forty-three acupuncture points were described, including EX-B2 *Huatuojiaji* points 夹脊穴 (14 studies), *ashi* points 阿是穴 (10 studies), LR3 *Taichong* 太冲 (8 studies), TE6 *Zhigou* 支沟 (8 studies), GB34 *Yanglingquan* 阳陵泉 (7 studies), ST36 *Zusanli* 足三里 (7 studies), LI4 *Hegu* 合谷 (6 studies), SP6 *Sanyinjiao* 三阴交 (5 studies), and EX-HN5 *Taiyang* 太阳 (5 studies). The most common approach was to treat the rash area (19 studies).

Nine studies used acupuncture therapies in combination with pharmacotherapy as integrative medicine (IM; S153, S159, S161, S162, S170, S172–S175). Comparators included antiviral drugs alone (S161, S167, S169, S170, S174–S176), antivirals plus pain management drugs (S163), antiviral drugs with other treatments such as vitamins (S153–S156, S160, S162, S164, S166, S171–S173, S177), antivirals plus pain management drugs plus other treatments such as vitamins (S152, S157, S158, S165, S168, S178), or other forms of pain management such as nerve blockers (S159). Antiviral treatment was administered at guideline-recommended doses in five studies (S153, S161, S169, S173, S175). None of the studies compared acupuncture therapies to sham/placebo treatment.

Risk of Bias

The methodological quality of included studies varied (see Table 7.1). Nine studies used a random number table or generator (S156–S159,

Table 7.1 Risk of Bias of Randomised Controlled Trials: Acupuncture and Related Therapies

Risk of Bias Domain	Low Risk n (%)	Unclear Risk n (%)	High Risk n (%)
Sequence generation	9 (33.3)	15 (55.6)	3 (11.1)
Allocation concealment	2 (7.4)	25 (92.6)	0 (0)
Blinding of participants	0 (0)	0 (0)	27 (100)
Blinding of personnel	2 (7.4)	0 (0)	25 (92.6)
Blinding of outcome assessor	2 (7.4)	25 (92.6)	0 (0)
Incomplete outcome data	25 (92.6)	2 (7.4)	0 (0)
Selective outcome reporting	1 (3.7)	26 (96.3)	0 (0)

S161, S166, S168, S169) or central randomisation to allocate participants (S155), and were judged as having low risk of bias for sequence generation (33.3% of all studies). Three studies (11.1%) allocated participants according to the order they arrived or visited (S152, S171, S175) and were judged as having high risk of bias while all other studies had unclear risk of bias for this domain. Two studies which used central allocation were judged as having low bias risk for allocation concealment (S155, S166). The majority of studies did not blind participants or personnel to group allocation and were considered to be at high risk of bias while the risk from a lack of blinding of outcome assessors was unclear in most studies. Two studies reported missing data; however, reasons were not provided and analysis was not performed to account for missing data (S166, S168). Both studies were therefore judged as having unclear risk of bias. One study reported reasons for missing data and performed appropriate analyses to account for the missing data (S155), and thus was judged as having low risk of bias. None of the other studies reported missing data and were assessed as having low risk of bias. The trial protocol was available for one study (S155) and specified outcomes were reported. For all other studies, there was no information of trial protocols or trial registration available and all were judged as having unclear risk of bias.

Acupuncture

Acupuncture, including manual acupuncture, surrounding acupuncture (needles inserted to surround lesions), and electro-acupuncture, was used in 19 studies (S153–S160, S162–S165, S167–S173). 1,746 participants were included and all studies were conducted in China.

Treatments were provided for seven (S172) to 28 days (S153), with 10 days as the median duration of treatment. Six studies reported a follow-up assessment (S158, S159, S163, S169–S171) which ranged from four weeks (S170) to 90 days (S158, S159, S163, S171). Syndrome differentiation was used in one study which reported Spleen deficiency with dampness encumbrance as well as *qi* stagnation and Blood stasis (S154).

Comparators included antivirals (S167, S169, S170), antivirals plus pain management drugs (S163), antiviral plus other treatments including vitamins and antihistamines (S153, S154, S156, S160, S162, S164, S171–S173), a combination of antivirals, pain management, and other treatments (S157, S158, S165, S168), and other pain management treatments such as a nerve block (S159). Three studies used antiviral therapies at doses recommended in clinical practice guidelines (S153, S169, S173).

Treatments most often were focused around the rash area (14 studies) and used EX-B2 *Huatuojiaji* 夹脊穴 (12 studies) or *ashi* 阿是穴 (10 studies) points. Other frequently used acupuncture points included LR3 *Taichong* 太冲 (7 studies), TE6 *Zhigou* 支沟 (7 studies), GB34 *Yanglingquan* 阳陵泉 (6 studies), LI4 *Hegu* 合谷 (6 studies), ST36 *Zusanli* 足三里 (6 studies), SP6 *Sanyinjiao* 三阴交 (5 studies), and EX-HN5 *Taiyang* 太阳 (5 studies).

Acupuncture Alone

Three studies compared acupuncture with pharmacotherapy (S155, S156, S157). Meta-analysis was possible for two studies which reported the visual analogue scale (VAS) pain score at the end of treatment (S155, S156). Data were reported in millimetres which were converted to centimetres for analysis. Compared with pharmacotherapy, acupuncture produced a greater reduction in pain score on the VAS by 1.17 cm at the end of treatment (2 studies, 249 participants; [95% confidence intervals −1.21, −1.12], I^2 = 0%). The reduction in pain seen at the end of treatment was also seen at a follow-up after 60 days in one study (S155), although the effect was not as great (MD −0.19 cm [−0.36, −0.03]).

Acupuncture improved two measures of rash healing in the same study (S155). The time from rash onset to crust formation was reduced by 0.78 days ([−0.89, −0.67]) and the time taken for resolution of the rash was reduced by 2.78 days ([−3.10, −2.46]). The time elapsed from rash onset to the cessation of formation of new lesions was less in those who received pharmacotherapy (MD 0.19 days [0.12, 0.26]) (S155). Another study reported on the time taken for crust formation and no new lesions (S157). As the time-point from which measurements were made was not specified, these data were not analysed. The incidence of post-herpetic neuralgia (PHN) one month after resolution of the rash was lower in those who received acupuncture (RR 0.25 [0.12, 0.50]). One study reported on adverse events (S155), with five cases of bleeding occurring in the acupuncture group.

Acupuncture as Integrative Medicine

Five studies used acupuncture as IM (S153, S159, S162, S172, S173). Two studies which did not specify the time-point from which measurements were made for incidence of PHN (S162) and cutaneous outcomes (S153) were excluded from analysis. Meta-analysis was not possible due to differences in the outcomes. When used with a nerve block, acupuncture reduced the pain score on the VAS at the end of treatment by 1.12 cm ([−1.62, −0.62]) but did not reduce the incidence of PHN three months from resolution of the rash (RR 0.29 [0.06, 1.29]) (S159).

Three studies reported effective rate (S159, S172, S173). However, one study reported effective rate based on descriptive criteria that does not permit accurate interpretation (S172) and the remaining two studies stated that effective rate was based on the 1994 guideline[2] but actually used different criteria. All studies were excluded from analysis.

The benefit of acupuncture as IM for herpes zoster remains unclear. Two studies reported on adverse events (S159, S162), with none occurring during the trials.

Acupuncture Plus Moxibustion Alone

Nine studies combined acupuncture with moxibustion to treat herpes zoster (S154, S155, S158, S160, S163, S165, S167–S169). Studies which did not specify the time-point for measurement of cutaneous outcomes were excluded from further analysis (S158, S160, S168). Meta-analysis was performed for incidence of PHN and effective rate as outcomes (see Table 7.2). The incidence of PHN one month after resolution of the rash was lower in those who received acupuncture plus moxibustion compared with pharmacotherapy (RR 0.29 [0.16, 0.53], $I^2 = 0\%$), although no difference was found when PHN was measured three months from resolution of the rash (RR 0.16 [0.02, 1.35], $I^2 = 0\%$).

Six studies reported outcomes based on effective rate and provided information about the definition of the effective rate (S154, S158, S165, S167–S169). One study stated that the effective rate was based on the 1994 guideline;[2] however, the criteria for assessment differed (S165) and this study was excluded from analysis. Data were

Table 7.2 Acupuncture plus Moxibustion *vs.* Pharmacotherapy: Incidence of Post-herpetic Neuralgia and Effective Rate

Outcome	No. of Studies (Participants)	Effect Size RR [95% CI] I^2	Included Studies
PHN: 1 month from resolution of rash	2 (251)	0.29 [0.16, 0.53]* 0%	S155, S169
PHN: 3 months from resolution of rash	2 (116)	0.16 [0.02, 1.35] 0%	S158, S163
Effective rate	5 (541)	2.67 [2.03, 3.52]* 43%	S154, S158, S167–S169

*Statistically significant.

Abbreviations: CI, confidence interval; RR, risk ratio.

pooled for five studies that reported effective rate according to the 1994 CM guideline[2] (S154, S158, S167–S169). The chance of achieving a 30% or greater reduction in symptoms and significant pain relief with acupuncture plus moxibustion was 2.67 that of pharmacotherapy ([2.03, 3.52], $I^2 = 43\%$).

Results from single studies showed that pain scores on the VAS were reduced by 0.83 cm at the end of treatment ([−1.24, −0.41]), although the effect was not sustained at the follow up after 60 days (MD −0.16 cm [−0.34, 0.01]) (S155). The time from pain onset to resolution occurred 6.59 days faster in those who received acupuncture plus moxibustion compared with oral and topical acyclovir ([−8.07, −5.11]) (S169).

Several single studies reported on cutaneous outcomes. The time from rash onset to crust formation was 1.42 days less with acupuncture plus moxibustion ([−1.52, −1.32]) compared with valacyclovir and vitamin B1 (S155). Similarly, the time from start of treatment to crust formation was 1.64 days less compared with oral and topical acyclovir ([−2.87, −0.41]) (S169). Two studies found that acupuncture plus moxibustion was superior to pharmacotherapy in reducing the time taken for cessation of new lesions from rash onset (MD −0.29 days [−0.35, −0.23]) (S155) and from start of treatment (MD −1.26 days [−2.16, −0.36]) (S169). The time from onset to resolution of the rash occurred 3.40 days faster in those who received acupuncture plus moxibustion ([−3.71, −3.09]) (S155).

Two studies reported on adverse events (S155, S158), with one study reporting no adverse events (S158) and the other reporting two cases of haematoma and five cases of bleeding in the intervention group, with no adverse events in the control group.

Acupuncture Plus Plum-blossom Needle Therapy as Integrative Medicine

One study combined acupuncture, plum-blossom needle therapy, and acyclovir in a study of 105 participants (S170). The study reported the time taken for crust formation and the time taken for cessation of new lesions, but due to not specifying the time-point at which measurements were made, these data were excluded from further analysis. The incidence of PHN one month after resolution of the rash was lower in those who received acupuncture, plum-blossom needle therapy and acyclovir compared with acyclovir alone (RR 0.11 [0.01, 0.83]). The study did not report on adverse events.

Acupuncture Plus Plum-blossom Needle Therapy Plus Moxibustion Alone

Two studies compared acupuncture, plum-blossom needle therapy, and moxibustion with valacyclovir, vitamin B1, and mecobalamin (a form of vitamin B12) (S164, S171). Both studies reported outcomes in terms of the pain score, time taken for crust formation, and time taken for cessation of new lesions. As neither specified the time-point from which measurements were made, some data were excluded from further analysis. Acupuncture, plum-blossom needle therapy, and moxibustion reduced the pain score on the VAS at the end of treatment by 1.73 cm (2 studies, 150 participants; [−2.91, −0.56], $I^2 =$ 89%) compared with valacyclovir, vitamin B1, and mecobalamin. There was statistical heterogeneity which could not be explored due to the small number of studies.

One study also reported on the incidence of PHN three months after resolution of the rash and effective rate according to the 1994 guideline[2] (S171). Acupuncture, plum-blossom needle therapy, and moxibustion did not significantly reduce the incidence of PHN compared with valacyclovir, vitamin B1, and mecobalamin (RR 0.14 [0.01, 2.63]). The number of people achieving a 30% or greater reduction in lesions and significant pain relief was not statistically different between the two groups (RR 1.20 [0.97, 1.48]). Neither study reported on adverse events.

Frequently Reported Points in Meta-analyses Showing Favourable Effects: Acupuncture

Studies included in analysis showing that acupuncture was beneficial were examined to identify the acupuncture points which may contribute to the effect. Studies were grouped according to outcome categories (see Chapter 5 for full details). Studies that used acupuncture alone or with other related therapies were pooled for analysis. Comparisons of acupuncture vs. pharmacotherapy and acupuncture as IM vs. pharmacotherapy were calculated separately. As no meta-analysis of acupuncture as IM produced a favourable result, this analysis could not be performed.

Two treatment approaches were common across all outcomes, which were to treat the rash area and use EX-B2 *Huatuojiaji* 夹脊穴 points (see Table 7.3). Acupuncture points which may have contributed

Table 7.3 Frequently Reported Points in Meta-analyses Showing Favourable Effects: Acupuncture

Outcome Category	No. of Meta-analyses	No. of Studies	Points	No. of Studies
Pain outcomes	2 (see Acupuncture alone; Acupuncture plus plum-blossom needle therapy alone)	4	Rash area	4
			EX-B2 Huatuojiaji 夹脊穴	2
			LI11 Quchi 曲池	2
			LI4 Hegu 合谷	2
			LR3 Taichong 太冲	2
			SI3 Houxi 后溪	2
			SP6 Sanyinjiao 三阴交	2
			ST36 Zusanli 足三里	2
			TE6 Zhigou 支沟	2
PHN	2 (see Acupuncture plus moxibustion alone)	4	Ashi points 阿是穴	3
			EX-B2 Huatuojiaji 夹脊穴	2
			Rash area	2
			TE6 Zhigou 支沟	2
Effective rate	2 (see Acupuncture plus moxibustion alone)	5	Rash area	4
			Ashi points 阿是穴	3
			EX-B2 Huatuojiaji 夹脊穴	2
			GB34 Yanglingquan 阳陵泉	2
			LR3 Taichong 太冲	2

Abbreviation: PHN, post-herpetic neuralgia.

to the treatment effects observed in RCTs include *ashi* points 阿是穴, TE6 *Zhigou* 支沟, and LR3 *Taichong* 太冲. The number of studies included in each outcome category was small, thus limiting the reliability of these findings.

Assessment Using Grading of Recommendations Assessment, Development and Evaluation

Grading of Recommendations Assessment, Development, and Evaluation (GRADE) approach was used to to evaluate the quality of evidence for the key comparisons and summarise the findings. After careful discussion, the comparison chosen by group consensus was acupuncture compared with antivirals plus pain management therapies. However, as none of the studies that evaluated acupuncture used antivirals plus pain management therapies as the comparator, it was not possible to prepare the summary of findings table. The quality of evidence for this comparison remains uncertain.

Moxibustion

Seventeen studies used moxibustion as the intervention, either alone (S152, S177, S178) or combined with acupuncture (S154, S155, S158, S160, S163, S165, S167–S169), acupuncture plus plum-blossom needling therapy (S164, S171), or plum-blossom needling therapy (S166). Two studies examined moxibustion as IM in comparison with the antiviral drug famciclovir (S161, S175). As the combinations of moxibustion with acupuncture and moxibustion with acupuncture plus plum-blossom needling therapy have been evaluated above, studies using these combinations are not included in subsequent analyses. As a result, six studies were included in this section (S152, S161, S166, S175, S177, S178).

All studies were conducted in China and included a total of 520 participants. Treatment was provided for five (S152) to 20 days (S177) and none of the studies reported syndrome differentiation. Four studies included a follow-up assessment either at 14 (S161, S175) or 30 days (S166, S178). Comparators included antiviral therapy alone

(S161, S175), antivirals plus other treatments such as vitamins (S166, S177), or antivirals plus pain management plus other treatments (S152, S178). The most frequently reported treatment approaches were to treat the rash area (3 studies) or use EX-B2 *Huatuojiaji* acupuncture points 夹脊穴 (2 studies).

Moxibustion Alone

Three studies compared moxibustion with pharmacotherapy, including antivirals plus other treatments (S177) and antivirals, pain management, and other treatments (S152, S178). All three studies reported on effective rate; however, one study reported effective rate data that was not in accordance with the 1994 guideline[2] and these results were not analysed (S178). Meta-analysis was performed for two studies that reported the effective rate according to the 1994 guideline[2] (S152, S177). Moxibustion resulted in a greater number of people achieving a 30% or greater reduction in lesions and significant improvement in pain compared with pharmacotherapy (2 studies, 158 participants; RR 1.19 [1.01, 1.41], $I^2 = 36\%$).

Two studies reported information on the incidence of PHN (S177, S178). One study reported assessing PHN one month from an unspecified time-point (S178) while the other did not provide details on when PHN was assessed (S177). As such, both studies were excluded from analysis for these outcomes. One study reported that no adverse events occurred during the trial (S178).

Moxibustion as Integrative Medicine

Two studies used moxibustion as IM with famciclovir at guideline-recommended doses (S161, S175). Both studies reported on the same outcomes: time taken for resolution of pain, time taken for crust formation, and time taken for cessation of new lesions. Neither study specified the time-point from which measurements were made. As such, data were excluded from analysis. The effect of moxibustion as IM remains unclear.

Moxibustion Plus Plum-blossom Needle Therapy Alone

One study compared moxibustion plus plum-blossom needle therapy with oral and topical acyclovir plus vitamin B1 (S166). Pain score at the end of treatment was 1.96 cm lower on the VAS with moxibustion plus plum-blossom needle therapy ([−2.40, −1.51]). Present pain intensity was also lower in those who received the intervention (MD −0.91 points [−1.09, −0.73]). Although the effective rate was described as following the 1994 guideline,[2] different levels of the treatment effect were reported which led to the exclusion of these results from further analysis. The study also reported six adverse events of dizziness, nausea, and diarrhoea, although the group in which these occurred was not specified.

Frequently Reported Points in Meta-analyses Showing Favourable Effects: Moxibustion

One meta-analysis was conducted with moxibustion as the intervention and effective rate was reported as the outcome. There were no overlaps in acupuncture points or treatment approaches used in both studies. As such, the particular points that may have produced beneficial effects with moxibustion could not be inferred.

Plum-blossom Needle Therapy

Six studies used plum-blossom needle therapy in the intervention group (S164, S166, S170, S171, S174, S176). Three studies used plum-blossom needle therapy with acupuncture (S164, S170, S171) and one study used plum-blossom needle therapy with moxibustion (S166); these have been described above. Two studies which used plum-blossom needle therapy are described here.

Plum-blossom needle therapy was compared with antivirals in two studies (S174, S176) with one using plum-blossom needle therapy as IM (S174). One hundred and twenty people were included, with both studies applying treatment around the rash area for one week. One study reported using plum-blossom needle therapy twice daily in severe cases and once daily in moderate cases (S176), while the other did not report the frequency of treatment. No CM syndromes were reported in either study.

Plum-blossom Needle Therapy Alone

One study (70 participants) compared plum-blossom needle therapy with intravenous and topical acyclovir (S176). The study stated that the effective rate reported was according to the 1994 guideline,[2] but the criteria described differed. These data were excluded from analysis. The study did not report on adverse events.

Plum-blossom Needle Therapy as Integrative Medicine

One study used plum-blossom needle therapy in combination with famciclovir and saline washes (S174). The study reported on time taken for crust formation and time taken for cessation of new lesions as the outcomes. However, the data was not presented in a way that allowed for re-analysis. The clinical evidence for plum-blossom needle therapy as IM remains uncertain. The study did not report on adverse events.

Acupuncture Therapies Compared with Guideline-recommended Doses of Antiviral Therapy

Five RCTs used antiviral therapies at doses recommended by international clinical practice guidelines[3,4] (S153, S161, S169, S173, S175). These studies are highlighted as they provide the best evidence for acupuncture therapies compared with recommended clinical practice. Interventions included acupuncture as IM (S153, S173), moxibustion as IM (S161, S175), and acupuncture plus moxibustion alone (S169).

Several studies reported on pain and cutaneous outcomes without specifying the time-point from which measurements were made, and these data were excluded from analysis (S153, S161, S175).

Further, one study stated that effective rate corresponded to the 1994 guideline[2] (S173) but described criteria that was different from the guideline, and these data were excluded from analysis. Data could be analysed for acupuncture plus moxibustion alone (S169).

Acupuncture plus moxibustion was compared with oral acyclovir (800 mg five times daily) and topical acyclovir (S169). The combination of acupuncture plus moxibustion decreased the time from start of treatment to resolution of pain by 6.59 days ([−8.07, −5.11]), the time taken for crust formation by 1.64 days ([−2.87, −0.41]), and the time taken for cessation of new lesions by 1.26 days ([−2.16, −0.36]). The study measured the effective rate in accordance with the 1994 guideline[2] and found that the chance of achieving a 30% or greater reduction in lesions and significant pain relief with acupuncture plus moxibustion was 3.23 that of oral and topical acyclovir ([1.86, 5.60]). Acupuncture plus moxibustion was not found to reduce the incidence of PHN one month after resolution of the rash (RR 0.16 [0.02, 1.22]).

Controlled Clinical Trials of Acupuncture and Related Therapies

Four CCTs of acupuncture therapies were eligible for inclusion (S179–S182). All studies were conducted in China. A total of 432 participants were recruited from hospital outpatient departments (S179, S181), inpatient departments (S180), or from both inpatient and outpatient departments (S182). Two studies reported the duration of herpes zoster which ranged from one hour to 14 days (S181). One study reported including participants within 72 hours of rash onset (S182) which is the time recommended for commencement of antiviral therapy.

More males than females were included in the studies that reported participant gender (255 compared with 177, respectively). Participant age ranged from 19 (S181) to 80 years (S182). Duration of treatment ranged from seven (S179–S181) to 10 days (S180, S182). None of the studies conducted follow-up assessments of participants.

None of the studies reported the CM syndrome involved. Interventions included acupuncture plus moxibustion (S181), plum-blossom needle therapy (S179), and moxibustion (S180, S182). One study combined acupuncture therapies with pharmacotherapy (S179). Three studies used antiviral therapy alone as the comparator (S179, S180, S182) and one combined antiviral therapy with analgesic medication (S181). None of the included studies used antiviral drugs at dosage levels recommended by clinical practice guidelines. Treating the rash area was a common approach in all studies and one study also used ST36 *Zusanli* 足三里 (S182). No other acupuncture points were reported in the four studies.

One study reported on pain and cutaneous outcomes but did not specify the time-point from which these measurements were made (S180). Data for these outcomes were not analysed. One study stated that the effective rate was measured according to the 1994 guideline[2] but described different criteria instead; thus, data for this outcome were not analysed (S179). It was only possible to analyse results for one study which reported effective rate according to the 1994 guideline (S181). Acupuncture plus moxibustion was not statistically different from ribavirin or interferon plus indomethacin in the number of people achieving a 30% or greater improvement in symptoms (RR 1.05 [0.96, 1.15]) (S181).

Three studies reported information on adverse events (S180–S182) with one study reporting that no adverse events occurred (S180). No adverse events were reported in the intervention groups. Thirty-three adverse events were reported in the pharmacotherapy groups, including 16 cases of nausea, epigastric discomfort, and other gastro-intestinal reactions, 16 cases of fever, fatigue, and other systemic symptoms, and one case of dizziness.

Non-controlled Studies of Acupuncture and Related Therapies

Acupuncture therapies were evaluated in 16 non-controlled studies which were eligible for inclusion. All studies were conducted in

China and a total of 680 people with herpes zoster were included. One study was a case report (S184) and the remaining studies were case series. Sample sizes ranged from one (S184) to 100 (S185) and the median sample size was 40.

Few studies reported information on CM syndromes. Two studies reported using syndrome differentiation for inclusion or for treatment, with one describing Liver-Gallbladder fire (S183) and the other describing dampness-heat (S184). Seven studies used acupuncture therapies alone (S183, S186–S191) while nine studies combined acupuncture with pharmacotherapy (S184, S185, S192–S198).

Acupuncture was the most common intervention and was either used alone (9 studies) (S183, S184, S186, S187, S190, S193–S196), with moxibustion (3 studies) (S188, S192, S197), or with plum-blossom needle therapy (1 study) (S191). Other interventions included moxibustion (2 studies) (S189, S198) and plum-blossom needle therapy (1 study) (S185). The most commonly reported treatment approaches were to treat the rash area (13 studies), use EX-B2 *Huatuojiaji* points 夹脊穴 (6 studies), or use other acupuncture points such as GB34 *Yanglingquan* 阳陵泉 (6 studies), LI11 *Quchi* 曲池, LI4 *Hegu* 合谷, LR3 *Taichong* 太冲, ST36 *Zusanli* 足三里 (3 studies each), *ashi* points 阿是穴, TE6 *Zhigou* 支沟, or TE5 *Waiguan* 外关 (2 studies each). Three studies reported that no adverse events occurred (S183, S185, S196).

Summary of Clinical Evidence for Acupuncture and Related Therapies

This review of clinical studies of acupuncture therapies for herpes zoster found variation in the interventions used, although little variation existed in the acupuncture points and treatment approaches used. Treatment durations were generally short (7–10 days), reflecting the transient nature of the disease. Few syndromes were reported which may be due to the predominantly symptomatic treatment of herpes zoster through using *ashi* points 阿是穴 and treating the rash area. Acupuncture and moxibustion were the most commonly used interventions and the most common treatment approaches were to treat the rash area, use local *ashi* points 阿是穴, or use acupuncture points such as EX-B2 *Huatuojiaji* 夹脊穴, GB34 *Yanglingquan* 阳陵泉, LR3 *Taichong* 太冲, ST36 *Zusanli* 足三里, and TE6 *Zhigou* 支沟.

Many studies reported on both pain and cutaneous outcomes. There is some promising evidence that some acupuncture therapies may help to reduce the intensity and duration of the condition. Practitioners can consider using acupuncture, moxibustion, and plum-blossom needle therapy to treat the symptoms of herpes zoster. The best evidence for the benefit of using acupuncture therapies compared with current management comes from the few studies using guideline-recommended antiviral treatments at recommended doses. Results from a single study found that acupuncture plus moxibustion resulted in greater reductions in pain compared with pharmacotherapies and also hastened rash healing time.

The interpretation of some results where the time taken for an event (e.g., resolution of pain, resolution of rash) was measured are limited by the lack of recording of the exact time-point that measurements were made. The baseline point for comparison could include onset of symptoms (rash or pain), status at randomisation, start of treatment, or other time-points and without this vital information, we cannot be certain of the effects of acupuncture therapies. Logically, the time-point from which measurement takes place should not be later than the day that treatment starts. It is possible that this lack of reporting may have led to an underestimation of the treatment effect of acupuncture therapies, although this cannot be confirmed.

As no minimal clinically important difference was determined for pain or cutaneous outcomes in herpes zoster, the clinical relevance of these findings remains uncertain. Some findings appear to be clinically important, such as a reduction in the time taken for pain resolution by 6.59 days, but as the reduction in time becomes smaller (e.g., one day or less), the less certain we can be about the importance of this reduction to patients. None of the included studies reported on disease-specific health-related quality of life. As herpes zoster is known to have a high health burden, this outcome must be included in future studies.

References

1. 郑春爱, 徐立. 艾灸治疗带状疱疹的临床随机对照试验 Meta 分析 [J]. 针灸临床杂志. 2011;11:48–50.
2. 国家中医药管理局. 中医病证诊断疗效标准. 南京大学出版社; 1994.
3. Gross G, Schofer H, Wassilew S, *et al.* Herpes zoster guideline of the German Dermatology Society (DDG). *J Clin Virol.* 2003; **26**(3): 277–89; discussion 91–3.
4. Dworkin RH, Johnson RW, Breuer J, *et al.* Recommendations for the management of herpes zoster. *Clin Infect Dis.* 2007; **44** (Suppl 1): S1–26.

8

Clinical Evidence for Combination Therapies — Herpes Zoster

OVERVIEW

The combination of two or more Chinese medicine therapies is common in clinical practice. Studies were assessed against rigorous inclusion criteria and 33 randomised controlled trials were selected for inclusion. The most common combination of interventions was acupuncture plus plum-blossom needle therapy and cupping. Analysis of results found some combinations of therapy to be beneficial and combination therapies appear to be well-tolerated by people with herpes zoster.

Introduction

Combination therapies are defined as two or more Chinese medicine (CM) interventions from different categories administered together, such as herbal medicine plus acupuncture or herbal medicine plus *qigong*. This approach is common in clinical practice. In this section, the clinical evidence from randomised controlled trials (RCTs) for combination therapies is evaluated.

Randomised Controlled Trials of Combination Therapies

Thirty-three RCTs involving 2,713 participants were included (see Figure 8.1). Studies were conducted in China and in either outpatient departments only or both inpatient and outpatient departments. One study included two treatment arms (S199), while the remainder used

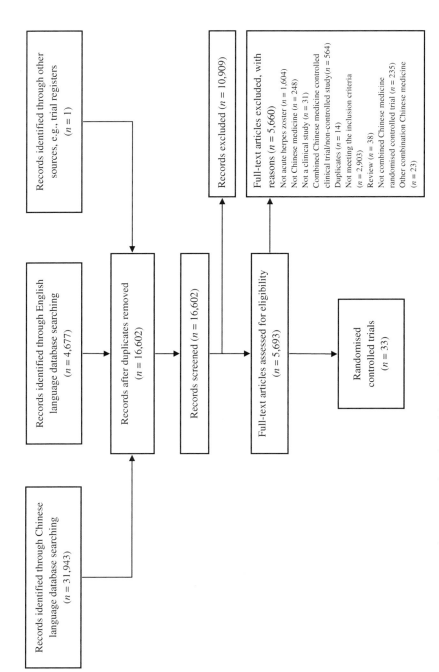

Figure 8.1 Flow chart of the study selection process: Combination therapies.

a two-arm design. The duration of herpes zoster ranged from one (S155, S158, S200–S211) to 14 (S212) days.

The studies included more males than females (1,359 and 1,245, respectively), although not all studies reported participant gender and some reported only for those who completed the study. The age of participants ranged from 18 (S155, S200, S201, S206, S208, S213–S215) to 85 years (S215), and in studies where the mean age was reported, the median of the mean was 48.9 years. Treatment duration ranged from one week (S202, S203, S211, S212, S216–S218) to 28 days (S203), and the median treatment duration was 10 days. Follow-up assessment after treatment had finished was conducted in 10 studies (S155, S158, S201, S204, S211, S212, S215, S219–S221) and ranged from two weeks (S220, S221) to 90 days (S158, S201, S212, S215).

Three studies report using CM syndromes for either diagnosis, treatment, or both (S201, S220, S221). All studies reported multiple syndromes and these included pattern/syndrome of *qi* stagnation and Blood stasis (3 studies) (S201, S220, S221), Spleen deficiency with dampness accumulation (2 studies) (S220, S221), dampness-heat accumulation (S201), and wind-fire toxin accumulation (S201).

Therapies included Chinese herbal medicine (CHM), acupuncture, moxibustion, plum-blossom needle therapy, and cupping in various combinations (see Table 8.1). The most common combination was acupuncture, plum-blossom needle therapy, and cupping which was tested in 10 studies (S155, S158, S199, S200, S202, S205, S209, S216–S218). One study reported combining CHM with an unspecified type of acupuncture therapy (S221) and this study was excluded from analysis. Combinations of CM therapies were used in conjunction with pharmacotherapy in five studies (S205, S211, S219, S222, S223).

In studies using CHM, six formulas or products were used in two or more studies. *Long dan xie gan tang* 龙胆泻肝汤 was used in five studies (S206, S211, S212, S220, S221), *Ji de sheng she yao pian* 季德胜蛇药片 in two studies (S207, S224), *ban lan gen* was used either in granular form 板蓝根颗粒 (S214) or as a topical application 板蓝根注射液 (S223) in two studies, *Chu shi wei ling tang* 除湿胃苓

Table 8.1   Summary of Combination Therapies Interventions

Combination Therapies	No. of Studies	Study References
Acupuncture + plum-blossom needle therapy + cupping	10	S155, S158, S199, S200, S202, S205, S209, S216–S218
CHM + acupuncture	4	S206, S211, S214, S220
CHM + plum-blossom needle therapy + cupping	3	S208, S225, S226
Acupuncture + moxibustion + cupping	3	S201, S204, S215
Plum-blossom needle therapy + cupping	3	S203, S219, S227
CHM + moxibustion	2	S212, S223
CHM + acupuncture + cupping	2	S222, S224
Acupuncture + plum-blossom needle therapy + moxibustion + cupping	2	S210, S213
Plum-blossom needle therapy + moxibustion + cupping	2	S228, S229
CHM + acupuncture therapy (NS)	1	S221
CHM + acupuncture + moxibustion + cupping	1	S207

Abbreviations: CHM, Chinese herbal medicine; NS, not specified.

汤 in two studies (S220, S221), *Chai hu shu gan san* 柴胡疏肝散 in two studies (S220, S221), and topical application of *Fu fang si huang wai xi ye* 复方四黄外洗液/*Fu fang si huang ye* 复方四黄液 in two studies (S220, S221). Four studies used multiple formulas (S211, S220, S221, S224) and a total of 44 herbs were used in all formulas. The most frequently reported herbs were *dang gui* 当归, *chai hu* 柴胡, *zhi zi* 栀子, and *gan cao* 甘草 (see Table 8.2).

The most common acupuncture therapy was acupuncture which was used in 21 studies. Cupping was the only other CM therapy used in included studies, and cupping was used in 25 studies. Across all studies, the most common treatment methods were to needle the rash area (24 studies), target the *ashi* points 阿是穴 (14 studies), or use the EX-B2 *Huatuojiaji* points 夹脊穴 (12 studies). Other common

Table 8.2   Frequently Reported Herbs in Clinical Studies of Combination Therapies

Most Common Herbs	Scientific Name	Frequency of Use
Dang gui 当归	*Angelica sinensis* (Oliv.) Diels	9
Chai hu 柴胡	*Bupleurum* spp	8
Zhi zi 栀子	*Gardenia jasminoides* Ellis	8
Gan cao 甘草	*Glycyrrhiza* spp	8
Ze xie 泽泻	*Alisma orientalis* (Sam.) Juzep.	7
Sheng di huang 生地黄	*Rehmannia glutinosa* Libosch.	7
Long dan cao 龙胆草	*Gentiana scabra* Bge.	7
Yan hu suo 延胡索	*Corydalis yanhusuo* W.T. Wang	5
Bai shao 白芍	*Paeonia lactiflora* Pall.	5
Che qian zi 车前子	*Plantago* spp	5
Da qing ye 大青叶	*Isatis indigotica* Fort.	4
Ban lan gen 板蓝根	*Isatis indigotica* Fort.	4
Chen pi 陈皮	*Citrus reticulata* Blanco	4
Huang qin 黄芩	*Scutellaria baicalensis* Georgi	4
Bai zhu 白术	*Atractylodes macrocephala* Koidz.	3
Chi shao 赤芍	*Paeonia* spp	3
Da huang 大黄	*Rheum* spp	3
Fu ling 茯苓	*Poria cocos* (Schw.) Wolf	3
Huang bai 黄柏	*Phellodendron chinense* Schneid.	3

acupuncture points were SP10 *Xuehai* 血海, ST36 *Zusanli* 足三里, and TE6 *Zhigou* 支沟 (3 studies each) (see Table 8.3).

Combinations of CM were compared with antiviral therapy alone (S204, S205, S211, S214, S226, S227) or with other treatments such as vitamins, cimetidine or carbamazepine (S155, S199, S200, S202, S206, S210, S213, S216–S219, S222–S225, S228, S229), antiviral therapy plus pain management medications (S201, S207, S215), and antiviral therapy plus pain management medications plus

Table 8.3 Frequently Used Points/Treatment Approaches in Clinical Studies of Combination Therapies

Most Common Points	No. of Studies
Rash area	24
Ashi points 阿是穴	14
EX-B2 Huatuojiaji points 夹脊穴	12
SP10 Xuehai 血海	4
ST36 Zusanli 足三里	4
TE6 Zhigou 支沟	4
BL17 Geshu 膈俞	3
GB34 Yanglingquan 阳陵泉	3
LI11 Quchi 曲池	3
LI4 Hegu 合谷	3

other treatments such as vitamins or carbamazepine (S158, S203, S208, S209, S212, S220, S221). Two studies used antiviral therapies at guideline-recommended doses (S205, S209).

Risk of Bias

The methodological quality of included studies was low to moderate (see Table 8.4). Eight studies used acceptable methods of randomisation and were judged as having low risk of bias (S155, S158, S203, S207, S209, S215, S219, S223). One study was judged as having low bias risk for allocation concealment as central randomisation (S155) was used. Due to the nature of the interventions, adequate blinding could not be achieved for participants and all studies were judged as having high bias risk. One study reported that personnel and outcome assessors were blind to group allocation and was assessed as having low risk of bias for these domains (S155). One study had missing data which was not explained or accounted for in analysis and was assessed as having unclear bias risk (S208). One study with missing data reported the reasons and accounted for this in analysis and was judged as having low bias risk (S155). One study registered the

Table 8.4   Risk of Bias in Randomised Controlled Trials: Combination Therapies

Risk of Bias Domain	Low Risk n (%)	Unclear Risk n (%)	High Risk n (%)
Sequence generation	8 (24.2)	22 (66.7)	3 (9.1)
Allocation concealment	1 (3.0)	32 (97.0)	0 (0)
Blinding of participants	0 (0)	0 (0)	33 (100)
Blinding of personnel	1 (3.0)	0 (0)	32 (97.0)
Blinding of outcome assessor	1 (3.0)	32 (97.0)	0 (0)
Incomplete outcome data	32 (97.0)	1 (3.0)	0 (0)
Selective outcome reporting	1 (3.0)	32 (97.0)	0 (0)

trial (S155) and reported on specified outcomes. All other studies were judged as having unclear risk of bias due to a lack of trial protocol or trial registration information.

Pain Score

Fourteen studies reported on the pain score at the end of treatment (S155, S200, S202, S204, S208, S209, S216, S217, S219–S221, S227–S229). Thirteen studies compared combination CM with pharmacotherapy (S155, S200, S202, S204, S208, S209, S216, S217, S220, S221, S227–S229). Visual analogue scale (VAS) scores that were reported in millimetres were converted to centimetres for inclusion in the main analysis. Meta-analyses were possible for two different combinations of CM therapies (see Table 8.5).

Compared with pharmacotherapy, benefits were seen in the VAS pain scores at the end of treatment for acupuncture plus plumblossom needle therapy plus cupping (mean difference MD −1.36 cm [95% confidence intervals −1.84, −0.88], I^2 = 92%) as well as plum-blossom needle therapy plus moxibustion plus cupping (MD −2.63 cm [−2.93, −2.32], I^2 = 6%). Statistical heterogeneity was noted for many analyses which was not always possible to explore through subgroup analyses due to the small number of included studies. Where subgroup analyses were possible, statistical

Table 8.5 Combination Therapies *vs.* Pharmacotherapy: Pain Score (Visual Analogue Scale)

Intervention	Group	No. of Studies (Participants)	Effect Size MD [95% CI] I^2	Included Studies
Acupuncture plus plum-blossom needle therapy plus cupping	All studies	6 (606)	−1.36 [−1.84, −0.88]* 92%	S155, S200, S202, S209, S216, S217,
	Subgroup: Antiviral plus other	5 (544)	−1.24 [−1.73, −0.75]* 91%	S155, S200, S202, S216, S217
Plum-blossom needle therapy plus moxibustion plus cupping	All studies	2 (192)	−2.63 [−2.93, −2.32]* 6%	S228, S229

*Statistically significant.
Abbreviations: CI, confidence interval; MD, mean difference.

heterogeneity was reduced when studies using the same comparator were analysed (see Table 8.5).

Results from single studies showed that some combination therapies were beneficial compared with pharmacotherapy in the pain score at the end of treatment. Benefit was seen for CHM plus acupuncture (MD −2.41 cm [−2.84, −1.98]) (S220), CHM plus plum-blossom needle therapy plus cupping (MD −2.02 cm [−2.35, −1.69]) (S208), and acupuncture plus moxibustion plus cupping (MD −3.04 cm [−4.39, −1.69]) (S204). Further, the reduction in pain was sustained at the follow up after 60 days with acupuncture plus plum-blossom needle therapy plus cupping (MD −1.89 cm [−3.52, −0.26]) (S155). No benefit was seen for plum-blossom needle therapy plus cupping (MD −0.46 cm [−1.44, 0.52]) (S227).

One study used combination therapies as integrative medicine (IM) (S219). The combination of plum-blossom needle therapy and cupping as IM with acyclovir also reduced the pain score by 2.31 cm ([−2.86, −1.76]) at the end of treatment, and by 3.23 cm ([−4.16, −2.30]) at follow up after 20 days compared with acyclovir alone (S219).

Time Taken for Resolution of Pain

Five studies reported on time taken for pain to resolve (S199, S201, S212, S216, S225), with all studies comparing combination CM with pharmacotherapy. One study reported data that did not allow for re-analysis (S201), three studies did not specify the time-point from which measurement was made (S199, S216, S225), and one study reported results that seemed unlikely given the nature of herpes zoster (S212). All studies were excluded from analysis. From the included studies, there is no evidence that combination therapies improve the time taken for the resolution of pain.

Time Taken for Crust Formation

Twelve studies reported on the time taken for the formation of crusts (S155, S158, S200, S204, S205, S207, S212, S213, S215,

S223, S225, S229). Combination CM therapies were compared with pharmacotherapy in 10 studies (S155, S158, S200, S204, S207, S212, S213, S215, S225, S229). One study measured time from rash onset to crust formation (S155), three studies measured the time from start of treatment to crust formation (S200, S212, S223), and eight did not specify the time-point from which measurement started (S158, S204, S205, S207, S213, S215, S225, S229). Data for these eight studies were excluded from analysis.

In single studies that compared combination therapies with pharmacotherapy, one study showed that the time from rash onset to crust formation was 0.46 days faster with acupuncture plus plum-blossom needle therapy plus cupping ([−0.59, −0.33]) (S155). When crust formation was measured from the time treatment started, crust formation occurred 3.88 days faster in people who received acupuncture plus plum-blossom needle therapy plus cupping ([−5.04, −2.72]) (S200) compared with acyclovir and vitamin C, and 0.88 days faster in people who received CHM plus moxibustion ([−1.25, −0.51]) compared with acyclovir, ibuprofen, and polyinosinic acid (S212).

One study which used combination therapies as IM was included in analysis (S223). The combination of CHM, moxibustion, acyclovir, interferon, and vitamin B1 reduced the time taken for crust formation by 1.20 days ([−1.81, −0.59]) compared with acyclovir, interferon, and vitamin B1 alone (S223).

Time Taken for Cessation of New Lesions

Eight studies reported on the amount of time elapsed until no new lesions developed (S155, S158, S204, S205, S207, S212, S214, S223), with six of these comparing combination therapies alone with pharmacotherapy (S155, S158, S204, S207, S212, S214). One study reported the time from rash onset to cessation of new lesions (S155) and three studies reported the time from the start of treatment to cessation of new lesions (S212, S214, S223). The remaining studies did not report the time-point from which measurements were made and data were excluded from analysis. Further, one study reported results which seemed unlikely given the nature of herpes zoster and was also excluded from analysis (S212). Meta-analysis was not possible.

One study that reported the time from rash onset to cessation of new lesions found that people who received acupuncture plus plum-blossom needle therapy plus cupping had a longer time taken for cessation of new lesions by 0.22 days ([0.15, 0.29]) (S155) compared with acyclovir, vitamin B1, and saline compresses. Whilst this result favours pharmacotherapy, the clinical significance of a five-hour difference in time taken for the cessation of new lesions is uncertain. In studies which reported the time from start of treatment to cessation of new lesions, no benefit was seen in people who received CHM plus acupuncture (MD 0.05 days [−0.44, 0.54]) (S214). One study found that CHM plus moxibustion as IM decreased the time from the start of treatment to cessation of new lesions by 1.40 days ([−1.99, −0.81]) (S223).

Time Taken for Resolution of Rash

Four studies reported on the time taken for the rash to resolve (S155, S204, S215, S225). One study reported time from rash onset to resolution (S155) while the remaining studies did not specify the time-point from which measurements were made. Data from these studies were excluded from analysis. Benefit with acupuncture plus plum-blossom needle therapy plus cupping compared with valacyclovir, vitamin B1, and wet skin compress was shown in one study which reported the time from onset to resolution of the rash (MD −3.21 days [−3.54, −2.88]) (S155).

Incidence of Post-herpetic Neuralgia

Eight studies reported on the incidence of post-herpetic neuralgia (PHN) and all studies measured the time of incidence from resolution of the rash (S155, S158, S201, S204, S209, S211, S212, S215). Two studies reported PHN one month after rash resolution (S155, S211), four studies reported PHN three months after rash resolution (S158, S201, S212, S215), and one reported PHN 60 days after rash resolution (S204). One study did not specify the time-point of measurement from resolution of the rash and was excluded from analysis (S209). Seven studies compared combination therapies with pharmacotherapy (S155, S158, S201, S204, S209, S212, S215). Two studies were included in meta-analyses (see Table 8.6). Acupuncture plus moxibustion plus cupping reduced the incidence of PHN measured at three months (risk ratio RR 0.08 [0.01, 0.63], $I^2 = 0\%$) compared with pharmacotherapy.

Single studies showed that when measured at three months after rash resolution, no benefit was seen with acupuncture plus plum-blossom needle therapy plus cupping (RR 0.33 [0.01, 7.87] (S158). CHM plus moxibustion also did not significantly decrease the chance of developing PHN measured at three months after rash resolution (RR 0.33 [0.04, 3.03]) (S212). When PHN was measured one month after resolution of the rash, acupuncture plus plum-blossom needle therapy plus cupping (RR 0.27 [0.14, 0.54]) (S155) decreased the risk of developing PHN.

Acupuncture plus moxibustion plus cupping was not found to reduce the chance of developing PHN at 60 days after the resolution of the rash (RR 0.17 [0.02, 1.30]) (S204). CHM plus acupuncture combined with acyclovir (as IM) reduced the incidence of PHN compared with acyclovir alone when measured at one month after the resolution of the rash (RR 0.07 [0.01, 0.51]) (S211).

Effective Rate

In total, 20 studies reported the effective rate with a definition provided (S158, S200, S202, S206–S210, S212, S213, S216, S218,

Table 8.6   Acupuncture plus Moxibustion plus Cupping *vs.* Pharmacotherapy: Post-herpetic Neuralgia (Three Months from Resolution of Rash)

No. of Studies	No. of Participants	Effect Size RR [95% CI] I^2	Included Studies
2	140	0.08 [0.01, 0.63]* 0%	S201, S215

*Statistically significant.

Abbreviations: CI, confidence interval; RR, risk ratio.

S222–S229). Diversity was seen in studies which used guidelines other than the 1994 guideline[1] and it was not possible to pool these studies for analysis. Therefore, only studies that reported the effective rate according to the 1994 guideline[1] are presented below. In addition, one study reported data which did not match the number of participants and was excluded from analysis (S228).

Seventeen studies reported the effective rate according to the specified guideline (S158, S199, S200, S202, S206–S210, S213, S216, S222–S226, S229). Fifteen studies compared combination CM therapies with pharmacotherapy (S158, S199, S200, S202, S206–S210, S213, S216, S224–S226, S229) and combination CM therapies were used as IM in two studies (S222, S223). Several meta-analyses were possible for studies where combination CM therapies were used alone (see Table 8.7). The number of people achieving a 30% reduction in lesions and improvements in pain was greater in those who received acupuncture plus plum-blossom needle therapy plus cupping (RR 1.20 [1.11, 1.30], $I^2 = 0\%$) or acupuncture plus plum-blossom needle therapy plus moxibustion plus cupping (RR 1.16 [1.05, 1.28], $I^2 = 0\%$) compared with pharmacotherapy. No benefit was seen when pharmacotherapy was compared with CHM plus plum-blossom needle therapy plus cupping (RR 1.13 [0.93, 1.37], $I^2 = 90\%$).

When CHM plus plum-blossom needle therapy plus cupping was compared with pharmacotherapy, substantial statistical heterogeneity was detected. Subgroup analyses were performed according to comparator type (antiviral therapy plus other treatment) and treatment duration (10 days or ≥14 days). Statistical heterogeneity was reduced in some analyses with favourable results seen. For CHM plus plum-blossom needle therapy plus cupping, treatment duration of 14 days produced a significant increase in the number of people achieving symptom improvement (RR 1.19 [1.06, 1.34], $I^2 = 37\%$).

When used alone, combinations of therapies in single studies showed no benefit over pharmacotherapy for:

- CHM plus acupuncture (RR 1.07 [0.94, 1.22]) (S206);
- CHM plus acupuncture plus moxibustion plus cupping (RR 1.19 [0.96, 1.46]) (S207);

Table 8.7 Combination Therapies *vs.* Pharmacotherapy: Effective Rate

Intervention	Group	No. of Studies (Participants)	Effect Size RR [95% CI] I^2	Included Studies
CHM plus plum-blossom needle therapy plus cupping	All studies	3 (400)	RR 1.13 [0.93, 1.37] 90%	S208, S224, S225
	Subgroup: Antiviral plus other	2 (300)	RR 1.07 [0.88, 1.29] 90%	S224, S225
	Subgroup: treatment duration 14d	2 (340)	RR 1.19 [1.06, 1.34]* 37%	S208, S225
Acupuncture plus plum-blossom needle therapy plus cupping	All studies	6 (410)	RR 1.20 [1.11, 1.30]* 0%	S158, S199, S200, S202, S209, S216
Acupuncture plus plum-blossom needle therapy plus moxibustion plus cupping	All studies	2 (170)	RR 1.16 [1.05, 1.28]* 0%	S210, S213

*Statistically significant.
Abbreviations: CHM, Chinese herbal medicine; CI, confidence interval; RR, risk ratio.

- CHM plus acupuncture plus cupping (RR 1.00 [0.94, 1.07]) (S224), and;
- Plum-blossom needle therapy plus moxibustion plus cupping (RR 1.08 [0.97, 1.19]) (S229).

Two studies evaluated effective rate according to the 1994 guideline[1] with combination therapies as IM (S222, S223). CHM and moxibustion with acyclovir, interferon, and vitamin B1 increased the number of people achieving a 30% or greater improvement in symptoms (RR 1.11 [1.01, 1.21] compared with acyclovir, interferon, and vitamin B1 alone (S223). No benefit was seen when CHM, acupuncture, and cupping were used as IM to oral and topical acyclovir and vitamins B1 and B12 compared with these medications alone (RR 1.18 [0.93, 1.49) (S222).

Combination Therapies Compared with Guideline-recommended Doses of Antiviral Therapy

Two studies compared various combinations of CM therapies with antiviral therapy at guideline-recommended dosages[2,3] (S205, S209). Outcomes included both pain and cutaneous outcomes, incidence of PHN, and effective rate. One study reported on cutaneous outcomes, but as the time-point from which measurement was made was not specified, data were excluded from analysis (S205). The study reported that adverse events did not occur during the trial.

In the remaining study, acupuncture plus plum-blossom needle therapy plus cupping reduced the VAS pain score at the end of treatment by 1.89 cm ([−2.34, −1.44]) compared with acyclovir (800 mg five times daily), indomethacin (25 mg three times daily), and topical acyclovir (five times daily) (S209). The incidence of PHN was measured from an unspecified time from rash resolution, and thus data were excluded from analysis. Finally, no effect was seen with this combination of interventions on the number of people achieving a 30% or greater reduction in symptoms (RR 1.20 [1.00, 1.44], p = 0.05).

Safety of Combination Therapies

Adverse events were reported in eight studies (327 participants in the combination therapy groups and 327 in the comparator groups) (S155, S158, S203–S205, S207, S214, S215). Five adverse events were reported in the combination therapy groups, which included five cases of bleeding (the intervention was acupuncture plus plum-blossom needle therapy plus cupping). Twenty-five adverse events were reported in the comparator groups, including seven cases of gastrointestinal discomfort, 10 cases of insomnia, one case of dizziness and nausea, and seven cases of unspecified events. Combination therapies appear to be well-tolerated based on the available data.

Summary of Combination Therapies Evidence

Many RCTs have evaluated combinations of CM therapies for herpes zoster, with acupuncture therapies and other CM therapies being used more commonly than CHM. The most common herbal formula was *Long dan xie gan tang* 龙胆泻肝汤 and the most common acupuncture approaches were to needle around the rash area, use *ashi* points 阿是穴, and target the acupuncture points EX-B2 *Huatuojiaji* 夹脊穴, SP10 *Xuehai* 血海, ST36 *Zusanli* 足三里, and TE6 *Zhigou* 支沟. Practitioners should consider syndrome diagnosis when formulating treatments using combinations of CM therapies.

The clearest benefit from the various combinations of CM therapies (i.e., those with statistically significant findings and acceptable levels of statistical heterogeneity) was seen for:

- Pain score (plum-blossom needle therapy plus moxibustion);
- Incidence of PHN (acupuncture plus moxibustion plus cupping);

- Effective rate (acupuncture plus plum-blossom needle therapy plus cupping, acupuncture plus plum-blossom needle therapy plus moxibustion plus cupping).

Based on the studies which reported adverse events, combination therapies were well-tolerated.

The combination of acupuncture, moxibustion, and cupping (with or without other interventions) was clearly effective for two outcomes. As both acupuncture and moxibustion are recommended in clinical practice guidelines, this combination of interventions may be a useful direction for future research. The best evidence was found for pain scores, incidence of PHN, and effective rate. Results from meta-analyses suggest that combination CM therapies may alleviate the acute pain reported with herpes zoster. However, statistical heterogeneity was seen in many meta-analyses and the overall findings remain uncertain in terms of alleviation of pain. Further research is needed.

Few of the included studies compared combinations of CM interventions with pharmacotherapy at guideline-recommended doses, with the vast majority administering antiviral and pain management treatments at doses less than recommended. This limits the applicability of the findings to clinical practice, particularly when the combination was used as IM. Future research must include antiviral therapy at internationally accepted doses in order to provide clinically relevant evidence for CM therapies.

Many studies reported on key outcomes relating to pain and rash healing, although several omitted details about the timing of measurement which limits the interpretation of the findings. Detailed reporting of outcome measures is critical to ensuring that the evidence can be interpreted in a meaningful way and can be translated into clinical practice. None of the studies reported outcomes in terms of health-related quality of life, which is also a similar issue for currently available RCTs of CHM, and acupuncture therapies. This is an important area for future research to address as the impact of herpes zoster on health-related quality of life is known to be high.

References

1. 国家中医药管理局. 中医病证诊断疗效标准. 南京大学出版社; 1994.

2. Gross G, Schofer H, Wassilew S, *et al.* Herpes zoster guideline of the German Dermatology Society (DDG). *J Clin Virol.* 2003; **26**(3): 277–89; discussion 91–3.

3. Dworkin RH, Johnson RW, Breuer J, *et al.* Recommendations for the management of herpes zoster. *Clin Infect Dis.* 2007; **44** (Suppl 1):S1–26.

9

Summary and Conclusions — Herpes Zoster

OVERVIEW

Many Chinese medicine treatments are used to manage symptoms of herpes zoster. Several have demonstrated benefits and further research is warranted. This chapter provides a 'whole evidence' analysis of the role of Chinese medicine from the classical literature, contemporary literature, and clinical studies.

Introduction

Herpes zoster is a self-limiting condition and, for many people, the rash and pain will resolve spontaneously with little consequence. For some, pain associated with the rash can have a considerable impact on quality of life and is associated with an increased risk of developing post-herpetic neuralgia (PHN).[1] Antiviral therapies are effective and can hasten rash healing. Clinical practice guidelines recommend their use in patients 50 years or older, immunocompromised patients, those with malignant disease, and patients with the zoster rash affecting more than one dermatome.[2] Chinese medicine (CM) treatments may be of value for these patients as well as for other patients who do not meet these criteria.

This monograph provides a 'whole evidence' analysis evaluating CM treatments for herpes zoster. Clinical practice guidelines and key CM textbooks have recommended a range of CM therapies which can be used for herpes zoster, including Chinese herbal medicine (CHM), various acupuncture techniques, and a range of other CM modalities. The systematic review of the classical literature provided the historical context of herpes zoster treatment, much of which is mirrored in contemporary practice. Findings from clinical evidence suggest that the demonstrated benefits of CHM, acupuncture, and moxibustion for herpes zoster are promising.

Chinese Herbal Medicine

The evidence referred to in this section can be found in Chapters 2, 3, 5, and 8. CHM has been used to treat herpes zoster for a long period of time. The earliest description of herpes zoster treatment identified in the review of classical literature was in *Hua Tuo Shen Fang* 华佗神方 (682 AD). Contemporary literature included in Chapter 2 recommends various formulas based on syndrome differentiation, including oral and topical formulas, herbal prescriptions, and manufactured products. The evidence for CHM has also been evaluated in 151 clinical studies, the majority of which were randomised clinical trials (RCTs).

In classical literature citations which described syndromes, these included Liver fire, wind-dampness, wind and heat in the Heart and Liver, disharmony between the Heart and Lung, and heat in the Spleen. Some overlap was seen with the syndromes described in Chapter 2, although terminology in the classical literature was more descriptive. Syndromes in clinical textbooks and guidelines in Chapter 2 include stagnated heat in the Liver meridian or dampness and heat in the Liver and Gallbladder, Spleen deficiency syndrome with dampness retention, and *qi* stagnation with Blood stasis. Common syndromes reported in clinical studies include excess heat in the Liver meridian, Liver-Gallbladder dampness-heat, *qi* stagnation and Blood stasis, and dampness-heat.

The herbal formula most frequently evaluated in clinical studies was *Long dan xie gan tang* (modified) 龙胆泻肝汤 (加减). This formula was also recommended in clinical guidelines in Chapter 2 and was the most frequently cited formula in the classical literature. Many of the most commonly reported herbs in clinical studies were consistent with those most commonly cited in the classical literature as well as those in guideline-recommended formulas in Chapter 2. These include *gan cao* 甘草, *huang qin* 黄芩, *chai hu* 柴胡, *zhi zi* 栀子, *sheng di huang* 生地黄 (*sheng di* 生地 in classical literature), *long dan cao* 龙胆草, *dang gui* 当归, *ze xie* 泽泻, *che qian zi* 车前子, *chuan xiong* 川芎, and *huang lian* 黄连. The extensive list of common herbs may reflect that little has changed in the management of herpes zoster over time. This may also be due to *Long dan xie gan tang* 龙胆泻肝汤 being heavily recommended in the contemporary literature (see Chapter 2) and also being the most cited formula in both classical literature and clinical studies. Nine of the above herbs are ingredients included in *Long dan xie gan tang* 龙胆泻肝汤 according to the *Guidelines for Diagnosis and Treatment of Common Diseases of Dermatology in Traditional Chinese Medicine.*[3]

Results from RCTs were available for many pain and cutaneous outcomes while few studies reported on health-related quality of life. The most promising evidence was for oral CHM, topical CHM, or a combination of the two, with benefits seen for some cutaneous outcomes. Oral CHM may also reduce the likelihood of incidence of PHN. *Long dan xie gan tang* 龙胆泻肝汤 produced positive effects on cutaneous outcomes and *Xiao chai hu tang* (modified) 加味小柴胡汤 was effective at reducing lesions by 30% or greater and producing significant reductions in pain (effective rate).

Limitations of clinical studies affect the interpretation of many findings and make the applicability of findings to clinical practice unclear (see Chapter 5 for a more detailed explanation of the limitations of included studies). The small number of adverse events seen with CHM (either alone or in combination with pharmacotherapy) was similar to that of pharmacotherapy. Thus, CHM can be considered safe for people with herpes zoster.

Chinese Herbal Medicine Formulas in Contemporary Literature, Classical Literature, and Clinical Studies

Many herbal formulas have been recommended in clinical practice guidelines in Chapter 2 and evaluated in clinical studies. Description and use of herbal formulas recommended in Chapter 2 are presented in Tables 9.1 and 9.2. *Long dan xie gan tang* 龙胆泻肝汤, which was

Table 9.1   Summary of Oral Chinese Herbal Medicine Formulas

Formula Name	Clinical Guidelines and Textbooks (Chapter 2)	Classical Literature (No. of Citations) (Chapter 3)	Clinical Studies* (Chapter 5)			Combination Therapies (Chapter 8)
			RCTs (No. of Studies)	CCTs (No. of Studies)	Non-controlled Studies (No. of Studies)	
Ban lan gen ke li 板蓝根颗粒	Yes	0	0	0	0	2
Chai hu shu gan san 柴胡疏肝散 plus Tao hong si wu tang 桃红四物汤 (加减) (modified)	Yes	0	0	0	1	0
Chu shi wei ling tang (modified) 除湿胃苓汤 (加减)	Yes	3	4	0	4	2
Da huang zhe chong wan 大黄蛰虫丸	Yes	0	0	0	0	0
Ji de sheng she yao pian 季德胜蛇药片	Yes	0	1	0	2	2
Liu shen wan 六神丸	Yes	0	2	0	3	0
Long dan xie gan tang (modified) 龙胆泻肝汤 (加减)	Yes	10	23	1	13	8
Long dan xie gan wan 龙胆泻肝丸	Yes	0	1	0	0	0
Qing kai ling kou fu ye 清开灵口服液	Yes	0	0	0	0	0
Shen ling bai zhu wan 参苓白术丸	Yes	0	0	0	0	0
Xin huang pian 新癀片	Yes	0	2	0	0	0
Xue fu zhu yu tang 血府逐瘀汤 plus Jin ling zi san 金铃子散 (加减) (modified)	Yes	0	0	0	0	0
Xue fu zhu yu pian 血府逐瘀片	Yes	0	0	0	0	0
Yuan hu zhi tong jiao nang 元胡止痛胶囊	Yes	0	0	0	0	0

*Some studies used two or more formulas. These are counted separately in this table.

Abbreviations: CCT, controlled clinical trial; RCT, randomised controlled trial.

Table 9.2 Summary of Topical Chinese Herbal Medicine Formulas

Formula Name	Clinical Guidelines and Textbooks (Chapter 2)	Classical Literature (No. of Citations) (Chapter 3)	Clinical Studies* (Chapter 5)			Combination Therapies (Chapter 8)
			RCTs (No. of Studies)	CCTs (No. of Studies)	Non-controlled Studies (No. of Studies)	
Bing shi san 冰石散	Yes	0	0	0	0	0
Dian dao san 颠倒散	Yes	0	0	0	0	0
Er wei ba du san 二味拔毒散	Yes	0	0	0	0	0
Fu fang huang bai ye 复方黄柏液	Yes	0	0	0	0	0
Huang lian gao 黄连膏	Yes	0	0	0	1	0
Huang ling dan 黄灵丹	Yes	0	0	0	0	0
Jin huang san 金黄散	Yes	0	0	0	0	0
Qing dai gao/oil 青黛膏/油	Yes	0	0	0	0	1
Qing liang ru ji 清凉乳剂	Yes	0	0	0	0	0
San huang xi ji 三黄洗剂	Yes	0	0	0	0	0
Shi run shao shang gao 湿润烧伤膏	Yes	0	1	0	0	0
Shuang bai san 双柏散	Yes	0	0	0	0	0
Si huang gao 四黄膏	Yes	0	0	0	0	0
Yu lu gao 玉露膏	Yes	0	0	0	0	0
Yun nan bai yao 云南白药	Yes	0	1	1	1	1
Zi cao oil 紫草油	Yes	0	0	0	0	0

*Some studies used two or more formulas. These are counted separately in this table.

Abbreviations: CCT, controlled clinical trial; RCT, randomised controlled trial.

also recommended in Chapter 2, was considered clinically important based on group consensus. As outlined above, *Long dan xie gan tang* 龙胆泻肝汤 has a long history of use, continues to be recommended in clinical texts and practice guidelines, and has clinical evidence which supports its use. *Chu shi wei ling tang* 除湿胃苓汤 has similarly remained a key formula for the treatment of herpes zoster.

For many of the oral and topical formulas recommended in key texts and guidelines in Chapter 2, there is a lack of historical data describing their application in herpes zoster and there was no clinical evidence which met the inclusion criteria for review. The few topical formulas which have been evaluated in clinical studies (see Table 9.2) were used in combination with an oral CHM formula. As such, there is currently no evidence available for the effects of these formulas when used alone. The potential benefit of many oral and topical formulas which are recommended in guidelines and clinical textbooks remains uncertain.

Acupuncture and Related Therapies

The evidence referred to in this section can be found in Chapters 2, 3, 7, and 8. Acupuncture and related therapies are another treatment option for CM practitioners to manage symptoms of herpes zoster. Acupuncture therapies have been described in the classical literature, many therapies are recommended in key textbooks and clinical guidelines included in Chapter 2, and 47 clinical studies have been conducted to verify the efficacy and safety of acupuncture therapies. Both acupuncture and moxibustion have been evaluated in clinical studies, are recommended in contemporary works in Chapter 2, and have been described in the classical literature. With the exception of acupuncture-point magnetic therapy, all interventions recommended in Chapter 2 have been evaluated in clinical studies. Plum-blossom needle therapy was evaluated in clinical studies but has not been recommended for use alone in key texts and clinical practice guidelines and was not described in the classical literature.

CM syndromes reported in clinical studies were similar to those in key textbooks and guidelines in Chapter 2. These include pattern/syndrome of *qi* stagnation and Blood stasis, Spleen deficiency with dampness encumbrance, excess heat in the Liver meridian, Liver-Gallbladder wind-fire, dampness-heat in the Spleen meridian, Liver-Gallbladder fire, and dampness-heat. The most frequently reported treatment approaches and acupuncture points used in clinical studies were to treat the rash area, stimulate EX-B2 *Huatuojiaji* points 夹脊穴, *ashi* points 阿是穴, and target other points such as GB34 *Yanglingquan* 阳陵泉, LR3 *Taichong* 太冲, ST36 *Zusanli* 足三里, TE6 *Zhigou* 支沟, LI11 *Quchi* 曲池, LI4 *Hegu* 合谷, and TE5 *Waiguan* 外关. Using acupuncture-related techniques around the rash area was described in contemporary texts in Chapter 2 and in the classical literature, and has also been evaluated in clinical studies. While there was some overlap in points described in Chapter 2 and those evaluated in Chapter 7, no acupuncture points were common to Chapters 2, 3, and 7. This is due to the absence of specified acupuncture points in the classical literature to treat herpes zoster.

While various acupuncture therapies were evaluated in clinical studies, consistency was seen in the acupuncture points and treatment approaches used. The best evidence from RCTs (from trials which used guideline-recommended doses of antiviral therapy) has shown that acupuncture combined with moxibustion decreased pain severity and enhanced rash healing. Acupuncture plus moxibustion combined with antiviral therapies reduced the amount of time from start of treatment to resolution of pain, crust formation and cessation of new lesions, and increased the number of people achieving a 30% or greater reduction in lesions and significant pain relief (effective rate).

The methodological quality of included studies was low to moderate and results should be interpreted in light of methodological shortcomings. Few adverse events were reported in clinical studies, although the proportion of studies which reported adverse events was low (11 out of 47 studies). Acupuncture therapies can be considered safe for people with herpes zoster.

Acupuncture Therapies in Contemporary Literature, Classical Literature, and Clinical Studies

Technological advances have meant that many new acupuncture therapies have become part of the clinical management of many diseases, including herpes zoster. For example, ear acupuncture and scalp acupuncture were developed in the 1950s[4] and 1970s,[5] respectively. Accordingly, such therapies would not be identified in the classical literature and few citations in the classical literature provided descriptions of herpes zoster treatment with acupuncture techniques. Acupuncture and moxibustion were consistently used across all evidence types (see Table 9.3), with many clinical studies evaluating these interventions separately or in combination.

Three interventions recommended in clinical guidelines and key texts in Chapter 2 were not evaluated in clinical studies included in

Table 9.3 Summary of Acupuncture Therapies

| | | | Clinical Studies* (Chapter 7) | | | |
| | | | | | | |
Intervention	Clinical Guidelines and Textbooks (Chapter 2)	Classical Literature (No. of Citations) (Chapter 3)	RCTs* (No. of Studies)	CCTs (No. of Studies)	Non-controlled Studies* (No. of Studies)	Combination Therapies (Chapter 8)*
Acupuncture (including electro-acupuncture)	Yes	4	25	1	15	36
Ear acupuncture	Yes	0	0	0	0	0
Scalp acupuncture	Yes	0	0	0	0	0
Moxibustion	Yes	3	19	3	2	10
Acupuncture-point magnetic therapy	Yes	0	0	0	0	0
Plum-blossom needle therapy	No	0	5	1	1	22

*Some studies used more than one intervention e.g. acupuncture plus moxibustion. These are counted separately in this table.

Abbreviations: CCT, controlled clinical trial; RCT, randomised controlled trial.

the review, and these were ear acupuncture, scalp acupuncture, and acupuncture-point magnetic therapy. Considering that one of the most common treatment approaches seen in clinical studies was to treat the rash area, the lack of inclusion of studies of ear acupuncture and scalp acupuncture was not surprising. However, the lack of evidence for acupuncture-point magnetic therapy is puzzling, especially since acupuncture-point magnetic therapy is often used for analgesia.

Finally, plum-blossom needle therapy was evaluated in six clinical studies and in 20 clinical studies as a combination therapy but has not been recommended for use in the key texts and guidelines identified in Chapter 2. Several studies in Chapter 7 combined plum-blossom needle therapy with acupuncture, moxibustion, or both. Plum-blossom needle therapy plus cupping is recommended in one key clinical practice guideline identified in Chapter 2,[6] and was evaluated in three studies in Chapter 8, with some benefit observed for pain alleviation. There is insufficient evidence from the included studies on the potential benefits of plum-blossom needle therapy alone for herpes zoster.

Implications for Practice

As health care shifts increasingly towards evidence-based practice, CM will rely on clinical research to provide the necessary evidence for contemporary practice. Although CM therapies can be used as stand-alone medication, they are increasingly being used as an adjunct to conventional medicine and should be given greater consideration in the context of medicine as a whole. As new evidence emerges, our understanding of how, and to what extent, CM treatments can improve herpes zoster is enriched. CM can contribute significantly to the overall care for people with herpes zoster.

The CM syndromes reported in key textbooks and guidelines (Chapter 2), in classical literature (Chapter 3), and in clinical evidence (Chapters 5, 7, 8 and 9) were generally consistent, with concepts of heat and fire, dampness and Spleen deficiency, and *qi* and Blood stagnation being reported in various ways. This consistency suggests that there has been little change in the understanding of herpes zoster over time. Further, there is consistent use of the formulas *Long dan xie gan tang* 龙胆泻肝汤 and *Chu shi wei ling tang* 除湿胃苓汤 as well as the interventions of acupuncture and moxibustion applied to the rash area. Again, there appears to be little change in the clinical management of herpes zoster over time.

Evidence from clinical studies suggests that some CHM formulas and some acupuncture therapies can be included in the overall healthcare plan for people with herpes zoster. Benefits were seen for pain and cutaneous outcomes as well as for the incidence of PHN. These therapies can be considered as adjunct therapy for patients over 50 years and those with compromised immune systems, malignant disease, or disseminated zoster, for whom pharmacological intervention is recommended.[2] Further, these therapies may be considered as a treatment option for patients at lower risk of complications and for whom pharmacological intervention is not recommended.

Many CHM formulas evaluated in clinical studies were investigator-developed formulas, with syndrome differentiation used either as an inclusion criterion or to guide treatment. This approach is reflective of clinical practice and allows for the translation of research findings into practice. For several therapies, there was insufficient evidence to support their use and thus clinicians should apply expert discretion for the use of these therapies on a case-by-case basis. Based on the included clinical studies, the number of adverse events with CM therapies was low. These therapies can be considered safe for people with herpes zoster.

Implications for Research

The number of clinical studies evaluating the efficacy and safety of CM treatments for herpes zoster is growing. There is encouraging evidence for some CHM formulas and acupuncture therapies, and more evidence is needed for other CM therapies recommended in clinical textbooks and practice guidelines. Two key issues that clinical research of CM therapies for herpes zoster needs to address are the definitions for outcomes and use of pharmacotherapies.

While many studies reported the same outcomes, such as time taken for resolution of pain or the rash, there was diversity in the time from which measurements were made and many studies did not specify this information. In the absence of validated outcome measures, detailed descriptions of outcome measures are needed to allow for appropriate synthesis of results from clinical studies.

Few studies included in the systematic reviews used antiviral therapies at doses recommended in internationally recognised clinical practice guidelines. The reasons for this are unclear. Regardless, in order to make appropriate and clinically relevant comparisons between CM and antiviral therapies, the dose of antiviral therapies must meet those specified in guidelines.

For some of the key herbs identified in clinical trials, there was experimental evidence to examine potential mechanisms. However, for others, there was little evidence and the mechanisms of action remain unclear. There is a need for more experimental evidence for many of the commonly used herbs used to treat herpes zoster. Further research is needed which addresses the following issues.

Many studies included in these reviews had methodological flaws and included small sample sizes. RCTs should be scientifically rigorous and adequately powered to detect important changes or differences between groups. Trial protocols were often not available and trial registrations could not identified for many included studies. Ensuring the publication or availability of these will increase transparency in reporting. Few included studies assessed health-related quality of life. Investigators should include health-related quality of life measures when planning the study design as the impact of herpes zoster on quality of life can be considerable. Studies including long-term follow up for incidence of PHN should use the generally accepted definition for PHN, which is the persistence of pain for three months or more after resolution of the rash.

Few, if any, studies reported reasons for why they selected the particular intervention that was used. The rationale for intervention and treatment details such as dosage and route of administration for CHM and the selection of acupuncture points for acupuncture interventions should be explained. Authentication of CHM formulas and ingredients should be undertaken and described. This should include the quantification of active constituents. While some studies included in these reviews described using CM syndromes, greater consideration should be given to the use of CM syndromes to guide clinical studies. Where possible and appropriate, these should be included in order to enhance translation to practice.

Many RCTs included in these reviews were judged to be at unclear risk of bias for many research method domains due to insufficient information. Reporting of key details such as randomisation and blinding are critical to enable appropriate interpretation of the reliability of the results. Research publications should follow the CONSORT statement with reference to the extension for herbal medicine,[7] acupuncture,[8] and moxibustion.[9] Several of the studies included in reviews reported that modifications were made to known formula or acupuncture points based on syndrome differentiation. Modifications should be reported in greater detail to assist translation to practice

Evidence is promising for many CM treatments, although the findings are limited by methodological shortcomings related to group allocation and blinding of participants and personnel. There is a lack of evidence for many interventions recommended in key texts and guidelines in the contemporary literature. Future research should therefore aim to provide high quality evidence either for or against the use of these interventions.

References

1. Volpi A, Gross G, Hercogova J, Johnson RW. Current management of herpes zoster: The European view. *Am J Clin Dermatol.* 2005; **6**(5):317–25.
2. Dworkin RH, Johnson RW, Breuer J, *et al.* Recommendations for the management of herpes zoster. *Clin Infect Dis.* 2007; **44** (Suppl 1):S1–26.
3. 中华中医药学会. 中医皮肤科常见病诊疗指南. 中国中医药出版社; 2012.
4. Gori L, Firenzuoli F. Ear acupuncture in European traditional medicine. *Evid Based Complement Alternat Med.* 2007; **4**(Suppl 1):13–6.
5. Allam H, ElDine NG, Helmy G. Scalp acupuncture effect on language development in children with autism: A pilot study. *J Altern Complement Med.* 2008; **14**(2):109–14.

6. 欧阳卫权. 皮肤病中医外治特色疗法精选[M]. 广州: 广东科技出版社; 2013.

7. Gagnier JJ, Boon H, Rochon P, *et al.* Reporting randomized, controlled trials of herbal interventions: An elaborated CONSORT statement. *Ann Intern Med.* 2006; **144**(5):364–7.

8. MacPherson H, Altman DG, Hammerschlag R, *et al.* Revised STandards for Reporting Interventions in Clinical Trials of Acupuncture (STRICTA): Extending the CONSORT statement. *J Evid Based Med.* 2010; **3**(3):140–55.

9. Cheng CW, Fu SF, Zhou QH, *et al.* Extending the CONSORT Statement to moxibustion. *J Integr Med.* 2013; **11**(1):54–63.

10

Introduction to Post-herpetic Neuralgia

OVERVIEW

This chapter provides an overview of the characteristics and symptoms of post-herpetic neuralgia, the economic burden of the disease, and impact on health-related quality of life, and also examines risk factors for the development of PHN. The pathological processes involved are described along with suggested management approaches from international clinical practice guidelines.

Definition of Post-herpetic Neuralgia

Post-herpetic neuralgia (PHN) is a common sequela of herpes zoster (for more information about herpes zoster, see Chapter 1). The primary characteristic of PHN is pain[1] that is usually experienced in the same dermatome affected by herpes zoster.[2] Pain may be intermittent or continuous and is described as burning, throbbing, intense itching, aching, lancinating, and electric shock-like.[1-3] Pain can be accompanied by numbness, tingling, and allodynia (pain response to a stimulus that would not normally elicit pain).[1-4] Pain can also be associated with other symptoms, such as sleep disturbance, chronic fatigue, loss of appetite and weight loss, and depression.[1]

The duration of PHN varies greatly[5] and symptoms may last for several years[6] or indefinitely.[7] In a longitudinal study, 48% of people were symptomatic one year after onset.[5] The likelihood of spontaneous remission after one year is limited.[3,6] Once established, effective management can be difficult and many patients are refractory to treatment.[8]

The definition of PHN varies from one to six months after resolution of the rash.[5] While the German Dermatology Society defines PHN as 'pain that persists for longer than four weeks or that occurs four weeks after a pain-free interval',[9, p281] the definition of pain persisting for ≥ 120 days after rash onset proposed by Dworkin and Portenoy[4] has been accepted as PHN for clinical and research purposes.[5,10] The various definitions have an impact on how PHN prevalence is calculated.

Epidemiology

Prevalence of PHN varies greatly depending on the definition used[8,10] including the time-point at which prevalence is measured and whether additional criteria for minimum levels of pain are applied. Data from Europe suggest that PHN incidence (based on the definition of pain lasting at least three months) is between 10% and 20% in patients over 50 years[11] but increases to nearly 80% in patients 80 years or older.[12] Similar results have been reported by Volpi *et al.*[8] who further state that PHN is rare in people under 40 years of age. The prevalence of PHN (60 days after developing herpes zoster) in people over 50 years was 27.4 times higher than in people under 50.[13] Many studies limit the assessment of PHN to three or six months after herpes zoster, and long-term data is lacking.[1]

Burden

The burden associated with PHN is substantial.[10] PHN is associated with significant loss of function, decreased quality of life (QoL), and economic burden,[3] with the main economic burden being the cost of pain relief.[8] Direct costs varied according to definitions used, with a mean direct cost of £341 for PHN at one month after herpes zoster diagnosis and £397 at three months after herpes zoster diagnosis.[14] Direct costs increase with pain severity.[14] Healthcare utilisation is much higher in PHN than in herpes zoster, with people with PHN making 11.9 and 12.0 visits to their GP based on one month and three month definitions, respectively.[15]

PHN can have a negative impact on physical wellbeing, with some patients experiencing chronic fatigue, loss of appetite and weight loss, sleep disturbances, reduced ability to perform activities of daily living, and reduced physical capacity.[16] People with PHN had worse scores on all domains of the Medical Outcome Study 36-item Short Form Health Survey (a general wellbeing questionnaire) compared to age-matched population norms and worse scores on the Self-Rated Health and Health State Index domains of the EuroQoL 5 dimensions questionnaire.[17] The health burden from PHN also includes mental wellbeing and relationships. Forty-three per cent of people with PHN reported moderate anxiety or depression.[18]

Risk Factors

Well-established risk factors for developing PHN after herpes zoster include advanced age, painful prodromal phase of herpes zoster, and more severe rash and pain with herpes zoster.[3,7,8,10] Other less predictable risk factors include fever during herpes zoster,[7,8] sensory dysfunction in affected dermatomes,[7] zoster opthalmicus,[9,19] gender (females are more susceptible than males),[8,9,20] presence of varicella zoster virus (VZV) in peripheral blood,[3] thoracic zoster,[2] trauma,[2] extended rash duration and cranial or sacral location of herpes zoster rash,[21,22] and psychological stress.[16,19,23]

Recent evidence has cast doubt on whether psychological stress is a risk factor for PHN.[24] Other possible factors include employment status, mobility at onset of herpes zoster, and the impact of pain on social relationships.[25] The risk of PHN is not increased in immunocompromised patients.[8,9]

Pathological Processes

The pathophysiology of PHN is not well understood.[19,26] As the nature of pain can vary over time and can differ from patient to patient,[27] several mechanisms have been proposed for neuropathic pain more broadly and for PHN specifically.[1,28,29] These include (1) nerve injury in the peripheral nervous system (PNS),[29,30] (2) sensitisation in the central nervous system (CNS),[29,30] and (3) continued viral replication leading to chronic ganglionitis.[28] The first two mechanisms are well-accepted as explanations for the pathophysiology of PHN while the third has not been reported frequently in the literature.

In the PNS, nerve injury due to inflammation produces hyperexcitability in nociceptors (cells that initiate the sensation of pain) which have a low threshold for activation. This can lead to increased excitability of central nociceptors in the dorsal horn.[31] Once central sensitisation has occurred, light touch induces pain. In the CNS, central sensitisation occurs due to the degeneration of nociceptive neurons.[1] Immunohistological studies have shown significant neuronal degeneration in people with constant pain from PHN[32] and loss of function in affected tissues.[33] A loss of C-fibre afferents in the skin have been found in the affected dermatome of people with PHN.[34]

A third hypothesis relates to the VZV. Gilden *et al.*[26] propose that people with PHN may experience pain due to persistent or low-grade infection in the ganglia. Post-mortem pathological studies of ganglia from patients with PHN have found the presence of inflammatory cells around the ganglia.[35,36] Further, virological findings in patients with chronic PHN found VZV deoxyribonucleic acid (DNA) in mononuclear cells (MNCs), which were seen neither in patients who did not develop PHN after herpes zoster nor in people with no history of herpes zoster.[37] In an elderly patient with a long history of PHN, VZV DNA in MNCs was found.[28] After treatment with famciclovir, repeated tests did not detect VZV DNA. Gilden *et al.*[26] suggest that the most likely explanation for the absence of VZV DNA after treatment with famciclovir is VZV ganglionitis.

Diagnosis

Diagnosis of PHN is based on clinical presentation with consideration to the various ways that PHN is defined. Some have argued that PHN should include only clinically important pain and a pain score of three or greater on a 10-point scale has been suggested.[38,39] This requirement has not yet been adopted in clinical practice guidelines.

In 2007, Robert Johnson called for a consensus on the definition of PHN[3] but this still has yet to happen at the time of this writing.

As diagnosis is based on clinical presentation, other potential causes of neuralgia need to be excluded. These include neoplastic, toxic, traumatic, and compressive causes.[2] Various tools such as the visual analogue scale (VAS), McGill Pain Questionnaire, and the disease-specific Zoster Brief Pain Inventory (ZBPI) can be used to measure and describe the nature of pain to facilitate diagnosis, and can also be used to monitor pain levels over time. In addition to clinical examination, quantitative sensory examination may also be considered to confirm pain of neuropathic origin. Tests may include assessment of response to light touch, temperature, pain, proprioception, and vibration.[40]

Management

Four clinical practice guidelines were identified which were relevant to PHN.[5,41–43] One guideline, produced by the American Academy of Neurology (AAN), is specific to PHN.[5] The other three are guidelines for the treatment of neuropathic pain but also specifically mention PHN. These are produced by the Neuropathic Pain Special Interest Group of the International Association for the Study of Pain (NeuPSIG),[42] the Canadian Pain Society (CPS),[43] and the European Federation of Neurological Societies Task Force (EFNS).[41]

Clinical practice guidelines provide treatment options for first, second, and third line therapies. However, the selection of appropriate treatments for PHN requires the consideration of several important factors. Dworkin *et al.*[42] suggest treatment selection should include a consideration of the potential for adverse effects, treatment of comorbidities such as depression and sleep disturbance, interactions with other medications, risk of misuse and abuse, and the cost of treatment. The issue of drug interactions is particularly important as polypharmacy is common in people with PHN[7] as they take an average of five different medications.[44] Combinations of treatments may be required to adequately manage pain as 'no one medication is universally effective'.[42, p59]

Prevention

As PHN is a sequela of herpes zoster, prevention of herpes zoster in the most vulnerable patients through vaccination is the first step in reducing the incidence of PHN. Active management of herpes zoster in the acute stage may prevent PHN.[3] Initiation of antiviral therapy within 72 hours of rash onset has been suggested to reduce the likelihood of developing PHN,[5] although findings from a recent Cochrane systematic review found oral acyclovir to have no benefit in reducing the incidence of PHN.[45] Whether other antivirals are beneficial in reducing PHN remains unclear.

Further, the well-cited requirement to commence antiviral therapy within 72 hours of rash onset is an arbitrary criterion developed from/for clinical trials that may not reflect the end of viral replication.[10] Although it is unclear whether antivirals that are commenced after 72 hours are beneficial, as antivirals are generally well-tolerated, they may be worth considering.[10]

Pharmacological Management

The AAN guideline categorises treatments into four groups according to their efficacy, the strength of evidence, and the level of side effects.[5] Group 1 treatments have medium to high efficacy with good strength of evidence and little side effects. Treatments recommended in this category include tricyclic antidepressants (TCAs), gabapentin, pregabalin, lidocaine patch, and controlled release oxycodone or morphine sulphate. Group 2 medications were aspirin in cream or ointment, topical capsaicin, and intrathecal methylprednisolone. These had lower efficacy than Group 1 medications as well as limited strength of evidence or have more negative side effects.

There is agreement across guidelines that TCAs, gabapentin, and pregabalin should be considered as the first line treatment for PHN (see Table 10.1). Variation exists in relation to opioid medications and tramadol which are recommended as either first[5] or second[41–43] line therapies. Further topical capsaicin has been recommended as either second[41] or third line therapy.[42]

Table 10.1   Summary of Guideline-recommended Treatments for Post-herpetic Neuralgia

Treatment Recommendation	AAN (2004)[5]	CPS (2014)[43]	EFNS (2010)[41]	NeuPSIG (2010)[42]
First line treatments	Gabapentin* Lidocaine patch* Oxycodone or morphine sulphate* Pregabalin* TCAs*	Gabapentin* Pregabalin* TCAs* SNRIs[≠]	Gabapentin* Lidocaine patch* Pregabalin* TCAs*	Gabapentin[≠] Lidocaine patch* Pregabalin[≠] TCAs (secondary amine TCAs)[≠]
Second line treatments	—	Tramadol[≠] Opioid analgesics*	Opioid analgesics* Capsaicin*	Opioid analgesics[≠] Tramadol[≠]
Third line treatments	—	Cannabinoids[≠]	—	Certain antidepressants[≠] Certain anticonvulsants[≠] (including carbamazepine) Topical low concentration capsaicin[≠] Dextromethorphan[≠] Memantine[≠] Mexiletine[≠]
Fourth line treatments	—	Methadone[≠] SSRIs[≠] Certain anticonvulsants[≠] Topical lidocaine* Miscellaneous agents*	—	—

*Recommendation for PHN; [≠]Recommendation for neuropathic pain.
Abbreviations: AAN, American Academy of Neurology; CPS, Canadian Pain Society; EFNS, European Federation of Neurological Societies Task Force; NeuPSIG, Neuropathic Pain Special Interest Group of the International Association for the Study of Pain; SNRIs, selective noradrenaline reuptake inhibitors; SSRIs, selective serotonin reuptake inhibitors; TCAs, tricyclic antidepressants.

Categories of key medications used to treat PHN include TCAs, anticonvulsants, opioid and opioid-like medications, and topical analgesics. Tricyclic antidepressants have been used for various types of neuropathic pain, although the mechanism of action is unknown.[46] The analgesic action of TCAs is thought to be due to the inhibited reuptake of noradrenaline and serotonin.[47] Amitryptiline, nortriptyline, desipramine, and maprotiline are effective for PHN,[5] although nortriptyline and desipramine have a better safety profile.[2]

Anticonvulsants pregabalin and gabapentin are calcium channel α_2-δ ligands which bind to voltage-gated calcium channels and inhibit the release of neurotransmitters.[42] Efficacy has been demonstrated compared with placebo and nortriptyline.[2] The pharmacokinetics of gabapentin are non-linear and titration is needed to reach levels of acceptable pain relief with tolerable side effects.[42] This may be overcome by using the newly formulated gabapentin enacarbil, a gabapentin pro-drug which is effective for PHN and provides sustained drug exposure.[48]

Opioid analgesics have diverse mechanisms of action in both the PNS and CNS.[10] The risk of side effects with long-term use and concerns about opioid misuse have been noted,[10,42] and consequently opioids are recommended as a second line treatment in the NeuPSIG guideline.[42] Tramadol is a synthetic drug which displays both opioid-like properties and mimics some of the properties of TCAs.[43] It is a weak μ-receptor agonist and interrupts the reuptake of noradrenaline and serotonin.[10,46] Topical lidocaine, a sodium channel blocker, provides effective pain relief with few systemic effects.[2,43]

Dosing regimens are described by Moulin *et al.*[43] and Dworkin *et al.*[42] Many drugs require titration to reach a dose that provides effective pain relief with acceptable side effects. Further, as much of the evidence is based on short duration trials (12 weeks or less),[42,49] there is little evidence on the long-term efficacy of pain medications for PHN.

Non-pharmacological Management

The AAN guideline describes non-pharmacological treatments for PHN, for which there is limited, insufficient, or no evidence of benefit.[5] NeuPSIG recommendations for interventional management recommend against sympathetic blocks for PHN.[50] Johnson *et al.*[3] acknowledge that a multi-modal approach is required for effective management of PHN. In addition to pain medications, education, counselling, and support may be beneficial. This includes general advice about physical activity, social interaction, use of ice packs, and clothing made from natural fibres.[3]

Pain management programmes exist for people who do not achieve adequate pain control through conventional or complementary therapies.[3] Patients with refractory PHN may also benefit from psychological support.[3]

Prognosis

The incidence of pain after resolution of the herpes zoster rash reduces as time passes, so for many people pain will resolve spontaneously. Between five and 10% of people continue to experience pain after 12 months. For these individuals, the chance of spontaneous resolution is limited[3] and pain is difficult to manage.[8] Individual response to pharmacological treatments is variable and 40-50% of people with PHN do not respond to any treatment.[12]

Even when under regular medical supervision with multiple pain medications, the majority of people with PHN continue to experience pain most or all of the time.[17] Specialised pain management services may provide some benefit for people who are resistant to treatment.[51] Effective pain relief is an unmet clinical need[1] and remains a challenge for patients and clinicians.

References

1. Johnson R. Zoster-associated pain: What is known, who is at risk and how can it be managed. *Herpes*. 2007; **14**(Suppl 2):30A–4A.
2. Tontodonati M, Ursini T, Polilli E, Vadini F, Di Masi F, Volpone D, *et al.* Post-herpetic neuralgia. *Int J Gen Med*. 2012; **5**:861–71.
3. Johnson RW, Whitton TL. Management of herpes zoster (shingles) and postherpetic neuralgia. *Expert Opin Pharmacother*. 2004; **5**(3):551–9.

4. Dworkin RH, Portenoy RK. Pain and its persistence in herpes zoster. *Pain*. 1996; **67**(2–3):241–51.

5. Dubinsky RM, Kabbani H, El-Chami Z, Boutwell C, Ali H. Practice parameter: Treatment of postherpetic neuralgia: An evidence-based report of the Quality Standards Subcommittee of the American Academy of Neurology. *Neurology*. 2004; **63**(6):959–65.

6. Dworkin RH, Gnann JW, Jr., Oaklander AL, Raja SN, Schmader KE, Whitley RJ. Diagnosis and assessment of pain associated with herpes zoster and postherpetic neuralgia. *J Pain*. 2008; **9**(Suppl 1):S37–44.

7. Kaye AD, Argoff CE. Postherpetic neuralgia. In: Kaye AD, Shah RV, (eds). Case Studies in Pain Management. Cambridge: Cambridge University Press; 2015.

8. Volpi A, Gross G, Hercogova J, Johnson RW. Current management of herpes zoster: The European view. *Am J Clin Dermatol*. 2005; **6**(5):317–25.

9. Gross G, Schofer H, Wassilew S, *et al*. Herpes zoster guideline of the German Dermatology Society (DDG). *J Clin Virol*. 2003; **26**(3):277–89; discussion 91–3.

10. Dworkin RH, Johnson RW, Breuer J, *et al*. Recommendations for the management of herpes zoster. *Clin Infect Dis*. 2007; **44**(Suppl 1): S1–26.

11. Mick G, Hans G. Postherpetic neuralgia in Europe: The scale of the problem and outlook for the future. *J Clini Gerontol Geriatr*. 2013; **4**:102–8.

12. Rowbotham MC, Petersen KL. Zoster-associated pain and neural dysfunction. *Pain*. 2001; **93**(1):1–5.

13. Choo PW, Galil K, Donahue JG, Walker AM, Spiegelman D, Platt R. Risk factors for postherpetic neuralgia. *Arch Intern Med*. 1997; **157**(11):1217–24.

14. Gauthier A, Breuer J, Carrington D, Martin M, Remy V. Epidemiology and cost of herpes zoster and post-herpetic neuralgia in the United Kingdom. *Epidemiol Infect*. 2009; **137**(1):38–47.

15. Gialloreti LE, Merito M, Pezzotti P, *et al*. Epidemiology and economic burden of herpes zoster and post-herpetic neuralgia in Italy: A retrospective, population-based study. *BMC Infect Dis*. 2010; **10**:230.

16. Schmader KE. Epidemiology and impact on quality of life of postherpetic neuralgia and painful diabetic neuropathy. *Clinical J Pain*. 2002; **18**(6):350–4.

17. Serpell M, Gater A, Carroll S, Abetz-Webb L, Mannan A, Johnson R. Burden of post-herpetic neuralgia in a sample of UK residents aged 50 years or older: Findings from the Zoster Quality of Life (ZQOL) study. *Health Qual Life Outcomes*. 2014; **12**:92.

18. Gater A, Uhart M, McCool R, Preaud E. The humanistic, economic and societal burden of herpes zoster in Europe: A critical review. *BMC Public Health*. 2015; **15**:193.

19. Jeon YH. Herpes Zoster and Postherpetic Neuralgia: Practical Consideration for Prevention and Treatment. *Korean J Pain*. 2015; **28**(3):177–84.

20. Jung BF, Johnson RW, Griffin DR, Dworkin RH. Risk factors for postherpetic neuralgia in patients with herpes zoster. *Neurology*. 2004; **62**(9):1545–51.

21. Forbes HJ, Thomas SL, Smeeth L, *et al*. A systematic review and meta-analysis of risk factors for postherpetic neuralgia. *Pain*. 2015.

22. Meister W, Neiss A, Gross G, *et al*. A prognostic score for postherpetic neuralgia in ambulatory patients. *Infection*. 1998; **26**(6):359–63.

23. Schmader K, Studenski S, MacMillan J, Grufferman S, Cohen HJ. Are stressful life events risk factors for herpes zoster? *J Am Geriatr Soc*. 1990; **38**(11):1188–94.

24. Harpaz R, Leung JW, Brown CJ, Zhou FJ. Psychological stress as a trigger for herpes zoster: Might the conventional wisdom be wrong? *Clin Infect Dis*. 2015; **60**(5):781–5.

25. Kawai K, Rampakakis E, Tsai TF, *et al*. Predictors of postherpetic neuralgia in patients with herpes zoster: A pooled analysis of prospective cohort studies from North and Latin America and Asia. *Int J Infect Dis*. 2015; **34**:126–31.

26. Gilden DH, Cohrs RJ, Mahalingam R. VZV vasculopathy and postherpetic neuralgia: Progress and perspective on antiviral therapy. *Neurology*. 2005; **64**(1):21–5.

27. Pappagallo M, Oaklander AL, Quatrano-Piacentini AL, Clark MR, Raja SN. Heterogenous patterns of sensory dysfunction in postherpetic neuralgia suggest multiple pathophysiologic mechanisms. *Anesthesiology*. 2000; **92**(3):691–8.

28. Gilden DH, Cohrs RJ, Hayward AR, Wellish M, Mahalingam R. Chronic varicella-zoster virus ganglionitis — a possible cause of postherpetic neuralgia. *J Neurovirol*. 2003; **9**(3):404–7.

29. Petersen KL, Fields HL, Brennum J, Sandroni P, Rowbotham MC. Capsaicin evoked pain and allodynia in post-herpetic neuralgia. *Pain.* 2000; **88**(2):125–33.

30. Wall PD. Neuropathic pain and injured nerve: Central mechanisms. *Br Med Bull.* 1991; **47**(3):631–43.

31. Tal M, Bennett GJ. Extra-territorial pain in rats with a peripheral mononeuropathy: Mechano-hyperalgesia and mechano-allodynia in the territory of an uninjured nerve. *Pain.* 1994; **57**(3):375–82.

32. Oaklander AL. The density of remaining nerve endings in human skin with and without postherpetic neuralgia after shingles. *Pain.* 2001; **92** (1–2):139–45.

33. Rowbotham MC, Fields HL. The relationship of pain, allodynia and thermal sensation in post-herpetic neuralgia. *Brain.* 1996; **119** (Pt 2):347–54.

34. Baron R, Saguer M. Mechanical allodynia in postherpetic neuralgia: Evidence for central mechanisms depending on nociceptive C-fiber degeneration. *Neurology.* 1995; **45**(12 Suppl 8):S63–5.

35. Smith FP. Pathological studies of spinal nerve ganglia in relation to intractable intercostal pain. *Surg Neurol.* 1978; **10**(1):50–3.

36. Watson CP, Deck JH, Morshead C, Van der Kooy D, Evans RJ. Postherpetic neuralgia: Further post-mortem studies of cases with and without pain. *Pain.* 1991; **44**(2):105–17.

37. Mahalingam R, Wellish M, Brucklier J, Gilden DH. Persistence of varicella-zoster virus DNA in elderly patients with postherpetic neuralgia. *J Neurovirol.* 1995; **1**(1):130–3.

38. Coplan PM, Schmader K, Nikas A, *et al.* Development of a measure of the burden of pain due to herpes zoster and postherpetic neuralgia for prevention trials: Adaptation of the brief pain inventory. *J Pain.* 2004; **5**(6):344–56.

39. Oxman MN, Levin MJ, Johnson GR, *et al.* A vaccine to prevent herpes zoster and postherpetic neuralgia in older adults. *N Eng J Med.* 2005; **352**(22):2271–84.

40. Votrubec M, Thong I. Neuropathic pain — a management update. *Aust Fam Physician.* 2013; **42**(3):92–7.

41. Attal N, Cruccu G, Baron R, *et al.* EFNS guidelines on the pharmacological treatment of neuropathic pain: 2010 revision. *Eur J Neurol.* 2010; **17**(9):1113-e88.

42. Dworkin RH, O'Connor AB, Audette J, *et al.* Recommendations for the pharmacological management of neuropathic pain: An overview and literature update. *Mayo Clin Proc.* 2010; **85**(3 Suppl):S3–14.

43. Moulin D, Boulanger A, Clark AJ, *et al.* Pharmacological management of chronic neuropathic pain: Revised consensus statement from the Canadian Pain Society. *Pain Res Manag.* 2014; **19**(6):328–35.

44. Gater A, Abetz-Webb L, Carroll S, Mannan A, Serpell M, Johnson R. Burden of herpes zoster in the UK: Findings from the zoster quality of life (ZQOL) study. *BMC Infect Dis.* 2014; **14**:402.

45. Chen N, Li Q, Yang J, Zhou M, Zhou D, He L. Antiviral treatment for preventing postherpetic neuralgia. *Cochrane Database of Systematic Reviews.* 2014(2).

46. Moulin DE, Clark AJ, Gilron I, *et al.* Pharmacological management of chronic neuropathic pain — consensus statement and guidelines from the Canadian Pain Society. *Pain Res Manag.* 2007; **12**(1):13–21.

47. Basbaum AI, Fields HL. Endogenous pain control mechanisms: Review and hypothesis. *Ann Neurol.* 1978; **4**(5):451–62.

48. Backonja MM, Canafax DM, Cundy KC. Efficacy of gabapentin enacarbil vs placebo in patients with postherpetic neuralgia and a pharmacokinetic comparison with oral gabapentin. *Pain Med.* 2011; **12**(7):1098–108.

49. Finnerup NB, Attal N, Haroutounian S, *et al.* Pharmacotherapy for neuropathic pain in adults: A systematic review and meta-analysis. *Lancet Neurol.* 2015; **14**(2):162–73.

50. Dworkin RH, O'Connor AB, Kent J, *et al.* Interventional management of neuropathic pain: NeuPSIG recommendations. *Pain.* 2013; **154**(11): 2249–61.

51. Gilron I, Bailey JM, Tu D, Holden RR, Weaver DF, Houlden RL. Morphine, gabapentin, or their combination for neuropathic pain. *N Eng J Med.* 2005; **352**(13):1324–34.

11

Post-herpetic Neuralgia in Chinese Medicine

OVERVIEW

This chapter describes the Chinese medicine syndrome differentiation and treatments recommended in clinical textbooks and guidelines that are most likely to relate to post-herpetic neuralgia. This chapter also describes some of the limitations to conducting searches of the classical Chinese medicine literature. Treatments in contemporary literature focus on syndrome differentiation, and commonly involve syndromes such as *qi* stagnation and Blood stasis, and Liver *yin* deficiency.

Introduction

As a common sequelae of herpes zoster, post-herpetic neuralgia (PHN) is frequently described in Chinese medicine (CM) discussions alongside herpes zoster. Indeed, CM textbooks and guidelines typically describe herpes zoster and PHN as two parts of the same condition with a degree of similarity and overlap in the syndromes and treatments used. If the cause of the pain is known to be herpes zoster, then PHN is referred to as *she chuan chuang* 蛇串疮, the same term used for herpes zoster. As such, no CM clinical textbook or guideline has been identified that specifically focuses on PHN. The information presented below comes from key CM contemporary texts and clinical guidelines for the clinical management of herpes zoster.

Pain arising from herpes zoster or PHN is often referred to as zoster-associated pain in conventional medicine, which reflects the continuum of pain symptoms from the onset of the rash to beyond rash resolution. Similarly, CM syndromes may also be seen as being on a continuum with syndromes persisting or transforming over time, particularly if untreated. The key syndromes and treatments seen in herpes zoster and PHN have been described in Chapter 2.

Aetiology and Pathogenesis

PHN can occur due to a lack of resolution of syndromes in the acute herpes zoster stage (see Chapter 2 for further information on aetiology for acute herpes zoster) or may present after a pain-free period following the resolution of herpes zoster. Pain may arise from emotional disturbance or pathogenic fire obstructing *qi* flow.[1] In addition to aetiology and pathogenesis of symptoms for herpes zoster, PHN may arise due to heat or fire consuming *yin*, emotional disturbance or overwork that depletes *qi*,[1] or Liver and Kidney *yin* deficiency.[2]

Syndrome Differentiation and Treatments

According to contemporary CM literature, treatment of PHN is based on syndrome differentiation according to presenting symptoms. The syndromes and treatments of herpes zoster and PHN are detailed in Chapter 2. While none of the reviewed guidelines specifically stated the syndromes which are related to PHN, the syndromes considered most likely to be PHN are (1) *qi* stagnation and Blood stasis and (2) Liver *yin* deficiency. The treatments for these syndromes are summarised in Table 11.1. These syndromes are described in the *Guidelines for Diagnosis and Treatment of Common Diseases of Dermatology in Traditional Chinese Medicine* published by the Chinese Medical Association in 2012[2] and the clinical text *Characteristic Diagnosis and Treatment of Diseases of Dermatology in Chinese Medicine*.[3] Both resources were used as references for the following section, in addition to other key textbooks and practice guidelines. Syndrome names were referenced to the standard terminologies published by the World Health Organisation.[4]

Note that the use of some herbs may be restricted in some countries. In addition, some herbs are restricted under the provisions of CITES. Readers are advised to comply with relevant regulations.

Chinese Herbal Medicine Treatment Based on Syndrome Differentiation

Qi Stagnation and Blood Stasis

Clinical manifestations: Purple macula is left on the skin after resolution of rashes and blisters with burning and pain in the local and nearby skin area; this pain can last for several months in severe cases and usually occurs in older people. Other symptoms include dizziness, fatigue, irritability, restlessness, and constipation; dark-purple tongue with petechia or spots, white coating, and taut and unsmooth pulse.[5–7]

Treatment principle: Regulate *qi*, promote Blood circulation, and activate meridians to stop pain.[5]

Formula: Modified *Chai hu shu gan san* 柴胡疏肝散 plus *Tao hong si wu tang* 桃红四物汤 (加减);[5–7] modified *Xue fu zhu yu tang* 血府逐瘀汤 plus *Jin ling zi san* 金铃子散 (加减).[2]

Herbs: *Chai hu shu gan san* 柴胡疏肝散 plus *Tao hong si wu tang* 桃红四物汤: *chai hu* 柴胡, *chi shao* 赤芍, *chuan xiong* 川芎, *zhi ke* 枳壳, *chen pi* 陈皮, *xiang fu* 香附, *gan cao* 甘草, *tao ren* 桃仁, *hong hua* 红花, *sheng di* 生地, *dang gui* 当归, *bai shao* 白芍, etc. (for modifications).

Xue fu zhu yu tang 血府逐瘀汤 plus *Jin ling zi san* 金铃子散: *tao ren* 桃仁, *hong hua* 红花, *dang gui* 当归, *chuan xiong* 川芎, *bai shao* 白芍, *dan shen* 丹参, *yu jin* 郁金, *wang bu liu xing* 王不留行, *yan hu suo* 延胡索, *chuan lian zi* 川楝子, *xiang fu* 香附, *chai hu* 柴胡, *chen pi* 陈皮, *zhi ke* 枳壳, *gan cao* 甘草 etc. (for modifications).

Main actions of herbs: *Chai hu shu gan san* 柴胡疏肝散 plus *Tao hong si wu tang* 桃红四物汤: *chen pi* 陈皮, *xiang fu* 香附, and *zhi ke*

枳壳 regulate *qi*. *Chi shao* 赤芍, *chuan xiong* 川芎, *hong hua* 红花, and *tao ren* 桃仁 regulate Blood. *Dang gui* 当归 and *bai shao* 白芍 tonify Blood, *chai hu* 柴胡 releases the exterior, *sheng di* 生地 clears heat, and *gan cao* 甘草 harmonises each herb.

Xue fu zhu yu tang 血府逐瘀汤 plus *Jin ling zi san* 金铃子散: *chen pi* 陈皮, *chuan lian zi* 川楝子, *xiang fu* 香附 and *zhi ke* 枳壳 regulate *qi*. *Chuan xiong* 川芎, *dan shen* 丹参, *hong hua* 红花, *tao ren* 桃仁, *wang bu liu xing* 王不留行, *yan hu suo* 延胡索, and *yu jin* 郁金 regulate Blood. *Dang gui* 当归 and *bai shao* 白芍 tonify Blood, *chai hu* 柴胡 releases the exterior, and *gan cao* 甘草 harmonises each herb.

Manufactured medicines: *Xin huang pian* 新癀片, *Xue fu zhu yu pian* 血府逐瘀片, *Da huang zhe chong wan* 大黄蛰虫丸, *Yuan hu zhi tong jiao nang* 元胡止痛胶囊.[2,8]

Liver Yin Deficiency

Clinical manifestations: Dull or stabbing pain in the chest after resolution of the rash, dry mouth and throat, dark/black tongue with grey or thin tongue coat, and thin/string pulse.[3]

Treatment principle: Nourish *yin* and soothe the Liver.[3]

Formula: *Yi guan jian* 一贯煎.[3]

Herbs: *Sheng di huang* 生地黄, *sha shen* 沙参, *mai dong* 麦冬, *gou qi zi* 枸杞子, *dang gui* 当归, *chuan lian zi* 川楝子.

Main actions of herbs: *Sheng di huang* 生地黄, *sha shen* 沙参, and *mai dong* 麦冬 nourish *yin*, *gou qi zi* 枸杞子 tonifies Kidney *yin* and nourishes Liver Blood, *dang gui* 当归 tonifies Blood, and *chuan lian zi* 川楝子 regulates *qi*.

Manufactured medicines: None identified.

For treatment principles and formula prescriptions for stagnated heat in the Liver meridian, dampness and heat in the Liver and Gallbladder, and Spleen deficiency syndrome with damp retention, see Chapter 2.

Table 11.1 Summary of Chinese Herbal Medicine Formulas for Post-herpetic Neuralgia

Syndrome Differentiation	Treatment Principle	Formula
Qi stagnation and Blood stasis 气滞血瘀	Regulate *qi* and promote Blood circulation, activate meridians to stop pain 理气活血, 通络止痛	Chai hu shu gan san 柴胡疏肝散 plus Tao hong si wu tang 桃红四物汤; Xue fu zhu yu tang 血府逐瘀汤 plus Jin ling zi san
Liver *yin* deficiency 肝阴亏虚	Nourish *yin*, soothe the Liver, activate meridians to stop pain 滋阴疏肝, 通络止痛	Yi guan jian 一贯煎

Acupuncture Therapies and Other Chinese Medicine Therapies

As many of the contemporary texts and guidelines describe herpes zoster and PHN as two parts of one disease, there is no identified guideline which specifically describes the management of PHN with acupuncture and other CM therapies. A review of the therapies recommended in selected clinical textbooks and guidelines for herpes zoster (see Chapter 2) found that all therapies were potentially relevant to PHN as well. The following sections describe the treatments recommended in clinical practice guidelines and textbooks for herpes zoster and PHN. Clinicians should exercise their judgment to determine the appropriateness of each intervention for patients with PHN.

Acupuncture therapies that can be used to treat PHN include acupuncture (body, ear, and scalp), moxibustion, and magnetic therapy. Point selection may be based on either specific functional points or *ashi* points 阿是穴 local to the pain site, or a combination of both approaches. The function of acupuncture points recommended in two or more clinical textbooks and guidelines are described below. Many other CM therapies have also been recommended for herpes zoster and may also be considered for PHN (see Chapter 2).

Analysis of acupuncture points:[9]

- LI11 *Quchi* 曲池 — Clears heat, resolves dampness, cools Blood, regulates nutritive *qi* and Blood, and expels exterior wind.
- PC6 *Neiguan* 内关 — Opens the chest, regulates and clears the Triple Energiser, calms the mind, and harmonises the Stomach.
- SP6 *Sanyinjiao* 三阴交 — Resolves damp, nourishes Blood and *yin*, cools Blood, stops pain, and strengthens the Spleen.
- ST36 *Zusanli* 足三里 — Tonifies *qi* and Blood, benefits the Stomach and Spleen, expels wind and damp, regulates nutritive and defensive *qi*, and dispels cold.

Other Management Strategies

Patients can be encouraged to participate in their own recovery. Lifestyle advice, dietary advice, and dietary therapy can be given to patients between clinic visits. Patients should be encouraged to focus on recuperating well from herpes zoster, dress appropriately for the weather, and pay attention to changes in the weather to prevent catching the common cold.[10] Maintaining a regular daily routine with adequate sleep is important to avoid fatigue.[10] Patients should avoid overwork and excessive mental stimulation, focus on mindfulness, and strive to maintain good health and a healthy immune system.

Patients should avoid excessive consumption of fatty, oily, or sweet foods, and seafood should also be avoided.[5] Diet should thus be light with plenty of fruits and vegetables.[5] Dietary therapy according to CM principles is another self-management strategy that patients can use. A broth can be prepared using 60g of *xi qian gen* 豨莶根 (the root of *xi qian cao* 豨莶草) stewed with a pig's hoof 猪蹄 and adding 100ml of rice wine 黄酒.[10] Although this broth can be used for all syndromes of herpes zoster and PHN, it is especially helpful for cases with severe pain and should be consumed twice daily. A liquid preparation can be made with 15g of *san qi* 三七 (also known as *tian qi* 田七) and 35g of *mu gua* 木瓜 soaked in wine in a sealed bottle for 15 days. A small amount can be drank daily to treat PHN, especially when severe pain is experienced.[10]

Post-herpetic Neuralgia in Classical Chinese Medicine Literature

Clinical management of herpes zoster and PHN has been discussed in CM contemporary literature. Searches of the classical CM literature were not practical to conduct as pain-related search terms would likely engender too many citations of pain causes unrelated to herpes zoster and PHN, and it is unlikely that pain following herpes zoster can be clearly distinguished from pain due to other causes. An alternative approach was taken to search within the herpes zoster citations identified in the classical literature (see Chapter 3 of *Herpes Zoster*) for passages that may be describing PHN. A review of citations related to herpes zoster found many that described pain as a symptom. However, all citations described pain in the acute stage of herpes zoster. No citation described pain persisting after resolution of the rash. As such, we were unable to identify citations describing CM treatments for PHN.

References

1. Shen DH, Wu XF, Wang N. Manual of Dermatology in Chinese Medicine. Seattle: Eastland Press Inc; 1995.
2. 中华中医药学会. 中医皮肤科常见病诊疗指南. 中国中医药出版社; 2012.
3. 黄尧洲. 皮肤病中医特色诊疗[M]. 人民军医出版社; 2008.
4. World Health Organization. Regional Office for the Western Pacific 2007, WHO International Standard Terminologies on Traditional Medicine in the Western Pacific Region. World Health Organization, Western Pacific Region, Geneva.
5. 李曰庆, 何清湖. 中医外科学[M]. 北京: 中国中医药出版社; 2012.
6. 陈德宇. 中西医结合皮肤性病学[M]. 北京: 中国中医药出版社; 2012.
7. 杨志波, 范瑞强, 邓丙戌. 中医皮肤性病学[M]. 北京: 中国中医药出版社; 2010.
8. 刘巧. 中医皮肤病诊疗学[M]. 北京: 人民卫生出版社; 2014.
9. Maciocia G. *The Foundations of Chinese Medicine*. Edinburgh, UK: Churchill Livingstone; 1989.
10. 陈达灿, 范瑞强. 皮肤性病科专病中医临床诊治[M]. 北京: 人民卫生出版社; 2013.

12

Methods for Evaluating Clinical Evidence — Post-herpetic Neuralgia

OVERVIEW

Post-herpetic neuralgia has been evaluated in many clinical studies. This chapter describes the methods used to identify and evaluate Chinese medicine therapies for treating post-herpetic neuralgia in clinical studies. Extensive searches of electronic databases were conducted, with results screened against rigorous inclusion criteria. An assessment of the methodological quality of the studies was made using standardised methods. Results from included studies were evaluated to provide an estimate of treatment effects as well as the safety of various Chinese medicine therapies for post-herpetic neuralgia.

Introduction

Clinical studies were reviewed following the methods outlined in Chapter 4 of *Herpes Zoster*. The search for herpes zoster and post-herpetic neuralgia (PHN) was conducted concurrently, with databases searched from their inception to February 2015. Citations of PHN were identified from these searches and eligibility was assessed according to the criteria below.

Inclusion Criteria

- Participants: adults (aged ≥ 18 years) with a diagnosis of PHN meeting one of the following criteria:

  - Pain persisting for one month/30 days after resolution of the rash;
  - Pain persisting for three months/90 days after resolution of the rash;
  - Pain persisting for two months/60 days from rash onset;
  - Pain persisting for four months/120 days from rash onset;
  - Other (see below).

- Interventions: Chinese herbal medicine (CHM), acupuncture and related therapies, or other Chinese medicine (CM) therapies used either alone or in combination with other CM therapies or pharmacotherapies (see Table 12.1). Studies combining CM therapies with pharmacotherapy were required to use the same pharmacotherapy in both the intervention and comparator groups.
- Comparators: no treatment, placebos, or pharmacotherapies that are recommended in international clinical practice guidelines for PHN[1] or for neuropathic pain.[2-4]
- Outcomes: studies reported at least one of the pre-specified outcome measures (see below and Table 12.2).

Studies using a definition of PHN other than those outlined above were reviewed to determine likelihood of PHN. Typical cases of herpes zoster are usually confined to one month from onset to resolution of rash. As such, we considered that studies of PHN defined as 'after rash resolution' where the reported duration of PHN was not less than one month were likely to meet one of the above criteria. Studies

Table 12.1 Chinese Medicine Interventions Included in Clinical Evidence Evaluation

Chinese herbal medicines (CHMs)	Oral or topical CHM
Acupuncture and related therapies	Acupuncture (including surrounding acupuncture and electro-acupuncture), moxibustion, and plum-blossom needle acupuncture

Table 12.2   Pre-specified Outcomes

Outcome Category	Outcome Measures	Scoring
Pain	1. Pain Visual Analogue Scale	1. 0–10 cm or 0–100 mm, lower is better
	2. McGill Pain Questionnaire[7]	2. 0–78 points, lower is better
	3. Other (e.g., verbal rating scale)	3. Various
Health-related Quality of Life	1. Zoster Brief Pain Inventory[8]	1. See Part 1, Chapter 4
	2. Zoster Impact Questionnaire[8]	2. See Part 1, Chapter 4
	3. SF-36[9]	3. 0–100 points per domain, higher is better
	4. EQ-5D[10]	4. See note
Symptom Assessment	1. Hamilton Rating Scale for Depression[11]	1. 0–50 points, lower is better
	2. Pittsburgh Sleep Quality Index[12]	2. 0–21 points, lower is better
	3. Other symptom assessment (with specified criteria)	3. As specified by study author
Adverse events	Adverse events reported by included studies	

Note: For description of scoring for EuroQoL 5 Dimensions questionnaire, see Chapter 4.

Abbreviations: EQ-5D, EuroQoL 5 Dimensions quality of life questionnaire; SF-36, Medical Outcome Study 36 item Short Form.

that described PHN as 'after rash resolution' but did not report the duration of PHN were excluded.

Pharmacotherapies recommended in clinical practice guidelines[1–4] include:

- Tricyclic antidepressants (TCAs), e.g., nortriptyline, amitriptyline, desipramine, maprotiline;
- Anticonvulsants, e.g., pregabalin, gabapentin, carbamazepine;
- Opioid medications, e.g., oxycodone, morphine;
- Tramadol;
- Topical lidocaine;
- Topical capsaicin;
- Intrathecal methylprednisolone.

Studies where guideline-recommended treatments were combined with other treatments were also included. Vitamins B1 and B12 are often used in China to aid nerve repair, although their efficacy in treating PHN is unknown.

Exclusion Criteria

- Studies of participants with herpes zoster or herpes zoster complications such as ophthalmic zoster, herpes zoster oticus (Ramsay Hunt syndrome), zoster encephalitis, zoster sine herpete, visceral herpes zoster, or disseminated herpes zoster;
- Studies of immunocompromised individuals such as human immunodeficiency virus (HIV) patients, cancer patients, patients with diabetes, or pregnant or breastfeeding women;
- Studies involving children (<18 years) or studies that included both adults and children where results were presented in aggregate;
- Studies using pain medications other than those recommended in international guidelines, herpes zoster vaccine, or CM as comparators.

Outcomes

The primary outcome was pain severity measured on the visual analogue scale or other scales such as verbal rating scales or the McGill Pain Questionnaire[7] (see Table 12.2). The visual analogue scale is frequently used to measure pain in PHN and is calculated either in millimetres or centimetres.

Secondary outcomes included health-related quality of life and adverse events. Outcome measures for health-related quality of life include the Zoster Brief Pain Inventory[8] and the Zoster Impact Questionnaire,[8] as well as general quality of life measures such as the Medical Outcome Study 36-item Short Form Health Survey[9] and EuroQoL 5 Dimensions questionnaire.[10] For more details on these health-related quality of life measures, see Chapter 4.

Other symptom-specific questionnaires include the Hamilton Rating Scale for Depression[11] and Pittsburgh Sleep Quality Index.[12] The Hamilton Rating Scale for Depression is a 17-item questionnaire which assesses symptoms of depression in the previous week.[11] Scores range from 0–50 with high scores indicating worse symptoms. Scores of between zero and seven are considered to be normal. The Pittsburgh Sleep Quality Index is a 24-item questionnaire which assesses sleep patterns and quality.[12] Scores are calculated for seven components: subjective sleep quality, sleep latency, sleep duration, habitual sleep efficiency, sleep disturbance, use of sleeping medication, and daytime dysfunction. Scores for each component are combined to give an overall score from zero to 21, with scores of five or greater indicating sleep disturbance.

Risk of Bias Assessment

The methodological quality of randomised controlled trials was assessed using the risk of bias tool of the Cochrane Collaboration.[5] For full details of the risk of bias domains and the judgment process, see Chapter 4.

Statistical Analyses

Frequency of CM syndromes, CHM formulas, herbs, and acupuncture points reported in included studies are presented using descriptive statistics. CM syndromes reported in two or more studies were presented. Where possible or available, the 20 most frequently reported CHM formulas and herbs and the top 10 acupuncture points that were used in at least two studies are presented, although for CHM formulas this was not always possible. Where data was limited, reports of single CM syndromes or acupuncture points were provided as a guide for the reader.

Definitions of statistical tests and results are provided in the glossary at the end of this monograph. For full details of statistical analyses, see Chapter 4. Subgroup analyses were planned where possible and appropriate and these included the duration of treatment, CM syndromes, CHM formula, and comparator type. Available case analysis with a random effects model was used in all analyses.

Assessment Using Grading of Recommendations Assessment, Development and Evaluation

The Grading of Recommendations Assessment, Development, and Evaluation approach was used to provide a summary of the results and quality of evidence for each of the important PHN outcomes.[6] The approach that was used for herpes zoster was also used for PHN. For full details of the process for assessing the quality of evidence, see Chapter 4.

References

1. Dubinsky RM, Kabbani H, El-Chami Z, Boutwell C, Ali H. Practice parameter: Treatment of postherpetic neuralgia: An evidence-based report of the Quality Standards Subcommittee of the American Academy of Neurology. *Neurology.* 2004; **63**(6):959–65.
2. Attal N, Cruccu G, Baron R, *et al.* EFNS guidelines on the pharmacological treatment of neuropathic pain: 2010 revision. *Eur J Neurol.* 2010; **17**(9):1113–e88.
3. Dworkin RH, O'Connor AB, Audette J, *et al.* Recommendations for the pharmacological management of neuropathic pain: An overview and literature update. *Mayo Clin Proc.* 2010; **85**(3 Suppl):S3–14.
4. Moulin D, Boulanger A, Clark AJ, *et al.* Pharmacological management of chronic neuropathic pain: Revised consensus statement from the Canadian Pain Society. *Pain Res Manag.* 2014; **19**(6):328–35.
5. Higgins JPT, Green S, (eds). Cochrane Handbook for Systematic Reviews of Interventions Version 5.1.0 [updated March 2011]. The Cochrane Collaboration, 2011. Available from www.cochrane-handbook.org. 2011.
6. Schunemann H, Brozek J, Guyatt G, Oxman A, editors. GRADE handbook for grading quality of evidence and strength of recommendations.

Group TGW, (eds). The GRADE Working Group: Available from www. guidelinedevelopment.org/handbook; 2013.

7. Melzack R. The McGill Pain Questionnaire: Major properties and scoring methods. *Pain.* 1975; **1**(3):277–99.

8. Coplan PM, Schmader K, Nikas A, *et al.* Development of a measure of the burden of pain due to herpes zoster and postherpetic neuralgia for prevention trials: Adaptation of the brief pain inventory. *J Pain.* 2004; **5**(6):344–56.

9. Ware JE, Jr., Sherbourne CD. The MOS 36-item short-form health survey (SF-36). I. Conceptual framework and item selection. *Med Care.* 1992; **30**(6):473–83.

10. Rabin R, de Charro F. EQ-5D: A measure of health status from the EuroQol Group. *Ann Med.* 2001; **33**(5):337–43.

11. Hamilton M. A rating scale for depression. *J Neurol Neurosurg Psychiatry.* 1960; **23**:56–62.

12. Buysse DJ, Reynolds CF, 3rd, Monk TH, Berman SR, Kupfer DJ. The Pittsburgh Sleep Quality Index: A new instrument for psychiatric practice and research. *Psychiatry Res.* 1989; **28**(2):193–213.

13

Clinical Evidence for Chinese Herbal Medicine — Post-herpetic Neuralgia

OVERVIEW

This chapter describes the evaluation of post-herpetic neuralgia clinical studies using scientific methods. More than 36,600 citations were identified, of which 20 studies were evaluated. Chinese herbal medicine may provide additional pain relief when used as an adjunct to guideline-recommended treatments and may additionally improve depressive symptoms.

Previous Systematic Reviews

No systematic reviews of Chinese herbal medicine (CHM) for post-herpetic neuralgia (PHN) could be identified in English language databases. Similarly in the Chinese literature, no systematic reviews were found that presented clinically meaningful comparisons.

Characteristics of Chinese Herbal Medicine Clinical Studies

A comprehensive search of nine English and Chinese language databases resulted in the identification of 36,621 potentially relevant citations. Full-text retrieval to assess eligibility was required for 5,639 citations and 20 clinical studies evaluating CHM for PHN met the inclusion criteria for review (see Figure 13.1). Eleven were

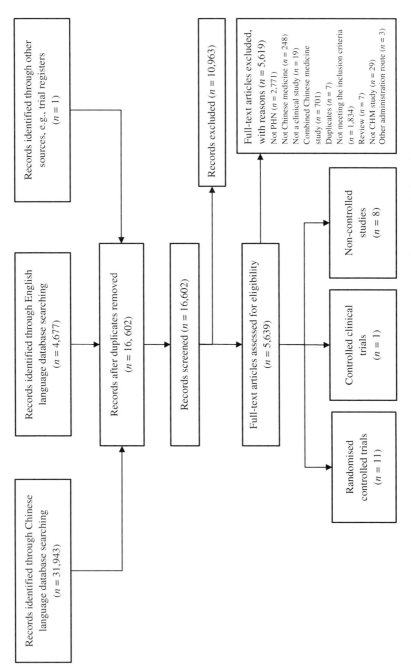

Figure 13.1 Flow chart of the study selection process: Chinese herbal medicine.

Table 13.1 Summary of Formulas in all Clinical Studies

Most Common Formulas	No. of Studies	Ingredients
Shen tong zhu yu tang 身痛逐瘀汤	2	Qin jiao 秦艽, chuan xiong 川芎, tao ren 桃仁, hong hua 红花, gan cao 甘草, qiang huo 羌活, mo yao 没药, dang gui 当归, ling zhi 灵脂, xiang fu 香附, niu xi 牛膝, di long 地龙

Note: Ingredients are referenced to the *Zhong Yi Fang Ji Da Ci Dian* 中医方剂大辞典 where available, or to the included study if not available.

randomised controlled trials (RCTs) (S230–S240), one was a controlled clinical trial (CCT) (S241), and eight were non-controlled studies (S242–S249). Controlled studies were evaluated to assess the efficacy and safety of CHM for PHN while details relating to the intervention and safety profile of non-controlled studies were described.

A total of 1,116 participants were included in the 20 studies. One study was conducted in Japan (S249) and the remaining studies were conducted in China. CHM was administered for between 10 (S238) and 30 days (S237). Few studies used Chinese medicine (CM) syndromes to select participants or to guide treatment. In studies that did report CM syndromes, these included the pattern/syndrome of *qi* stagnation and Blood stasis (S232, S243, S244) and *qi* deficiency and Blood stasis (S246).

Several studies described two or more formulas in the intervention group (S237, S240, S241, S244). Oral administration of CHM was most common and was used in all 20 studies (S230–S247, S249). Two studies also used topical administration of CHM (S244, S248). Two studies used *Shen tong zhu yu tang* 身痛逐瘀汤 (S235, S243); this aside, there was no overlap in formulas evaluated in clinical studies (see Table 13.1). A total of 76 different herbs were used and the most commonly used herbs in all clinical studies included *dang gui* 当归, *yan hu suo* 延胡索, and *hong hua* 红花 (see Table 13.2).

Table 13.2   Frequently Reported Herbs in all Clinical Studies

Most Common Herbs	Scientific Name	Frequency of Use
Dang gui 当归	*Angelica sinensis* (Oliv.) Diels	11
Yan hu suo 延胡索	*Corydalis yanhusuo* W.T. Wang	9
Hong hua 红花	*Carthamus tinctorius* L.	8
Chai hu 柴胡	*Bupleurum* spp	7
Chuan xiong 川芎	*Ligusticum chuangxiong* Hort.	7
Gan cao 甘草	*Glycyrrhiza* spp	7
Tao ren 桃仁	*Prunus* spp	7
Bai shao 白芍	*Paeonia lactiflora* Pall.	6
Chi shao 赤芍	*Paeonia* spp	6
Huang qi 黄芪	*Astragalus membranaceus* spp	6
Yu jin 郁金	*Curcuma* spp	6
Dan shen 丹参	*Salvia miltiorrhiza* Bge.	5
Di long 地龙	*Pheretima* spp	4
Quan xie 全蝎	*Buthus martensii* Karsch	4
Ru xiang 乳香	*Boswellia* spp	4
Shu di huang 熟地黄	*Rehmannia glutinosa* Libosch.	4
Xiang fu 香附	*Cyperus rotundus* L.	4

Randomised Controlled Trials of Chinese Herbal Medicine

After examining the full-text articles identified from the search, 11 RCTs met the eligibility criteria for this review (S230–S240). One three-arm study included two CHM treatment arms (S233), while another four-arm study included two CHM arms and one arm which combined CHM with acupuncture (S234). The results for the arm that combined CHM with acupuncture are presented in Chapter 16.

Two studies defined PHN as pain persisting for three months or more after resolution of the rash (S233, S240), eight studies defined PHN as pain persisting for one month or more after resolution of the rash (S230–S232, S234–S236, S238), and two studies defined PHN as pain persisting after rash resolution without reference to a time-point

(S237, S239). As both studies reported the duration of PHN to be at least one month, both studies were included in this review.

All studies were conducted in China and included a total of 799 participants. The majority of studies were conducted in outpatient departments (9 studies) (S230–S232, S234–S238, S240). Participant age ranged from 33 (S236) to 85 years (S230, S238), and the median of the age means was 59.8 years in studies that reported the mean age. There was a similar number of males and females in the studies (390 males and 379 females). PHN duration ranged from one month (S231, S232, S235, S236, S238, S239) to two years (S236). Treatment with CHM was provided for between 10 (S237, S238) and 30 days (S237). Follow-up assessments were made at four weeks (S232) and three months (S231).

CM syndrome differentiation was used as an inclusion criterion and to guide treatment in one study (S232), which described the pattern/syndrome of *qi* stagnation and Blood stasis. All studies provided CHM for oral use, with eight studies using oral CHM as integrative medicine (IM) (S231, S233–S238, S240). Both multiple arm studies had one treatment arm as oral CHM alone and the other as oral CHM as IM, and results for these were analysed separately. Comparators included opioid medications alone (S236), tricyclic anti depressants (TCAs) alone (S232, S235) or with other treatments (S230, S231, S237, S239), TCAs with opioid medications (S238), and anticonvulsants alone (S233, S240) or with other treatments (S234). Other treatments typically included vitamins B1 or B12 (or derivatives).

Many formulas were investigator-developed and as such there was no overlap in formulas used across studies. Fifty-seven different herbs were used in the 11 studies. The most common herbs were *dang gui* 当归 (9 studies), *yan hu suo* 延胡索 (7 studies), *chai hu* 柴胡, *gan cao* 甘草, and *hong hua* 红花 (6 studies) (see Table 13.3).

Risk of Bias

The methodological quality of included studies was assessed by identifying potential sources of bias. The overall quality of evidence derived from the included studies was low to moderate (see Table 13.4). All studies were described as randomised, but only one

Table 13.3   Frequently Reported Herbs in Randomised Controlled Trials

Most Common Herbs	Scientific Name	Frequency of Use
Dang gui 当归	*Angelica sinensis* (Oliv.) Diels	9
Yan hu suo 延胡索	*Corydalis yanhusuo* W.T. Wang	7
Chai hu 柴胡	*Bupleurum* spp	6
Gan cao 甘草	*Glycyrrhiza* spp	6
Hong hua 红花	*Carthamus tinctorius* L.	6
Chuan xiong 川芎	*Ligusticum chuangxiong* Hort.	5
Tao ren 桃仁	*Prunus* spp	5
Bai shao 白芍	*Paeonia lactiflora* Pall.	5
Huang qi 黄芪	*Astragalus membranaceus* spp	5
Dan shen 丹参	*Salvia miltiorrhiza* Bge.	4
Chi shao 赤芍	*Paeonia* spp	4
Yu jin 郁金	*Curcuma* spp	4
Ru xiang 乳香	*Boswellia* spp	3
Di long 地龙	*Pheretima* spp	3
Xiang fu 香附	*Cyperus rotundus* L.	3

Note: The use of some herbs may be restricted in some countries. Readers are advised to comply with relevant regulations.

Table 13.4   Risk of Bias of Randomised Controlled Trials: Chinese Herbal Medicine

Risk of Bias Domain	Low Risk n (%)	Unclear Risk n (%)	High Risk n (%)
Sequence generation	1 (9.1)	10 (90.9)	0 (0)
Allocation concealment	0 (0)	11 (100)	0 (0)
Blinding of participants	0 (0)	0 (0)	11 (100)
Blinding of personnel	0 (0)	0 (0)	11 (100)
Blinding of outcome assessor	0 (0)	11 (100)	0 (0)
Incomplete outcome data	11 (100)	0 (0)	0 (0)
Selective outcome reporting	0 (0)	11 (100)	0 (0)

study (8.3%) described using a random number table to allocate participants (S238) and was assessed as having low risk of bias. None of the studies described details of allocation concealment and all were judged as having unclear risk of bias. None of the studies stated that participants or personnel were blind to group allocation and all were judged as having high bias risk for these domains. No details were provided for whether outcome assessors were blind to group allocation and all studies were thus assessed as having unclear bias risk for this domain. There was no missing data due to participant attrition and all studies were considered to pose low risk of bias in terms of incomplete outcome assessment. Finally, as none of the studies published trial protocols or registered trial details with trial registries, all were assessed as having unclear bias risk for selective outcome reporting.

Oral Chinese Herbal Medicine

Eleven studies evaluated oral CHM for PHN. Five treatment arms evaluated oral CHM alone (S230, S232–S234, S239) and eight treatment arms used oral CHM as IM (S231, S233–S238, S240). Most studies reported the pain score on the visual analogue scale (VAS) and meta-analyses for this outcome were possible.

Pain Score

Oral Chinese Herbal Medicine Alone

Two studies reported the VAS pain score (S232, S234). Oral CHM alone did not produce a statistically different reduction in pain scores at the end of treatment compared with pharmacotherapy (2 studies, 117 participants; MD –0.30 cm [–1.12, 0.52], $I^2 = 0\%$).

Oral Chinese Herbal Medicine as Integrative Medicine

Five studies using oral CHM as IM evaluated pain score on the VAS (S231, S234–S236, S240). Pain score on the VAS at the end of treatment

Table 13.5 Oral Chinese Herbal Medicine as Integrative Medicine *vs.* Pharmacotherapy: Pain Score (Visual Analogue Score)

Outcome	No. of Studies (Participants)	Effect Size MD [95% CI] I²	Included Studies
Pain score (cm)	5 (318)	−1.88 [−3.34, −0.42]* 98%	S231, S234–S236, S240
Subgroup: treatment duration 4 weeks	3 (188)	−1.09 [−1.37, −0.81]* 0%	S231, S234, S236
Subgroup: treatment duration < 4 weeks	2 (130)	−2.85 [−6.65, 0.96] 99%	S235, S240
Subgroup: PHN ≥ 1 month after rash resolution	4 (350)	−1.01 [−1.22, −0.80]* 0%	S231, S234–S236

*Statistically significant.
CI: Confidence interval; MD, mean difference; PHN, post-herpetic neuralgia.

was 1.88 cm less in those who received oral CHM as IM compared with pharmacotherapy ([−3.34, −0.42], I² = 98%) (see Table 13.5). Statistical heterogeneity was explored through subgroup analyses. As all studies used different comparators, subgroup analysis according to comparator type was not possible. When treatment effect according to the duration of treatment was explored, studies which used oral CHM as IM for four weeks resulted in a VAS pain score that was 1.09 cm lower than pharmacotherapy ([−1.37, −0.81]) with no statistical heterogeneity (I² = 0%). In studies which used oral CHM as IM for less than four weeks, no treatment effect was observed and there was high statistical heterogeneity. Finally, studies using the same definition of PHN (one month or more after resolution of the rash) favoured CHM as IM with no statistical heterogeneity (MD −1.01 cm [−1.22, −0.80], I² = 0%).

Hamilton Rating Scale for Depression

Oral Chinese Herbal Medicine Alone

One study reported outcomes according to the Hamilton Rating Scale for Depression (HAM-D) (S232). No difference was observed between those who received oral CHM and those who received amitriptyline in HAM-D scores at the end of treatment (MD −1.49 points [−3.23, 0.25]).

Oral Chinese Herbal Medicine as Integrative Medicine

Two studies reported outcomes in terms of emotional wellbeing from the HAM-D (S231, S235). Oral CHM as IM reduced depression scores by 2.45 points compared with pharmacotherapy (2 studies, 128 participants; [−3.70, −1.20], I^2 = 13%).

Frequently Reported Orally Administered Herbs in Meta-analyses Showing Favourable Effects

Studies that were included in meta-analyses were examined to identify herbs which may have contributed to the favourable effects observed. Subgroup analyses were not included in calculations. Outcomes were grouped according to three categories:

(1) Pain outcomes: VAS pain score, verbal rating scale;
(2) Health-related quality of life: Medical Outcome Study 36-item Short Form Health Survey, EuroQoL 5 Dimensions, Zoster Brief Pain Inventory (ZBPI), Zoster Impact Questionnaire;
(3) Symptom severity: HAM-D, Pittsburgh Sleep Quality Index.

Studies which reported two or more outcomes in the same category were counted only once in the analysis. If no meta-analysis was able to be conducted or if there was no overlap in herbs across studies (i.e., each herb in included studies has a frequency of one), the results are not presented. The highest frequency herbs that are reported in at least two studies were selected to be presented. Related meta-analyses are noted in the table.

Three herbs, *dang gui* 当归, *gan cao* 甘草, and *hong hua* 红花, were seen in meta-analyses which showed favourable outcomes with oral CHM for both pain outcomes and symptom severity (see Table 13.6). These herbs may have contributed to the positive results

Table 13.6 Frequently Reported Herbs in Meta-analyses Showing Favourable Effects: Oral Chinese Herbal Medicine *vs.* Pharmacotherapy

Herbs	Scientific Name	Frequency of Use
Pain outcomes: 1 meta-analysis, 5 RCTs (Table 13.5)		
Dang gui 当归	*Angelica sinensis* (Oliv.) Diels	5
Gan cao 甘草	*Glycyrrhiza* spp	5
Hong hua 红花	*Carthamus tinctorius* L.	4
Chai hu 柴胡	*Bupleurum* spp	3
Bai shao 白芍	*Paeonia lactiflora* Pall.	3
Chuan xiong 川芎	*Ligusticum chuangxiong* Hort.	3
Tao ren 桃仁	*Prunus* spp	3
Symptom severity: 1 meta-analysis, 2 RCTs (see HAM-D)		
Dang gui 当归	*Angelica sinensis* (Oliv.) Diels	2
Hong hua 红花	*Carthamus tinctorius* L.	2
Gan cao 甘草	*Glycyrrhiza* spp	2

Note: The use of some herbs may be restricted in some countries. Readers are advised to comply with relevant regulations.

Abbreviations. HAM-D: Hamilton Rating Scale for Depression.

shown and thus should be considered when formulating a CHM prescription.

Safety of Oral Chinese Herbal Medicine for Post-herpetic Zoster

Oral Chinese Herbal Medicine Alone

All five studies (143 participants in the intervention group and 139 in the comparator group) which evaluated oral CHM reported information on adverse events (S230, S232–S234, S239). One study reported that no adverse events occurred while the trial was conducted (S233). Twelve cases of adverse events were reported in the intervention groups and these included five cases of diarrhoea, three cases of discomfort associated with the taste of the CHM, two cases of upper abdominal discomfort, and one case each of nausea and vomiting. Sixty-eight adverse events were reported in the comparator groups and these included drowsiness (16 cases), dry mouth (15 cases), constipation (9 cases), blurred vision with drowsiness and sweating (9 cases), poor appetite plus dizziness (9 cases), nausea plus acid reflux (3 cases), difficulty in urination (3 cases), dizziness (2 cases), sweating (1 case), and orthostatic hypotension (1 case).

Oral Chinese Herbal Medicine as Integrative Medicine

Seven studies (275 participants in the intervention group and 261 in the comparator group) reported information on adverse events (S231, S233–S235, S237, S238, S240). Three studies reported that no adverse events occurred during the trial (S233, S237, S240). There were slightly more adverse events with oral CHM as IM compared with pharmacotherapy (18 vs. 16). Adverse events in the intervention group included eight cases of poor appetite and dizziness, three cases of nausea and acid reflux, two cases of gastrointestinal reactions, two cases of mild nausea, and one case each of nausea plus vomiting, mild diarrhoea, and mild dizziness. Adverse events in the pharmacotherapy groups included nine cases of poor appetite and dizziness, three cases of mild dizziness, three cases of nausea and acid reflux, and one case of mild nausea.

Assessment Using Grading of Recommendations Assessment, Development and Evaluation

The interventions considered to be important to clinical practice were selected based on panel consensus and assessed using the Grading of Recommendations Assessment, Development, and Evaluation (GRADE; see Chapter 4) approach. The panel nominated three comparisons — oral CHM as IM with gabapentin, oral CHM as IM with pregabalin, and oral CHM as IM with TCAs. None of the included studies compared oral CHM as IM with pregabalin and the quality of the evidence for this comparison remains unclear.

Oral Chinese Herbal Medicine plus Gabapentin vs. Gabapentin

- The quality of the evidence for oral CHM plus gabapentin vs. gabapentin was low (see Table 13.7). Oral CHM plus gabapentin was found to produce greater reductions in pain severity than gabapentin alone. No study reported on outcomes from the ZBPI.

Oral Chinese Herbal Medicine plus Tricyclic Anti depressants vs. Tricyclic Anti depressants

- Evidence for oral CHM plus TCAs vs. TCAs was also of low quality (see Table 13.8). Oral CHM combined with TCAs also reduced pain severity at the end of treatment. No studies reported outcomes in terms of the ZBPI.

Randomised Controlled Trial Evidence for Formulas Commonly Used in Clinical Practice

Two studies used formulas that are recommended in clinical textbooks and guidelines (see Chapter 12). One study used *Xue fu zhu yu tang* 血府逐瘀汤 alone (S240) which differs from the guideline recommendation to use the formula in combination with *Jin ling zi san* 金铃子散加减. As such, the results are not presented. One three-arm study compared *Liu shen wan* 六神丸 alone and as IM with carbamazepine (S233). The study did not report on pain outcomes and safety was the sole outcome relevant to this review. The study reported that no adverse events occurred during the trial.

Controlled Clinical Trials of Chinese Herbal Medicine

One CCT was identified which met the inclusion criteria (S241). The study was conducted in an outpatient department in China and included 90 participants who had PHN (defined as after rash resolution) for between two and six months (mean 3.4 months). The mean

Table 13.7 GRADE: Oral Chinese Herbal Medicine plus Gabapentin *vs.* Gabapentin

Outcomes (Treatment duration)	No of Participants (Studies)	Quality of the Evidence (GRADE)	Relative Effect (95% CI)	Anticipated Absolute Effects	
				Risk with Gabapentin	Risk Difference with Oral CHM plus Gabapentin
Pain severity (VAS) (14 days)	68 (1 RCT)	⊕⊕◯◯ LOW[1,2]	—	The mean pain severity was **6.68** cm	MD **4.79 cm lower** (5.27 lower to 4.31 lower)
Adverse events	68 (1 RCT)	No adverse events			

The risk in the intervention group (and its 95% confidence interval) is based on the assumed risk in the comparison group and the relative effect of the intervention (and its 95% CI).

Abbreviations: CI, confidence interval; CHM, Chinese herbal medicine; GRADE, Grading of Recommendations Assessment, Development and Evaluation; MD, mean difference; RCT, randomised controlled trial; VAS, visual analogue scale.

1. High risk of bias from blinding
2. Uncertainty in results because of small sample size

<u>Study References</u>

Pain severity (VAS): S240
Adverse events: S240

Table 13.8   GRADE: Oral Chinese Herbal Medicine plus Tricyclic Anti depressants *vs.* tricyclic Anti depressants

Outcomes (Treatment duration)	No of Participants (Studies)	Quality of the Evidence (GRADE)	Relative Effect (95% CI)	Anticipated Absolute Effects	
				Risk with TCAs	Risk difference with CHM plus TCAs
Pain severity (VAS) (3 weeks)	62 (1 RCT)	⊕⊕◯◯ LOW[1,2]	—	The mean pain was **3.05 cm**	MD **0.91 cm** lower (1.23 lower to 0.59 lower)
Adverse events	62 (1 RCT)	Adverse events in the intervention group included one case of nausea and vomiting. No adverse events in the TCA group.			

The risk in the intervention group (and its 95% confidence interval) is based on the assumed risk in the comparison group and the relative effect of the intervention (and its 95% CI).

Abbreviations: CI, confidence interval; GRADE, Grading of Recommendations Assessment, Development and Evaluation; MD, mean difference; RCT, randomised controlled trial; TCAs, tricyclic anti depressants; VAS, visual analogue scale.

1. High risk of bias from blinding may influence results
2. Uncertainty in results because of small sample size

Study References
Pain severity (VAS): S235
Adverse events: S235

age of participants was 63.4 years and more females were included than males (54 females and 36 males). Treatment with oral CHM was provided for 30 days and no follow-up assessment was made after treatment ceased.

The study did not report syndrome differentiation. The CHMs evaluated were two investigator-developed formulas and herbs included *ban lan gen* 板蓝根, *chi shao* 赤芍, *chuan xiong* 川芎, *da qing ye* 大青叶, *dang gui* 当归, *hong hua* 红花, *quan xie* 全蝎, *tao ren* 桃仁, *wu gong* 蜈蚣, *yan hu suo* 延胡索, and *yu jin* 郁金. CHM was compared with doxepin, vitamin B1, and vitamin B12.

Although the study reported assessing the pain score on the VAS, no data was actually presented. Adverse events were reported in both intervention and comparator groups. Adverse events in the CHM group included two cases of diarrhoea and one case each of nausea and dizziness. Adverse events in those who received doxepin and vitamins B1 and B12 included three cases of nausea and one case each of dizziness and diarrhoea.

Non-controlled Studies of Chinese Herbal Medicine

Eight non-controlled studies evaluating CHM for PHN were included (S242–S249). One study was conducted in Japan (S249) while the rest were conducted in China. All non-controlled studies were case series and included a total of 227 participants. Sample sizes ranged from 12 (S249) to 38 (S247) and the median sample size was 30.

One study included people with pain persisting for three months or more after resolution of the rash (S247) and four used a definition of pain persisting for one month or more after resolution of the rash (S242–S244, S248). Two reported PHN after rash resolution (no time-point specified) and duration of PHN was two months or more (S246, S249). Both studies were considered likely to be PHN and were included. Similarly, one study which did not specify a definition of PHN but which reported the persistence of pain for a duration of three months or more was also included (S245).

Three studies reported using CM syndrome differentiation as an inclusion criterion and for treatment (S243, S244, S246). Two studies reported the pattern/syndrome of *qi* stagnation and Blood stasis (S243, S244) and one study reported *qi* deficiency and Blood stasis (S246). Four studies used CHM in combination with various pharmacotherapies (S244, S247–S249). Six studies administered CHM orally (S242, S243, S245–S247, S249) and two studies administered CHM topically (S244, S248). There was no overlap across studies in the formulas used. The herbs most frequently reported included *tao ren* 桃仁 (5 studies), *xiang fu* 香附 (5 studies), *hong hua* 红花 (4 studies), and *dang gui* 当归 (4 studies) (see Table 13.9).

Seven studies (189 participants) reported information on adverse events (S242–S246, S248, S249) with four studies reporting that no

Table 13.9   Frequently Reported Herbs in Non-controlled Studies

Most Common Herbs	Scientific Name	Frequency of Use
Tao ren 桃仁	*Prunus* spp	5
Xiang fu 香附	*Cyperus rotundus* L.	5
Dang gui 当归	*Angelica sinensis* (Oliv.) Diels	4
Hong hua 红花	*Carthamus tinctorius* L.	4
Gan cao 甘草	*Glycyrrhiza* spp	3
Mo yao 没药	*Commiphora* spp	3
Quan xie 全蝎	*Buthus martensii* Karsch	3
Yu jin 郁金	*Curcuma* spp	3
Bai shao 白芍	*Paeonia lactiflora* Pall.	2
Chuan xiong 川芎	*Ligusticum chuangxiong* Hort.	2
Dan shen 丹参	*Salvia miltiorrhiza* Bge.	2
Di long 地龙	*Pheretima* spp	2
Huang qi 黄芪	*Astragalus membranaceus* spp	2
Ji xue teng 鸡血藤	*Spatholobus suberectus* Dunn	2
Mu dan pi 牡丹皮	*Paeonia suffruticosa* Andr.	2
Yan hu suo 延胡索	*Corydalis yanhusuo* W.T. Wang	2
Zhi ke 枳壳	*Citrus aurantium* L.	2

Note: The use of some herbs may be restricted in some countries. Readers are advised to comply with relevant regulations.

adverse events occurred (S243, S245, S246, S248). In the other studies, adverse events occurred which included five cases of mild gastrointestinal discomfort, three cases of hot flashes and gastric discomfort, and one case of dizziness.

Summary of Clinical Evidence for Chinese Herbal Medicine

Compared with herpes zoster, the number of clinical studies that have examined the benefits of CHM for PHN is small. While few studies reported CM syndromes, those that were reported were consistent with those described for herpes zoster and included *qi* stagnation or deficiency and Blood stasis. Most studies evaluated oral CHM which reflects clinical textbooks and guidelines. Many studies used investigator-developed formulas. As such, there was little overlap in formulas used across studies. One formula, *Shen tong zhu yu tang* 身痛逐瘀汤, was used in one RCT and one non-controlled study. Practitioners should consider syndrome differentiation when prescribing CHM for patients and may consider using formulas that include *dang gui* 当归, *gan cao* 甘草, *hong hua* 红花, *chai hu* 柴胡, *bai shao* 白芍, *chuan xiong* 川芎, and *tao ren* 桃仁.

When the efficacy of CHM in RCTs was evaluated, little benefit was found in terms of the VAS pain score and emotional wellbeing as measured by the HAM-D when CHM was used alone. However, CHM as IM was effective in reducing VAS pain scores and improving emotional wellbeing as measured by the HAM-D and was also well-tolerated by participants. The herbs that may have contributed to these benefits provide some direction for further research and guidance for clinicians. As there was no overlap in formulas used in RCTs, there is no evidence for the potential effects of specific formulas.

The duration of treatment with CHM ranged from 10 to 30 days. Considering that the duration of PHN in patients resistant to treatment can range from several months to many years,[1] the short duration of treatment reported by these studies was surprising. This may be due to both the definition of PHN used in the study and the duration of PHN experienced by included participants. For example, studies that used the PHN definition of pain persisting for one month or more after resolution of the rash may have included more people with shorter durations of PHN. For this group, a short duration of treatment may be clinically appropriate. The majority of studies reported the duration of PHN as a range, without presenting the mean and standard deviation. Without knowing the mean duration of PHN, the appropriateness of the treatment duration is unclear.

While various definitions of PHN have been suggested in the literature, the definition generally used in clinical practice and research is pain persisting for three months or more after the resolution of the rash.[2] The most common definition of PHN used in included studies was pain persisting for one month or more after resolution of the rash. Further, few studies reported follow-up after cessation of treatment. While short-term benefits were seen with CHM as IM, the long term efficacy in chronic PHN, and in patients refractory to treatment, remains unclear.

As was seen for herpes zoster, many studies combined guideline-recommended treatments with other non-guideline-recommended treatments such as vitamins B1 and B12. Vitamins B1 and B12 and other derivatives are often used in China to aid nerve repair. The evidence for these therapies is scant and any synergistic or antagonistic actions when used with guideline-recommended pain management therapies are unknown. As such, the findings from this review should be considered in light of their use.

References

1. Dworkin RH, Schmader KE. Treatment and prevention of postherpetic neuraglia. *Clin Infect Dis.* 2003; **36**(7):877–82.
2. Dubinsky RM, Kabbani H, El-Chami Z, Boutwell C, Ali H. Practice parameter: Treatment of postherpetic neuralgia: An evidence-based report of the Quality Standards Subcommittee of the American Academy of Neurology. *Neurology.* 2004; **63**(6):959–65.

14

Pharmacological Actions of Common Herbs — Post-herpetic Neuralgia

OVERVIEW

Clinical trials of Chinese herbal medicine provide experimental evidence for the potential action mechanisms of many herbs. The pathological processes involved in post-herpetic neuralgia have been described in Chapter 10. This chapter describes a selection of laboratory studies of the ten most frequently used herbs in randomised controlled trials.

Introduction

As described in Chapter 10, several mechanisms have been proposed for neuropathic pain and pain in post-herpetic neuralgia (PHN). These include nerve injury in the peripheral nervous system,[1,2] sensitisation in the central nervous system (CNS),[2,3] and varicella zoster virus replication leading to ganglionitis.[1] Nitric oxide (NO), tumour necrosis factor-α (TNF-α), interleukin (IL)-1β, and IL-6 have all been implicated in neuropathic pain[4-6] and may play a role in PHN.

One of the most common models of neuropathic pain is the chronic constrictive injury (CCI)[7] model where four ligations of the L5 nerve are made. This model is commonly used to evaluate mechanical allodynia using the von Frey test and thermal hyperalgesia using the Hargreave's test. In the von Frey test in rodents, a von Frey filament is applied to the central plantar region until buckling or paw withdrawal occurs.[8] The threshold of force required to elicit paw withdrawal is calculated from the lowest three out of five consecutive tests from which paw withdrawal is provoked. The Hargreave's test uses progressive light intensity which applies heat to the left and right hind paws until animals voluntarily withdraw the paws.[9,10] Repeated measures are made with a minimum of five minutes between paw evaluations.

This section evaluates potential mechanisms for eleven of the most frequently used herbs in randomised controlled trials (RCTs) of Chinese herbal medicine (CHM) (see Chapter 13). The methodology described in Chapter 6 was followed to identify relevant studies.

Methods

This chapter provides a general overview of the experimental evidence relating to the pharmacology of herbs and their constituent compounds for post-herpetic neuralgia. The constituent compounds were identified by searching herbal monographs, high quality reviews of CHM, herbal medicine encyclopedia, materia medica and/or PubMed. To identify preclinical publications a literature search of PubMed and/or CNKI was undertaken. The search strategy included the terms for each herb and their constituent compounds. Relevant data were extracted and a summary of the findings is reported here.

Experimental Studies on *Dang Gui* 当归

Many compound groups have been identified in *dang gui* 当归 (*Angelica sinensis* (Oliv.) Diels) and these include volatile oils, amino acids, sterols, and sugars.[11] *Dang gui* and its compounds have antinociceptive and anti-inflammatory properties.[12-16] Vanillin, a volatile oil, alleviated allodynia in the von Frey test but did not influence thermal hyperalgesia on the Hargreave's test.[12]

Other compounds of *dang gui* have been implicated in the inflammatory response. Four hydrosoluble fractions of *dang gui* time-dependently increased the production of inducible nitric oxide synthase (iNOS) and subsequently NO, both markers of inflammation, in murine peritoneal macrophage cells.[13] An increase in NO production mediated by iNOS expression was also seen in murine macrophages with a polysaccharide of *dang gui,* both *in vitro* and *in vivo.*[16] In the same study, a polysaccharide of *dang gui* stimulated macrophages to produce tumour necrosis-α (TNF-α), a pro-inflammatory cytokine.

Conversely, n-Butylidenephthalide, a polysaccharide of *dang gui*, was found to decrease TNF-α production in lipopolysaccharide (LPS) stimulated murine dendritic cells DC2.4.[14] Production of the pro-inflammatory cytokine IL-6 was also inhibited by n-Butylidenephthalide. Ligustilide, a volatile oil of *dang gui,* inhibited iNOS expression in LPS-stimulated murine RAW 264.7 cells and also inhibited the production of NO, TNF-α, and prostaglandin E_2 (PGE_2, an inflammatory mediator).[15]

Experimental Studies on *Yan Hu Suo* 延胡索

Alkaloids are the most abundant compounds in *yan hu suo* 延胡索 (*Corydalis yanhusuo* W.T. Wang).[11] *Yan hu suo* has been shown to have anti-nociceptive and anti-inflammatory properties.[17–20] Extracts of *yan hu suo* were evaluated using the CCI model of neuropathic pain in rats.[17] High doses of *yan hu suo* in the treatment and maintenance phases decreased mechanical allodynia using von Frey filaments. *Yan hu suo* decreased the time taken for paw withdrawal in tests of thermal hyperalgesia in the maintenance phase but not in the induction phase. The same study also found that *yan hu suo* decreased nerve injury-induced phosphorylation of the *N*-methyl-D-aspartate (NMDA) receptor subunit NR1 (pNR1 or pGluN1) in the superficial dorsal horn and nucleus proprius during the induction phase, suggesting that NMDA pNR1 modulation may be the mechanism for anti-nociception.

Extracts of *yan hu suo* have been evaluated to determine their potential for thermal hyperalgesia.[19] After injecting the inflammatory agent Complete Freund's adjuvant (CFA) into the hind paws of rats, *yan hu suo* extract produced a greater reduction in paw withdrawal latency in the Hargreave's test than saline treated rats 24 hours after inflammation was induced. An alkaloid of *yan hu suo*, dehydrocorybulbine, attenuated mechanical allodynia in the von Frey test and hyperalgesia in the Hargreave's test at a non-sedative dose.[20] The anti-nociceptive effect seen with dehydrocorybulbine in the neuropathic component of the formalin assay, which examines acute, inflammatory, and neuropathic pain responses, was dose-dependent and produced effects similar to those induced by high doses of morphine. Dehydro-corybulbine also inhibited the production of pro-inflammatory cytokines IL-1β and IL-6 in LPS-stimulated mouse RAW 264.7 macrophages.[18]

Experimental Studies on *Hong Hua* 红花

Hong hua 红花 (*Carthamus tinctorius* L.) contains many groups of compounds such as phenolic compounds, volatile oils, fixed oils, and various other constituents including arabinose, β-sitosterol, and mannose.[11] Few studies have examined the effect of *hong hua* or its compounds in neuropathic pain or inflammatory models, with those that have been conducted showing anti-inflammatory properties.[21,22] Extracts of *hong hua* inhibited the production of NO in LPS-stimulated RAW 264.7 cells to a greater extent than curcumin (positive control) and LPS control.[21]

Hydroxysafflor yellow A is a phenolic compound of *hong hua* which may reduce or repair inflammatory neuronal damage. Research on ischaemic stroke found that hydroxysafflor yellow A attenuated the expression of toll-like receptor 4 (TLR-4) in LPS-stimulated mouse microglia.[22] This resulted in less neuronal damage occurring shortly after LPS stimulation. As TLR-4 plays a key role in the induction of inflammatory responses, this mechanism may be relevant for neuropathic pain including PHN.

Experimental Studies on *Gan Cao* 甘草

Gan cao 甘草 (*Glycyrrhiza uralensis* Fisch; *Glycyrrhiza inflata* Bat.; *Glycyrrhiza glabra* L.) contains triterpene saponins, flavonoids, and coumarin derivatives.[11] *Gan cao* is often described as an herb that har-monises the actions of other herbs, but it has many other therapeutic properties including anti-nociceptive actions.[7,23,24] *Gan cao* dose-dependently and time-dependently induced anti-allodynic and anti-hyperalgesic effects in CCI-induced neuropathic pain in rats.[7] The effects were greater at higher doses and when *gan cao* was combined with another herb, *bai shao* 白芍. The actions of *gan cao* may be due to the decreased expression of sirtuin 1 (Sirt1), an enzyme with various roles including inflammatory regulation, in the dorsal root ganglion when *gan cao* and *bai shao* were administered together.

Compound 5 (olean-11,13(18)-dien-3β,30-*O*-dihemiphthalate) of glycyrrhetinic acid reduced thermal hyperalgesia in a sciatic nerve CCI-induced neuropathic pain model in rats.[23] Another compound, liquiritigenin, dose-dependently reduced mechanical, thermal, and cold hyperalgesia with no effects on motor performance.[24]

Experimental Studies on *Chuan Xiong* 川芎

Many compounds have been identified from *chuan xiong* 川芎 (*Ligusticum chuangxiong* Hort.) including groups of phthalides, biphthalides, alkaloids, amino acid derivatives, amines, organic acids, esters, and lactones.[11] However, few of these compounds have been evaluated for their effects on chronic or neuropathic pain. The anti-inflammatory actions of ligustilide, which is common to both *chuan xiong* and *dang gui*, and limonene, which is a volatile oil found in both *chuan xiong* and *chai hu*, have been described above.

Two compounds present in *chuan xiong*, α-pinene and linalool, decreased thermal hyperalgesia in the formalin-inflamed mouse hind paw inflammatory model.[25] Vanillic acid, the oxidised form of vanillin, inhibited CFA-induced mechanical hyperalgesia in mice and inhibited the production of IL-1β, TNF-α, and IL-33 in the carrageenan-induced inflammatory pain model.[26]

Experimental Studies on *Bai Shao*
白芍 and *Chi Shao* 赤芍

The two herbs *bai shao* 白芍 (*Paeonia lactiflora* Pall.) and *chi shao* 赤芍 (*Paeonia lactiflora* Pall.; *Paeonia veitchii* Lynch) share a common source in *Paeonia lactiflora* Pall. and there is considerable overlap in the identified constituents. The experimental evidence for both herbs, which are commonly referred to as peony, are presented here. The key compound groups of peony include glycosides, tannins, and volatile oils.[11] Many experimental studies have demonstrated the anti-inflammatory effects of peony compounds.[7,27–30] A key compound, paeonol, has been shown to dose-dependently inhibit the production of TNF-α, IL-1β, IL-6,[27,28] IL-10,[27] NO, and PGE_2[28] in LPS-stimulated RAW 264.7 cells.

Paeoniflorin inhibited NO and IL1-β production in microglial cells[29] and also inhibited NO, PGE_2, TNF-α, and IL-6 in LPS-stimulated RAW 264.7 cells.[30] In the same study, albiflorin also produced similar levels of inhibition in the production of NO, PGE_2, TNF-α, and IL-6. In the CCI model of neuropathic pain, total glycosides of peony (extracted active compounds) reduced both mechanical allodynia and thermal hyperalgesia at sufficiently high doses.[7]

Experimental Studies on *Huang Qi* 黄芪

Huang qi 黄芪 (*Astragalus membranaceus* (Fisch.) Bge. var. mongholicus (Bge.) Hsiao; *Astragalus membranaceus* (Fisch.) Bge) contains many groups of compounds including triterpensaponins, flavonoids, polysaccharides, and other constituents.[11] *Huang qi* has been shown to have anti-inflammatory effects.[31–34] *Huang qi* reduced iNOS, COX-2, IL-6, IL-1β, and TNF-α expression and also inhibited the production of NO in LPS-stimulated RAW 264.7 cells.[33]

An active fraction of *huang qi* inhibited the expression of iNOS, down-regulated cyclooxygenase- (COX) 2 expression, and decreased the production of PGE_2, IL-1β, and IL-6 in LPS-stimulated RAW 264.7 cells.[31] The compounds isoliquiritigenin and calycosin inhibited IL-6 and IL-12 production in LPS-stimulated bone marrow-derived dendritic cells,[32] and isoliquiritigenin also inhibited TNF-α production.[32] Conversely, a polysaccharide of *huang qi* was found to increase the level of TNF-α and production of NO in LPS-stimulated RAW 264.7 cells.[34] This may suggest that different compounds produce different physiological effects.

Experimental Studies on *Chai Hu* 柴胡

Two key groups of compounds have been identified from *chai hu* 柴胡 (*Bupleurum chinense* DC.; *Bupleurum scorzonerifolium* Willd.) — triterpene saponins and volatile oils.[11] Limonene, a volatile oil of *chai hu*, has been shown to have anti-inflammatory actions in RAW 264.7 macrophage cell lines. D-Limonene dose-dependently inhibited LPS-induced NO and PGE_2 expression while decreasing the expression of iNOS and COX-2 proteins.[35] D-limonene also decreased the expression of IL-1β, IL-6, and TNF-α in the same cells.[35]

Another compound of *chai hu*, saikosaponin, reversed mechanical allodynia and thermal hyperalgesia in rats, with effects seen in higher doses three days after sciatic nerve CCI surgery.[36] The highest dose (25mg/kg) provided the greatest pain relief. Saikosaponin-a also inhibited or reduced the expression of TNF-α, IL-1β, and IL-2 pro-inflammatory cytokines, p38 mitogen-activated protein kinase, and nuclear factor-κB (NF-κB) in the spinal cord.

Experimental Studies on *Dan Shen* 丹参

Dan shen 丹参 (*Salvia miltiorrhiza* Bge.) includes the compound groups quinones, diterpene ketones and lactones, phenols, and other constituents such as baicalin and β-sitosterol.[11] Compounds of *dan shen* have shown anti-nociceptive and anti-inflammatory effects.[37–39] In a spinal nerve ligation (SNL) pain model in rats, the quinone tanshinone IIA inhibited SNL-induced mechanical allodynia in a dose-dependent manner.[37] Tanshinone IIA also reduced the expression of pro-inflammatory cytokines TNF-α and IL-1β, increased superoxide dismutase (an anti-oxidant marker of oxidative stress), and decreased malondialdehyde (a pro-oxidant marker of oxidative stress).

Baicalin, isolated from *huang qin* 黄芩 but also present in *dan shen*, was found to attenuate allodynia and thermal hyperalgesia in a SNL pain model in rats and acted synergistically with morphine to enhance anti-nociceptive effects.[38] Baicalin also inhibited histone-H3 acetylation and expression of histone deacetylase 1 in the dorsal horn of the spinal cord on the same side. Another *dan shen* compound, salvianolic acid B, reduced mechanical hyperalgesia in the CCI neuropathic pain model in rats.[39]

Experimental Studies on *Tao Ren* 桃仁

Tao ren 桃仁 (*Prunus persica* (L.) Batsch; *Prunus davidiana* (Carr.) Franch.) contains glycosides, fixed and volatile oils, flavonoids, and triterpenes.[11] Limonene is found in *tao ren*, *chuan xiong*, and *chai hu* and its actions have been described above. Other studies have demonstrated the anti-nociceptive and anti-inflammatory actions of *tao ren*.[40–44] The flavonoid naringenin was found to reduce thermal hyperalgesia on the Hargreave's test, mechanical hyperalgesia using a pin prick test, and cold water-induced allodynia in the CCI model of neuropathic pain.[40] Further, naringenin reduced the production of NO in CCI rats. In another study, naringenin alleviated the pain induced by formalin, capsaicin, and CFA.[42] As reduction in pain-related behaviours were seen in both stages of the formalin assay, naringenin may have both anti-nociceptive and anti-inflammatory properties.

Epigallocatechin-3-gallate and two of its compounds (23 and 30) were evaluated in the CCI model of neuropathic pain.[44] Both epigallocatechin-3-gallate and compound 30 reduced thermal hyperalgesia, with greater effects seen with compound 30. No benefit was seen with compound 23. Kaempferol also reduced thermal hyperalgesia and mechanical allodynia compared with vehicle-treated groups in a rat model of diabetic neuropathic pain.[43] Kaempferol suppressed the release of NO and PGE$_2$ while attenuating the expression of iNOS, TNF-α, and COX-2 in LPS and sodium nitroprusside-stimulated RAW 264.7 cells and peritoneal macrophages.[41]

Summary of Pharmacological Actions of the Frequently Reported Herbs Used to Treat Post-herpetic Neuralgia

Some similarities were seen between the herbs used for PHN and the herbs used for herpes zoster (see Chapter 6). The herbs *gan cao*, *chai hu*, *dang gui*, and *yan hu suo* were common to both conditions.

Many experimental studies have demonstrated the anti-nociceptive properties of the herbs *dang gui, yan hu suo, gan cao, chuan xiong, bai shao/chi shao, chai hu, dan shen,* and *tao ren.* Anti-inflammatory properties were also commonly observed which may explain the mechanism of action of these herbs in the treatment of PHN. As the interest in natural products for the discovery of medicinal drugs grows, it is likely that more research will be conducted which will further elucidate the benefits of CHM for PHN.

References

1. Gilden DH, Cohrs RJ, Hayward AR, Wellish M, Mahalingam R. Chronic varicella-zoster virus ganglionitis — a possible cause of postherpetic neuralgia. *J Neurovirol.* 2003; **9**(3):404–7.
2. Petersen KL, Fields HL, Brennum J, Sandroni P, Rowbotham MC. Capsaicin evoked pain and allodynia in post-herpetic neuralgia. *Pain.* 2000; **88**(2):125–33.
3. Wall PD. Neuropathic pain and injured nerve: Central mechanisms. *Br Med Bull.* 1991; **47**(3):631–43.
4. Leung L, Cahill CM. TNF-α and neuropathic pain — a review. *J Neuroinflammation.* 2010; **7**:27.
5. Levy D, Zochodne DW. NO pain: Potential roles of nitric oxide in neuropathic pain. *Pain Pract.* 2004; **4**(1):11–8.
6. Sommer C, Kress M. Recent findings on how proinflammatory cytokines cause pain: Peripheral mechanisms in inflammatory and neuropathic hyperalgesia. *Neurosci Lett.* 2004; **361**(1–3):184–7.
7. Zhang J, Lv C, Wang HN, Cao Y. Synergistic interaction between total glucosides and total flavonoids on chronic constriction injury induced neuropathic pain in rats. *Pharm Biol.* 2013; **51**(4):455–62.
8. Vachon P, Masse R, Gibbs BF. Substance P and neurotensin are up-regulated in the lumbar spinal cord of animals with neuropathic pain. *Can J Vet Res.* 2004; **68**(2):86–92.
9. Guenette SA, Ross A, Marier JF, Beaudry F, Vachon P. Pharmacokinetics of eugenol and its effects on thermal hypersensitivity in rats. *Eur J Pharmacol.* 2007; **562**(1–2):60–7.
10. Hargreaves K, Dubner R, Brown F, Flores C, Joris J. A new and sensitive method for measuring thermal nociception in cutaneous hyperalgesia. *Pain.* 1988; **32**(1):77–88.

11. Bensky D, Clavey S, Stoger E. *Chinese Herbal Medicine Materia Medica.* 3rd ed. Seattle, US: Eastland Press, Inc; 2004.

12. Beaudry F, Ross A, Lema PP, Vachon P. Pharmacokinetics of vanillin and its effects on mechanical hypersensitivity in a rat model of neuropathic pain. *Phytother Res.* 2010; **24**(4):525–30.

13. Chen Y, Duan JA, Qian D, Guo J, Song B, Yang M. Assessment and comparison of immunoregulatory activity of four hydrosoluble fractions of Angelica sinensis in vitro on the peritoneal macrophages in ICR mice. *Int Immunopharmacol.* 2010; **10**(4):422–30.

14. Fu RH, Hran HJ, Chu CL, *et al.* Lipopolysaccharide-stimulated activation of murine DC2.4 cells is attenuated by n-butylidenephthalide through suppression of the NF-kappaB pathway. *Biotechnol Lett.* 2011; **33**(5):903–10.

15. Su YW, Chiou WF, Chao SH, Lee MH, Chen CC, Tsai YC. Ligustilide prevents LPS-induced iNOS expression in RAW 264.7 macrophages by preventing ROS production and down-regulating the MAPK, NF-kappaB and AP-1 signaling pathways. *Int Immunopharmacol.* 2011; **11**(9):1166–72.

16. Yang X, Zhao Y, Wang H, Mei Q. Macrophage activation by an acidic polysaccharide isolated from Angelica sinensis (Oliv.) Diels. *J Biochem Mol Biol.* 2007; **40**(5):636–43.

17. Choi JG, Kang SY, Kim JM, *et al.* Antinociceptive effect of Cyperi rhizoma and Corydalis tuber extracts on neuropathic pain in rats. *Korean J Physiol Pharmacol.* 2012; **16**(6):387–92.

18. Ishiguro K, Ando T, Maeda O, Watanabe O, Goto H. Dehydrocorydaline inhibits elevated mitochondrial membrane potential in lipopolysaccharide-stimulated macrophages. *Int Immunopharmacol.* 2011; **11**(9): 1362–7.

19. Wei F, Zou S, Young A, Dubner R, Ren K. Effects of four herbal extracts on adjuvant-induced inflammation and hyperalgesia in rats. *J Altern Complement Med.* 1999; **5**(5):429–36.

20. Zhang Y, Wang C, Wang L, *et al.* A novel analgesic isolated from a traditional Chinese medicine. *Curr Biol.* 2014; **24**(2):117–23.

21. Liao H, Banbury L, Liang H, *et al.* Effect of honghua (Flos Carthami) on nitric oxide production in RAW 264.7 cells and alpha-glucosidase activity. *J Tradit Chin Med.* 2014; **34**(3):362–8.

22. Lv Y, Qian Y, Ou-Yang A, Fu L. Hydroxysafflor yellow A attenuates neuron damage by suppressing the lipopolysaccharide-induced TLR4 pathway in activated microglial cells. *Cell Mol Neurobiol.* 2016.

23. Akasaka Y, Sakai A, Takasu K, *et al.* Suppressive effects of glycyrrhetinic acid derivatives on tachykinin receptor activation and hyperalgesia. *J Pharmacol Sci.* 2011; **117**(3):180–8.

24. Chen L, Chen W, Qian X, Fang Y, Zhu N. Liquiritigenin alleviates mechanical and cold hyperalgesia in a rat neuropathic pain model. *Sci Rep.* 2014; **4**:5676.

25. Li XJ, Yang YJ, Li YS, Zhang WK, Tang HB. α-Pinene, linalool, and 1-octanol contribute to the topical anti-inflammatory and analgesic activities of frankincense by inhibiting COX-2. *J Ethnopharmacol.* 2016; **179**:22–6.

26. Calixto-Campos C, Carvalho TT, Hohmann MS, *et al.* Vanillic acid inhibits inflammatory pain by inhibiting neutrophil recruitment, oxidative stress, cytokine production, and NF-κB activation in mice. *J Nat Prod.* 2015; **78**(8):1799–808.

27. Chen N, Liu D, Soromou LW, *et al.* Paeonol suppresses lipopolysaccharide-induced inflammatory cytokines in macrophage cells and protects mice from lethal endotoxin shock. *Fundam Clin Pharmacol.* 2014; **28**(3):268–76.

28. Himaya SW, Ryu B, Qian ZJ, Kim SK. Paeonol from Hippocampus kuda Bleeler suppressed the neuro-inflammatory responses *in vitro* via NF-κB and MAPK signaling pathways. *Toxicol In.* 2012; **26**(6):878–87.

29. Nam KN, Yae CG, Hong JW, Cho DH, Lee JH, Lee EH. Paeoniflorin, a monoterpene glycoside, attenuates lipopolysaccharide-induced neuronal injury and brain microglial inflammatory response. *Biotechnol Lett.* 2013; **35**(8):1183–9.

30. Wang QS, Gao T, Cui YL, Gao LN, Jiang HL. Comparative studies of paeoniflorin and albiflorin from Paeonia lactiflora on anti-inflammatory activities. *Pharm Biol.* 2014; **52**(9):1189–95.

31. Lai PK, Chan JY, Wu SB, *et al.* Anti-inflammatory activities of an active fraction isolated from the root of Astragalus membranaceus in RAW 264.7 macrophages. *Phytother Res.* 2014; **28**(3):395–404.

32. Li W, Sun YN, Yan XT, *et al.* Flavonoids from Astragalus membranaceus and their inhibitory effects on LPS-stimulated pro-inflammatory cytokine production in bone marrow-derived dendritic cells. *Arch Pharm Res.* 2014; **37**(2):186–92.

33. Ryu M, Kim EH, Chun M, *et al.* Astragali Radix elicits anti-inflammation via activation of MKP-1, concomitant with attenuation of p38 and Erk. *J Ethnopharmacol.* 2008; **115**(2):184–93.

34. Zhao LH, Ma ZX, Zhu J, Yu XH, Weng DP. Characterization of polysaccharide from Astragalus radix as the macrophage stimulator. *Cell Immunol.* 2011; **271**(2):329–34.

35. Yoon WJ, Lee NH, Hyun CG. Limonene suppresses lipopolysaccharide-induced production of nitric oxide, prostaglandin E_2, and pro-inflammatory cytokines in RAW 264.7 macrophages. *J Oleo Sci.* 2010; **59**(8):415–21.

36. Zhou X, Cheng H, Xu D, *et al.* Attenuation of neuropathic pain by saikosaponin a in a rat model of chronic constriction injury. *Neurochem Res.* 2014; **39**(11):2136–42.

37. Cao FL, Xu M, Wang Y, Gong KR, Zhang JT. Tanshinone IIA attenuates neuropathic pain via inhibiting glial activation and immune response. *Pharmacol Biochem Behav.* 2015; **128**:1–7.

38. Cherng CH, Lee KC, Chien CC, *et al.* Baicalin ameliorates neuropathic pain by suppressing HDAC1 expression in the spinal cord of spinal nerve ligation rats. *J Formos Med Assoc.* 2014; **113**(8):513–20.

39. Isacchi B, Fabbri V, Galeotti N, *et al.* Salvianolic acid B and its liposomal formulations: Anti-hyperalgesic activity in the treatment of neuropathic pain. *Eur J Pharm Sci.* 2011; **44**(4):552–8.

40. Kaulaskar S, Bhutada P, Rahigude A, Jain D, Harle U. Effects of naringenin on allodynia and hyperalgesia in rats with chronic constriction injury-induced neuropathic pain. Zhong xi yi jie he xue bao = *Journal of Chinese integrative medicine.* 2012; **10**(12):1482–9.

41. Kim SH, Park JG, Lee J, *et al.* The dietary flavonoid Kaempferol mediates anti-inflammatory responses via the Src, Syk, IRAK1, and IRAK4 molecular targets. *Mediators Inflamm.* 2015;904142.

42. Pinho-Ribeiro FA, Zarpelon AC, Fattori V, *et al.* Naringenin reduces inflammatory pain in mice. *Neuropharmacology.* 2016.

43. Raafat K, El-Lakany A. Acute and subchronic *in-vivo* effects of Ferula hermonis L. and Sambucus nigra L. and their potential active isolates in a diabetic mouse model of neuropathic pain. *BMC Complement Altern Med.* 2015; **15**:257.

44. Xifro X, Vidal-Sancho L, Boadas-Vaello P, *et al.* Novel epigallocatechin-3-gallate (EGCG) derivative as a new therapeutic strategy for reducing neuropathic pain after chronic constriction nerve injury in mice. *PloS One.* 2015; **10**(4):e0123122.

15

Clinical Evidence for Acupuncture and Related Therapies — Post-herpetic Neuralgia

OVERVIEW

The efficacy of acupuncture and related treatments has been examined by many clinical studies and these findings have been published in English and Chinese language scientific journals. This chapter provides an assessment of the evidence for acupuncture therapies from clinical studies. An extensive search of English and Chinese language databases identified more than 36,000 citations which were screened against inclusion criteria. A total of 14 clinical studies were included for review. Their analyses showed that acupuncture may reduce post-herpetic neuralgia in the short term.

Introduction

Acupuncture is part of a family of techniques aimed at stimulating the body's acupuncture points to correct imbalances of energy and restore health to the body. Methods of stimulating acupuncture points include:

- Acupuncture: insertion of an acupuncture needle into acupuncture points. This includes manual acupuncture (manual stimulation of acupuncture needles), surrounding acupuncture (needles inserted in the area surrounding a lesion or rash site), and electro-acupuncture (stimulation of the needle by an electrical stimulating device);

- Moxibustion: burning of herbs (usually *ai ye* 艾叶, *artemesia* spp) close to or on the skin to induce a warming sensation;
- Plum-blossom needle therapy: application of a plum-blossom needle containing a bundle of short embedded needles which is usually tapped lightly on the skin.

Previous Systematic Reviews

No systematic reviews of acupuncture therapies were found in English language databases. Similarly, no systematic reviews comparing commonly used acupuncture or other Chinese medicine (CM) therapies with pharmacotherapy or systematic reviews investigating the efficacy of acupuncture, moxibustion, or plum-blossom needle therapy could be identified.

Characteristics of Clinical Studies of Acupuncture and Related Therapies

More than 36,600 citations were identified from searches of English and Chinese clinical research databases with the full text of over 5,000 articles assessed for eligibility. After reviewing these articles against inclusion criteria, 14 clinical studies were selected for evaluation (see Figure 15.1). Seven of these were randomised controlled trials (RCTs) (S250–S256) and seven were non-controlled studies (S257–S263). No controlled clinical trials were identified. The findings from RCTs were evaluated for efficacy and safety while details of non-controlled studies are described.

Two studies were conducted in the USA (S262, S263) and the remainder was conducted in China. A total of 722 participants were enrolled in these studies. A range of definitions of post-herpetic neuralgia (PHN) were used, with the most common definition being one month or more after the resolution of the rash. Few studies reported details on CM syndromes, with one study each reporting

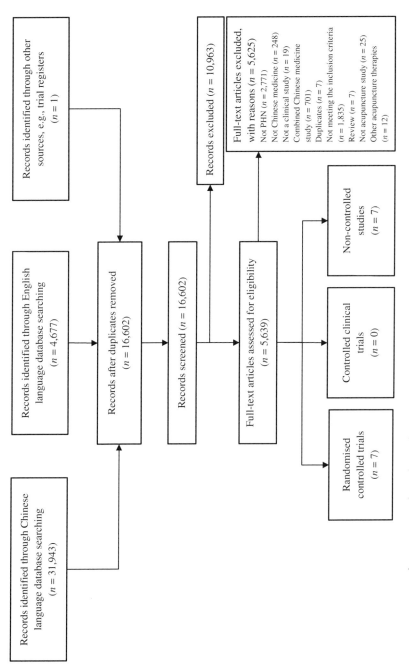

Figure 15.1 Flow chart of the study selection process: Acupuncture and related therapies.

qi or Blood stagnation (S262) and another reporting *bi* syndrome and *wei* syndrome (S263).

The most common intervention was acupuncture which was used in 12 studies (S251–S261, S263). Other interventions that were evaluated included moxibustion (S250) and plum-blossom needle therapy (S262). Comparators included anticonvulsants alone (S252, S254, S256) or with other treatments (S251), tricyclic antidepressants (TCAs) plus other treatments (S250), opioid medications alone (S255), and tramadol with other treatments (S253).

Forty-four different acupuncture points or treatment approaches were described in all clinical studies with the most common approaches using EX-B2 *Huatuojiaji* points 夹脊穴 or *ashi* points 阿是穴 (8 studies each). Other commonly used acupuncture points included ST36 *Zusanli* 足三里, LR3 *Taichong* 太冲, and LI4 *Hegu* 合谷 (4 studies each), as well as SP6 *Sanyinjiao* 三阴交 and TE6 *Zhigou* 支沟 (3 studies each).

Randomised Controlled Trials of Acupuncture and Related Therapies

Seven RCTs including 469 participants evaluated acupuncture therapies for PHN pain reduction (S250–S256). One study was a three-arm trial which evaluated two interventions and only one arm was relevant to this review (S253). Data for the second arm was not analysed.

One study used a definition of PHN of three months or more after resolution of the rash (S250) and four studies defined PHN as occurring one month or more after the resolution of the rash (S251, S252, S254, S256). One study included people with PHN after rash resolution without a specified time-point (S255) and the duration of PHN was reported to be more than four weeks for all participants. As the acute phase of herpes zoster is considered to be 28 days, it is likely that this study included people with PHN according to the definition of one month after rash resolution or more. As such, the study was considered eligible for inclusion.

Participants ranged in age from 34 (S251) to 80 years (S253). The mean age of participants was reported in all but one study (S255) and the median of the mean age was 57.7 years. The number of males and females was approximately similar (237 males, 226 females) in studies which stated the gender of participants. Duration of PHN ranged from one month (S252, S254, S256) to 48 months (S256). Treatment was provided for seven days (S251) to four weeks (S250) and the median duration of treatment was 14 days. None of the studies reported providing follow-up assessments of participants.

CM syndrome differentiation was not described in these studies. The most frequently evaluated intervention was acupuncture (S251–S253, S254–S256) and one study used moxibustion as the intervention (S250). The most common treatment approach was to focus on EX-B2 *Huatuojiaji* points 夹脊穴 (5 studies). Other common approaches were to use *ashi* points 阿是穴 (4 studies), treat the area around the herpes zoster rash (2 studies), and use acupuncture points LI4 *Hegu* 合谷, LR3 *Taichong* 太冲, SP6 *Sanyinjiao* 三阴交, and ST36 *Zusanli* 足三里 (2 studies each).

Guideline-recommended comparators included TCAs (S250), anticonvulsants (alone or combined with other treatments) (S251, S252, S254, S256), opioid medications (S255), and tramadol with other treatments (S253). Several studies combined guideline-recommended treatments with other treatments, such as non-steroidal anti-inflammatory drugs (NSAIDs) (S250, S251, S253), cimetidine (S250), and vitamins (S253).

Risk of Bias

Studies were assessed to determine their methodological quality (see Table 15.1). Two studies used a random number table for group allocation and were judged as having low risk of bias (S251, S253). One study allocated participants according to the order of visit and was judged as having high bias risk (S256). All the remaining studies provided insufficient information about allocation and were judged as having unclear risk of bias. All studies were judged as having unclear

Table 15.1   Methodological Quality of Included Randomised Controlled Trials: Acuncture and Related Therapies

Risk of Bias Domain	Low Risk n (%)	Unclear Risk n (%)	High Risk n (%)
Sequence generation	2 (28.5)	4 (57.1)	1 (14.3)
Allocation concealment	0 (0)	7 (100)	0 (0)
Blinding of participants	0 (0)	0 (0)	7 (100)
Blinding of personnel	0 (0)	0 (0)	7 (100)
Blinding of outcome assessor	0 (0)	7 (100)	0 (0)
Incomplete outcome data	4 (57.1)	3 (42.8)	0 (0)
Selective outcome reporting	0 (0)	7 (100)	0 (0)

risk of bias for allocation concealment due to insufficient information. All studies were judged as having high bias risk for blinding of both participants and personnel.

Insufficient information was provided to determine whether outcome assessors were blinded to group allocation and thus all studies were assessed as having unclear bias risk for this domain. Three studies reported participant withdrawals (S250–S252) and while one study described the reasons for withdrawal (S251), none of the studies accounted for the missing data in analyses. All three studies were judged as having unclear risk of bias for incomplete outcome data. None of the included studies published their trial protocols or provided details of trial registration and thus all were judged as having unclear risk of bias for selective outcome reporting.

Acupuncture

Six studies used acupuncture to treat PHN (S251–S256). All studies were conducted in China and included a total of 409 participants. Treatments were provided for between seven days (S251) and four weeks (S250). None of the studies followed-up participants after treatments ended.

CM syndrome differentiation was not described in these studies. Acupuncture was used either alone (S251–S253) or as integrative medicine (IM) (S254–S256). Comparators included anticonvulsants alone (S252, S256) or in combination with other treatments such as NSAIDs (S251) and tramadol plus NSAIDs plus vitamin B1 (S253). The most commonly used treatment approach was to apply treatment to EX-B2 *Huatuojiaji* 夹脊穴 (5 studies) or *ashi* 阿是穴 points (4 studies), or to use LI4 *Hegu* 合谷 (2 studies).

Acupuncture Alone

Three studies compared acupuncture with pharmacotherapy (S251–S253). When used alone, acupuncture reduced the pain score on a visual analogue scale (VAS) by 2.55cm (2 studies, 140 participants; [–2.96, –2.13], I^2 = 72%) (S251, S252) compared with pharmacotherapy when PHN was assessed one month after resolution of the rash. While statistical heterogeneity was high, it was not possible to conduct subgroup analyses due to the small number of included studies. The reliability of this finding remains unclear.

Results from a single study showed that the itch score on a five-point scale (0–4; a higher score means worse itch) was reduced in people who received acupuncture compared with carbamazepine (mean difference MD –0.39 [95% confidence intervals –0.74, –0.04]) (S252). One study (66 participants) reported that no adverse events occurred during the trial (S253).

Acupuncture as Integrative Medicine

Three studies compared acupuncture as IM with guideline-recommended treatments (S254–S256). One study combined acupuncture with pregabalin to treat 77 people with PHN (S256). The definition used for PHN was pain one month after resolution of the rash. As IM, acupuncture reduced the pain score on the VAS by 1.50 cm ([–2.32, –0.68]). All three studies reported information on adverse events. Adverse events in the intervention groups included six cases of dizziness and drowsiness, two cases of dizziness, and an unspecified number of cases of transdermal fentanyl use, mild drowsiness, constipation, bloating, and difficult urination. Adverse events in the comparator groups included five cases of dizziness and drowsiness, two cases of fatigue, one case of dizziness, and an unspecified number of cases of transdermal fentanyl use, mild drowsiness, constipation, bloating, and difficult urination.

Assessment Using Grading of Recommendations Assessment, Development and Evaluation

The comparisons for the summary-of-findings tables were determined by group consensus. Panelists selected acupuncture, both alone and as IM, to be compared with gabapentin, pregabalin, and TCAs. The included studies did not include the comparison of acupuncture with pregabalin, gabapentin, or TCAs, or the comparison of acupuncture plus TCAs with TCAs alone. Thus, no summary-of-findings tables could be prepared for these comparisons.

Acupuncture plus Gabapentin vs. Gabapentin

- The quality of evidence from one study of acupuncture plus gabapentin compared with gabapentin was low (see Table 15.2). The study did not report outcomes for pain severity on the VAS or the Zoster Brief Pain Inventory.

Acupuncture plus Pregabalin vs. Pregabalin

- The quality of the evidence for acupuncture plus pregabalin compared with pregabalin was low (see Table 15.3). Acupuncture plus pregabalin produced a greater reduction in pain severity at the end of treatment than pregabalin alone. No study reported on the Zoster Brief Pain Inventory.

Frequently Reported Points in Meta-analyses Showing Favourable Effects: Acupuncture

To identify which acupuncture points may have contributed to the favourable effects shown in meta-analyses, acupuncture studies were examined in further detail with the same approach used for the

Table 15.2   GRADE: Acupuncture plus Gabapentin *vs.* Gabapentin

Outcomes	No of Participants (Studies)	Quality of the Evidence (GRADE)	Relative Effect (95% CI)	Anticipated Absolute Effects	
				Risk with Gabapentin	Risk Difference with Acupuncture plus Gabapentin
Adverse events	61 (1 RCT)			Adverse events in the intervention group included two cases of dizziness. Adverse events in the control group included two cases of fatigue and one case of dizziness.	

The risk in the intervention group (and its 95% confidence interval) is based on the assumed risk in the comparison group and the relative effect of the intervention (and its 95% CI).

Abbreviations: CI, confidence interval; GRADE, Grading of Recommendations Assessment, Development and Evaluation; RCT, randomised controlled trial.

<u>Study References</u>
Adverse events: S254

Table 15.3   GRADE: Acupuncture plus Pregabalin *vs.* Pregabalin

Outcomes (Treatment duration)	No of Participants (Studies)	Quality of the Evidence (GRADE)	Relative Effect (95% CI)	Anticipated Absolute Effects	
				Risk with Pregabalin	Risk Difference with Acupuncture plus Pregabalin
Pain severity (VAS) (2 weeks)	77 (1 RCT)	⊕⊕◯◯ LOW[1,2]	—	The mean pain was **3.9 cm**	MD **1.5 cm** lower (2.32 lower to 0.68 lower)
Adverse events	77 (1 RCT)	Adverse events in the intervention group were six cases of drowsiness and dizziness, and in the control group included five cases of drowsiness and dizziness.			

The risk in the intervention group (and its 95% confidence interval) is based on the assumed risk in the comparison group and the relative effect of the intervention (and its 95% CI).

Abbreviations: CI, confidence interval; GRADE, Grading of Recommendations Assessment, Development and Evaluation; MD, mean difference; RCT, randomised controlled trial; VAS, visual analogue scale.

1. High risk of bias from blinding
2. Uncertainty in results because of small sample size

Study References
Pain severity (VAS): S256
Adverse events: S256

examination of CHM studies (see Chapter 13). Acupuncture alone produced results superior to pharmacotherapy for pain severity on the VAS. Two acupuncture points/treatment approaches were common in both the studies included in the meta-analysis: *ashi* 阿是穴 points and EX-B2 *Huatuojiaji* 夹脊穴. These two approaches may have contributed to the effects reported.

Moxibustion

One study evaluated moxibustion in people with PHN (S250). The study, which included 60 participants, compared moxibustion with doxepin, ibuprofen, and cimetidine. The definition of PHN was three months or more after resolution of the rash (S250). Treatment was provided for four weeks and the study did not report any follow-up assessments once treatment ceased. No CM syndrome was reported. Moxibustion was applied to the rash area, the auricular points CO12 Liver 肝, TF4 *Shenmen* 神门, and AH6a Sympathetic 交感, and the body points LR3 *Taichong* 太冲, SP6 *Sanyinjiao* 三阴交, ST36 *Zusanli* 足三里, LI10 *Shousanli* 手三里, and PC6 *Neiguan* 内关.

The pain score on the VAS after four weeks of treatment was 1.79 cm lower in those who received moxibustion compared with doxepin, ibuprofen, and cimetidine ([−2.19, −1.39]) (S250). The study also reported two cases of burns in the intervention group.

Controlled Clinical Trials of Acupuncture and Related Therapies

No eligible studies that evaluated acupuncture therapies in controlled clinical trials were identified.

Non-controlled Studies of Acupuncture and Related Therapies

Seven studies evaluated a range of acupuncture therapies to treat PHN (S257–S263). Two case reports were conducted in the USA

(S262, S263) and the remaining five studies, which were case series, were conducted in China. A total of 253 people with PHN participated in these studies and the sample size ranged from one (S262, S263) to 87 (S260), with 36 as the median sample size.

One study used a PHN definition of three months or more after resolution of the rash (S261), five studies defined PHN as pain persisting for one month or more after resolution of the rash (S257–S260, S263), and one study was included based on PHN specified as after the resolution of rash with a 13-month history of PHN (S262).

Acupuncture was the most common intervention and was used in six studies (S257–S261, S263). The remaining study used plum-blossom needle therapy (S262). Two studies combined acupuncture therapy with pharmacotherapy (S257, S261).

CM syndromes were used to guide treatment in two studies (S262, S263) and these included *qi* or Blood stagnation (S262), *bi* syndrome, and *wei* syndrome (S263). The most common treatment approaches were to needle the *ashi* 阿是穴 points (4 studies) or to use EX-B2 *Huatuojiaji* points 夹脊穴 (3 studies). Acupuncture points used in two studies included BL17 *Geshu* 膈俞, BL18 *Ganshu* 肝俞, LI4 *Hegu* 合谷, LR14 *Qimen* 期门, LR3 *Taichong* 太冲, SP10 *Xuehai* 血海, ST36 *Zusanli* 足三里, and TE6 *Zhigou* 支沟.

Among the four studies that reported on adverse events (S257, S258, S260, S262), two studies stated that no adverse events occurred (S258, S262) while the other two studies recorded one case of fainting in participants who received electro-acupuncture (S260) and an unspecified number of cases of mild dizziness, fatigue, drowsiness, and nausea in people who received acupuncture (S257).

Summary of Clinical Evidence for Acupuncture and Related Therapies

While there was a diversity of interventions used to treat PHN in clinical studies, acupuncture was the most commonly used intervention. Few CM syndromes were reported with only one matching those described in clinical textbooks and clinical guidelines (*qi* or

Blood stagnation).[1-3] The acupuncture points used were broadly consistent with those recommended in textbooks and guidelines (see Chapter 11) and were similar to those used in the management of herpes zoster in the acute stage. Practitioners should use their clinical judgment in selecting acupuncture interventions to treat PHN. Based on the evidence, *ashi* points 阿是穴 and EX-B2 *Huatuojiaji* 夹脊穴 appear to contribute to pain relief and are appropriate.

Treatment duration in included RCTs was short, with only one study reporting a treatment duration of four weeks. Although this is surprising, the short timeframe may be due to the definitions of PHN that were used. As the majority of studies defined PHN as pain persisting only one month or more after the resolution of the rash, chronicity may not have been established in included participants yet.

Evidence from meta-analyses of acupuncture alone suggest that acupuncture may reduce pain scores on the VAS. However, considerable statistical heterogeneity was detected which could not be explored through subgroup analysis. While the evidence is promising, further research is needed to clarify the potential benefits of acupuncture therapies for PHN, especially through the use of established measures that assess health-related quality of life.

Not surprisingly, pain scores as measured on the VAS was the most commonly reported outcome. Many studies and meta-analyses showed that VAS pain scores with acupuncture therapies was 1–2 cm less than with pain management medications. As no minimum clinically important difference has been established for pain scores on the VAS in people with PHN, the clinical importance of these results remains uncertain.

References

1. 李曰庆, 何清湖. 中医外科学[M]. 北京: 中国中医药出版社; 2012.
2. 陈德宇. 中西医结合皮肤性病学[M]. 北京: 中国中医药出版社; 2012.
3. 杨志波, 范瑞强, 邓丙戌. 中医皮肤性病学[M]. 北京: 中国中医药出版社; 2010.

16

Clinical Evidence for Combination Therapies — Post-herpetic Neuralgia

OVERVIEW

The clinical application of Chinese medicine often involves combining various treatments. Studies of combination therapies were screened against rigorous inclusion criteria which resulted in the inclusion of 10 randomised controlled trials. The most frequently tested combination was Chinese herbal medicine with acupuncture. Analyses showed that several combinations of CM therapies can reduce pain and improve emotional wellbeing. Combination therapies were well-tolerated, with fewer adverse events reported compared with pharmacotherapy.

Introduction

Combination therapies are defined as two or more Chinese medicine (CM) interventions from different categories administered together, such as Chinese herbal medicine (CHM) plus acupuncture or CHM plus *qigong*. This approach is common in clinical practice. In this section, the clinical evidence for combination therapies from randomised controlled trials (RCTs) is evaluated.

Randomised Controlled Trials of Combination Therapies

Ten RCTs involving 1,246 participants were included for further analyses after reviewing available clinical studies against inclusion criteria (S264–S273) (see Figure 16.1). All studies were published in

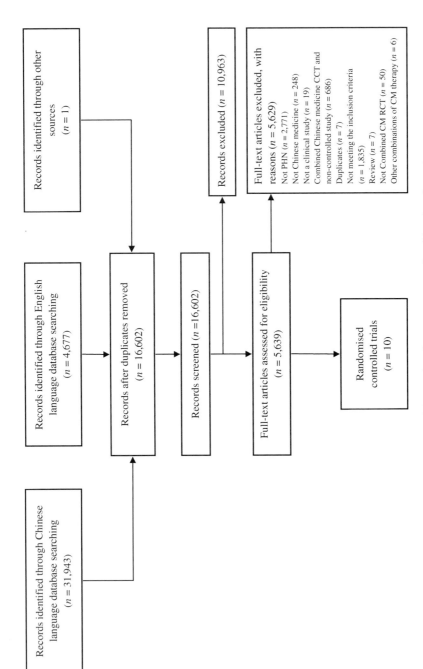

Figure 16.1 Flow chart of the study selection process: Combination therapies.

Chinese and all but one study (S272) used a two-arm parallel study design. The remaining study (S272) included three treatment arms, one of which was included in this chapter. Two studies were conducted in outpatient departments (S272, S273), six were conducted in both inpatient and outpatient departments (S264, S267–S271), and two did not specify the setting (S265, S266).

Various definitions of PHN were used. Four studies defined PHN as pain persisting at three months or more past the resolution of the rash (S265, S267, S269, S270) and five studies defined PHN as pain persisting at one month or more past the resolution of the rash (S266, S268, S271–S273). One study included people with pain after rash resolution without specifying a time-point (S264). As the lower range for the duration of PHN was more than two months, this study was included.

Participants were aged between 18 (S271) and 84 years old (S265), and the median of the mean age was 61.7 years. Slightly more males were included than females (389 males and 349 females). The durations of PHN recorded were one month or more (S267, S272, S273), with one study reporting an upper range of 37 months (S267). Treatment was provided for between two weeks (S268, S270) and 45 days (S266). None of the studies reported on follow-up assessments after the end of treatment.

CM syndrome differentiation was not described in these studies. Treatments included CHM, acupuncture, moxibustion, plumblossom needle therapy, and cupping (see Table 16.1). The most common combination was CHM plus acupuncture and was used in six studies (S264, S267, S268, S270, S272, S273). Three studies used combinations of CM as IM (S270, S272, S273).

In studies using CHM as the intervention, there were no overlaps in formulas. Forty-nine different herbs were used and the most common were *dang gui* 当归 (8 studies), *chuan xiong* 川芎 (6 studies), and *hong hua* 红花 (6 studies) (see Table 16.2). Many studies using acupuncture and other CM therapies applied treatments to acupuncture points and also used other approaches. In total, 36 acupuncture points were described across all clinical studies. The most common

Table 16.1 Summary of Combination Therapies Interventions

Combination Therapies	No. of Studies	Study References
CHM + acupuncture	6	S272, S264, S267, S268, S270, S273
CHM + moxibustion	1	S266
CHM + plum-blossom needle therapy + cupping	1	S271
CHM + plum-blossom needle therapy + moxibustion + cupping	1	S269
Acupuncture + plum-blossom needle therapy + cupping	1	S265

Table 16.2 Frequently Reported Herbs in Randomised Controlled Trials

Most Common Herbs	Scientific Name	Frequency of Use
Dang gui 当归	*Angelica sinensis* (Oliv.) Diels	8
Chuan xiong 川芎	*Ligusticum chuangxiong* Hort.	6
Hong hua 红花	*Carthamus tinctorius* L.	6
Chai hu 柴胡	*Bupleurum* spp	5
Tao ren 桃仁	*Prunus* spp	5
Gan cao 甘草	*Glycyrrhiza* spp	5
Bai shao 白芍	*Paeonia lactiflora* Pall.	5
Shui zhi 水蛭	*Whitmania* spp; *Hirudo nipponica* Whitman	4
Wu gong 蜈蚣	*Scolopendra subspinipes mutilans* L. Koch	4
Quan xie 全蝎	*Buthus martensii* Karsch	3
Ru xiang 乳香	*Boswellia* spp	3
Di long 地龙	*Pheretima* spp	3
Zhi ke 枳壳	*Citrus aurantium* L.	3
Mo yao 没药	*Commiphora* spp	3
Chi shao 赤芍	*Paeonia* spp	3

Table 16.3   **Frequently Reported Points in Randomised Controlled Trials**

Most Common Points	No. of Studies
Ashi 阿是穴	6
LR3 Taichong 太冲	5
EX-B2 Huatuojiaji 夹脊穴	5
LI4 Hegu 合谷	4
Location of pain	3
SP6 Sanyinjiao 三阴交	3
ST7 Xiaguan 下关	3
LI11 Quchi 曲池	3
ST36 Zusanli 足三里	3
GB14 Yangbai 阳白	3
GB34 Yanglingquan 阳陵泉	3

approaches included using the *ashi* points 阿是穴 (6 studies), LR3 *Taichong* 太冲, and EX-B2 *Huatuojiaji* 夹脊穴 (5 studies each) (see Table 16.3).

Combinations of CM were most frequently compared with anti-convulsant medications, either alone (S267, S270, S271, S273) or in combination with other treatments such as vitamins (S269), vitamin B1/B12 or derivatives plus non-steroidal anti-inflammatory drugs (NSAIDs) (S264, S268), vitamins plus valacyclovir (S265), and NSAIDs plus dipyridamole (S272). One study used trocyclic antidepressants (TCAs) plus other treatments as the comparator (S266).

Risk of Bias

The methodological quality of studies was assessed to identify potential sources of bias (see Table 16.4). The overall quality of included studies was low to moderate. Three studies (31.3%) were assessed as having low risk of bias for sequence generation as they used a random number table to allocate participants to groups (S268, S269,

Table 16.4   Risk of Bias of Randomised Controlled Trials: Combination Therapies

Risk of Bias Domain	Low Risk n (%)	Unclear Risk n (%)	High Risk n (%)
Sequence generation	3 (30)	7 (70)	0 (0)
Allocation concealment	0 (0)	10 (100)	0 (0)
Blinding of participants	0 (0)	0 (0)	10 (100)
Blinding of personnel	0 (0)	0 (0)	10 (100)
Blinding of outcome assessor	0 (0)	10 (100)	0 (0)
Incomplete outcome data	10 (100)	0 (0)	0 (0)
Selective outcome reporting	0 (0)	10 (100)	0 (0)

S271). The remaining studies were described as being randomised, but no description of the randomisation process was provided. Thus, these studies were assessed as having unclear risk of bias. None of the studies reported the method of allocation concealment and all were assessed as having unclear risk of bias. Neither participants nor personnel were blinded to group allocation in all studies and thus all were judged as having high risk of bias for blinding of participants and personnel.

There was insufficient information to assess whether outcome assessors were blinded to group allocation and again all studies were assessed as having unclear risk of bias for blinding of outcome assessors. None of the studies reported loss to follow up and all were assessed as having low risk of bias for incomplete outcome data. Lastly, study protocols were not available for any of the included studies and none reported trial registration; thus, all were judged as having unclear risk of bias for selective outcome reporting.

Pain Score

Nine studies reported outcomes in terms of pain scores based on the visual analogue scale (VAS) at the end of treatment (S264–S269, S271–S273). Meta-analysis was possible for the interventions CHM

Table 16.5   Chinese Herbal Medicine plus Acupuncture vs. Pharmacotherapy: Pain Score (Visual Analogue Score)

Intervention	No. of Studies (Participants)	Effect Size MD [95% CI] I²	Included Studies
CHM + acupuncture alone	3 (211)	−1.46 [−1.78, −1.15]* 0%	S264, S267, S268
CHM + acupuncture as IM	2 (217)	−1.58 [−1.93, −1.23]* 0%	S272, S273

*Statistically significant.

Abbreviations: CI, confidence interval; CHM, Chinese herbal medicine; IM, integrative medicine; MD, mean difference.

plus acupuncture alone and CHM plus acupuncture as IM (see Table 16.5). CHM plus acupuncture resulted in VAS pain scores that were 1.46 cm less than pharmacotherapy ([−1.78, −1.15], I² = 0%) and CHM as IM resulted in VAS pain scores that were 1.58 cm lower than pharmacotherapy ([−1.58, −1.23], I² = 0%).

Results from single studies showed that combination therapies were beneficial in terms of reducing VAS pain scores, with:

- CHM plus moxibustion compared with doxepin, vitamin B1, and adenosylcobalamin (a form of vitamin B12) (mean difference MD −2.14 cm [−2.82, −1.46) (S266);
- CHM plus plum-blossom needling therapy and cupping compared with carbamazepine (MD −4.00 cm [−4.87, −3.13]) (S271);
- CHM plus plum-blossom needling therapy, moxibustion, and cupping compared with pregabalin and mecobalamin (MD −1.88 cm [−2.35, −1.41]) (S269), and;
- Acupuncture plus plum-blossom needling therapy and cupping compared with carbamazepine, valacyclovir, and vitamin B12 (MD −1.76 cm [−1.83, −1.68]) (S265).

Time Taken for Resolution of Pain

One study reported the time taken for pain to resolve in 160 participants (S273). However, as the time-point from which measurement was made was not reported, the data for this outcome were not analysed.

Pittsburgh Sleep Quality Index

One study assessed the sleep quality of people with PHN (S264). CHM plus acupuncture resulted in a Pittsburgh Sleep Quality Index score that was 1.53 points lower compared with carbamazepine, mecobalamin, and ibuprofen ([−2.62, −0.44]) (S264).

Frequently Reported Herbs and Points in Meta-analyses Showing Favourable Effects

Additional analyses were conducted to identify the herbs and points which may have contributed to the positive effects seen in meta-analyses. The process for this has been described in Chapter 13. When CHM and acupuncture were used alone, seven herbs were used in two studies each (see Table 16.6). These herbs may have contributed to the positive effects observed. The most frequently reported acupuncture points in the same analysis include LI4 *Hegu* 合谷 and EX-B2 *Huatuojiaji* 夹脊穴 (3 studies each), and SP6 *Sanyinjiao* 三阴交, ST7 *Xiaguan* 下关, LI11 *Quchi* 曲池, LR3

Table 16.6 Frequently Reported Herbs in Meta-analyses Showing Favourable Effects: Chinese Herbal Medicine plus Acupuncture Alone *vs.* Pharmacotherapy

Herbs	Scientific Name	Frequency of Use
Pain outcomes: 1 meta-analysis, 3 RCTs (Table 16.5)		
Chai hu 柴胡	*Bupleurum* spp	2
Chuan xiong 川芎	*Ligusticum chuangxiong* Hort.	2
Dang gui 当归	*Angelica sinensis* (Oliv.) Diels	2
Hong hua 红花	*Carthamus tinctorius* L.	2
Shui zhi 水蛭	*Whitmania pigra* Whitman, *Hirudo nipponica* Whitman, *Whitmania acranulata* Whitman	2
Tao ren 桃仁	*Prunus* spp	2
Zhi qiao 枳壳	*Citrus aurantium* L.	2

Taichong 太冲, GB14 *Yangbai* 阳白, and *ashi* points 阿是穴 (2 studies each). Clinicians may consider using these points for the treatment of PHN.

When CHM and acupuncture was used as IM, only *dang gui* 当归 was common to both studies that reported on the VAS pain score. This herb may have contributed to the positive effects observed with CHM plus acupuncture as IM. As the number of studies included in this meta-analysis was small (2 studies), this finding should be interpreted with caution. The acupuncture or other CM therapy approach of treating the painful area was common to both studies included in the meta-analysis. This is unsurprising as it is a common approach in clinical practice.

Safety of Combination Therapies for Post-herpetic Neuralgia

Adverse events were reported in six studies (210 participants in the intervention groups and 217 participants in the comparator groups) (S266, S267, S269–S272), with one study reporting that no adverse events occurred during the trial (S267). Eleven adverse events were reported in the intervention groups, including five cases of fever and three cases of mild diarrhoea with CHM plus moxibustion (S266), one case of abnormal liver function with CHM plus plum-blossom needle therapy, moxibustion, and cupping (S269), and two cases of diarrhoea with CHM plus acupuncture as IM with carbamazepine, indomethacin, and dipyridamole (S272).

The number of adverse events in those who received guideline-recommended treatments was higher than in those who received combination therapy (29 events compared with 11 events with combination therapies). Adverse events in the guideline-recommended treatment groups included nine cases of loss of appetite and dizziness, six cases of gastrointestinal symptoms, three cases of abnormal liver function, three cases of nausea and acid reflux, two cases of muscle soreness and fatigue, and one case each of abnormal urine (details not specified), rash, renal dysfunction, mild drowsiness, and depression. In addition, there was an unspecified number of cases of mild dizziness, fatigue, drowsiness, and nausea.

Summary of Clinical Evidence for Combination Therapies

Combination therapies have been found to be beneficial in reducing pain due to PHN. The best evidence for effective pain reduction comes from multiple studies that used CHM in combination with acupuncture (alone or as IM), for which meta-analyses were possible. Results from single studies suggest that other combinations of treatments may also be beneficial both for pain and for improving emotional wellbeing. Combination therapies were well-tolerated, with fewer adverse events reported compared with those who received pharmacotherapy.

Although none of the studies reported syndrome differentiation, it appears that the approach for treating PHN in clinical studies is consistent. The herbs and acupuncture approaches used when treatments were combined were similar to those seen in reviews of treatments used alone. For example, 12 of the herbs most frequently used in CHM clinical studies were also frequently used in studies of combination therapies. Similarly, six acupuncture points or treatment approaches which were frequently reported in acupuncture clinical studies were also commonly used in studies of combination therapies.

Clinicians should exercise their judgment when selecting interventions for use in combination. Herbs such as *chai hu* 柴胡, *chuan xiong* 川芎, *dang gui* 当归, *hong hua* 红花, *shui zhi* 水蛭, *tao ren* 桃仁, and *zhi qiao* 枳壳 can be considered for herbal prescriptions. Acupuncture points LI4 *Hegu* 合谷, EX-B2 *Huatuojiaji* 夹脊穴, SP6 *Sanyinjiao* 三阴交, ST7 *Xiaguan* 下关, LI11 *Quchi* 曲池, LR3 *Taichong* 太冲, GB14 *Yangbai* 阳白, and *ashi* points 阿是穴 may be considered when combining CHM with acupuncture therapies or other CM therapies.

17

Summary and Conclusions — Post-herpetic Neuralgia

OVERVIEW

This chapter describes the 'whole evidence' analysis of Chinese medicine therapies in the management of post-herpetic neuralgia. Evidence from clinical studies are summarised and reviewed against the recommendations from contemporary texts and guidelines in Chapter 11. Few interventions recommended in contemporary literature have evidence to support their use in clinical practice. In light of these findings, directions for further research are suggested.

Introduction

In people with post-herpetic neuralgia (PHN), persistent and intractable pain can cause considerable discomfort and have a significant impact on daily life.[1] Despite the availability and demonstrated effects of various pain management medications, individual treatment response can vary[2] and many people continue to report pain most or all of the time.[3] Chinese medicine (CM) may provide a viable alternative treatment option for patients.

This monograph provides a 'whole-evidence' analysis of the evaluation of CM treatment for PHN. Recommendations from contemporary literature, including clinical practice guidelines and key CM texts, have been described in Chapter 11. Due to the complexity of identifying cases or discussions of PHN in the classical literature, this source of evidence was unable to be reviewed. However, it is likely that discussions of PHN treatment in classical CM works exist. Clinical studies have provided evidence that was evaluated to assess the treatment effects of various CM therapies for PHN (see Chapters 13, 15, and 16). Promising benefits were observed for Chinese herbal medicine (CHM) as an adjunct to pharmacological management, as were the potential benefits of acupuncture alone or as an adjunct to pharmacotherapy.

Chinese Herbal Medicine

The evidence referred to in this section can be found in Chapters 11, 13 and 16. CHM has been recommended in clinical textbooks and guidelines in Chapter 11 to treat syndromes considered likely to be PHN. CHM was also evaluated in 20 clinical studies which were included in this review. The syndromes described in key textbooks in Chapter 11 and those seen in the evidence from clinical studies had similarities. Key textbooks describe syndromes of *qi* stagnation and Blood stasis and Liver *yin* deficiency. While the syndrome of Liver *yin* deficiency was not documented in clinical studies, both *qi* stagnation and Blood stasis and *qi* deficiency with Blood stasis were reported.

None of the formulas recommended in contemporary literature were evaluated in clinical studies (see Table 17.1). One formula, *Xue fu zhu yu tang* 血府逐瘀汤, is recommended by the contemporary literature to be used in combination with *Jin ling zi san* 金铃子散. Although *Xue fu zhu yu tang* 血府逐瘀汤 was used in one randomised controlled trial (RCT), it was not used in combination with *Jin ling zi san* 金铃子散 and thus the clinical evidence for the guideline-recommended treatment remains uncertain.

The five most frequently reported herbs in all included clinical studies were *dang gui* 当归, *yan hu suo* 延胡索, *hong hua* 红花, *chai hu* 柴胡, and *chuan xiong* 川芎. Three of these herbs (*dang gui* 当归, *hong hua* 红花, and *yan hu suo* 延胡索) are ingredients of formulas recommended by clinical texts and guidelines in Chapter 11 for treating *qi* stagnation and Blood stasis. This may suggest that clinical studies are following the treatment principle of regulating *qi* and promoting Blood circulation despite not explicitly describing the treatment principle in the study report.

Table 17.1   Summary of Chinese Herbal Medicine Formulas

| Formula Name | Clinical Guidelines and Textbooks (Chapter 11) | Clinical Studies (Chapter 13) | | | Combination Therapies (Chapter 16) |
		RCTs (No. of Studies)	CCTs (No. of Studies)	Non-controlled Studies (No. of Studies)	
Chai hu shu gan san 柴胡疏肝散 plus Tao hong si wu tang 桃红四物汤 (加减) (modified)	Yes	0	0	0	0
Xue fu zhu yu tang 血府逐瘀汤 plus Jin ling zi san 金铃子散 (加减) (modified)	Yes	0	0	0	0
Xin huang pian 新癀片	Yes	0	0	0	0
Xue fu zhu yu pian/tang 血府逐瘀片/汤	Yes	0	0	0	1
Da huang zhe chong wan 大黄蛰虫丸	Yes	0	0	0	0
Yuan hu zhi tong jiao nang 元胡止痛胶囊 (capsules)	Yes	0	0	0	0
Dan shen zhu she ye 丹参注射液	Yes	0	0	0	1

Abbreviations: CCT, controlled clinical trial; RCT, randomised controlled trial.

Few clinical studies met the eligibility criteria for inclusion. This was largely due to not meeting the pre-specified definition of PHN (i.e., pain persisting for one month or more after resolution of the rash). A consensus on the definition of PHN is lacking, and such a definition would provide greater clarity about the benefits of oral CHM on chronic PHN. Evidence from included studies showed that CHM when used alone could reduce pain, although the number of studies was low. Evidence is more promising for CHM as an adjunct to pain management medication with a reduction in pain score by 1.88 cm on the pain visual analogue scale (VAS). Statistical heterogeneity was noted which limits the certainty of the findings.

Further, oral CHM may help reduce depressive symptoms when combined with pain management medications. The number of adverse events was lower in participants who received oral CHM compared with those who received pain management treatments. Based on included studies, oral CHM can be considered a safe adjunct to conventional medical management.

Chinese Herbal Medicine Formulas in Contemporary Literature and Clinical Studies

The comparison of CHM treatments across evidence types is limited to the contemporary literature described in Chapter 11 and clinical studies discussed in Chapters 13 and 16. Herbal formulas and manufactured products that are recommended for syndromes most likely to relate to PHN are described in Table 17.1. Unlike herpes zoster, there was no evidence from clinical studies where these CHM were used alone or as integrative medicine (IM) to confirm or refute the recommendations in key clinical texts. Two studies which combined CHM with acupuncture or other CM therapies used formulas recommended in key textbooks and guidelines. There is a need for high quality, well-designed clinical studies to evaluate these recommended treatments in order to inform clinical practice.

Acupuncture and Related Therapies

The evidence referred to in this section can be found in Chapters 11, 15 and 16. Many acupuncture and related therapies have been recommended in clinical practice guidelines and other key contemporary texts in Chapters 2 and 11 to treat syndromes of herpes zoster and PHN. Although acupuncture and moxibustion were described in the classical literature to treat conditions most likely to be herpes zoster, whether these therapies were also used for PHN remains unclear. The intervention most commonly evaluated in clinical studies was acupuncture, which was used in 12 of the 14 included studies.

Few clinical studies reported the CM syndromes of included participants. Of the studies that did, two syndromes were reported, specifically *qi* or Blood stagnation and *bi* and *wei* syndrome. While *qi* or Blood stagnation is similar to one of the key syndromes reported for herpes zoster and PHN, none of the reviewed guidelines or textbooks described *bi* or *wei* syndrome as specifically relating to PHN. This is likely due to the approach for diagnosis in CM where *bi* or *wei* syndrome is diagnosed as a condition and further differentiation is made to distinguish the syndrome. In this case, a patient may have *bi* syndrome with *qi* or Blood stagnation. It is notable that the Liver *yin* deficiency syndrome, which is described in a clinical monograph, was not described in any of the included studies.

The most common approaches in clinical studies of acupuncture therapies for PHN were similar to those used for herpes zoster. Acupuncture applied to EX-B2 *Huatuojiaji* points 夹脊穴 or *ashi* points 阿是穴 was used in eight of the 14 studies. Other commonly used acupuncture points included ST36 *Zusanli* 足三里, LR3 *Taichong* 太冲, LI4 *Hegu* 合谷, SP6 *Sanyinjiao* 三阴交, and TE6 *Zhigou* 支沟. This is largely reflective of the acupuncture points recommended in Chapter 11.

Due to the diversity of interventions and comparators in clinical studies, few meta-analyses were possible. Acupuncture used alone produced greater reductions in pain severity measured on the VAS than pharmacotherapy, although statistical heterogeneity was detected. Results for other interventions are primarily from single studies and further research is needed to examine their potential benefits for PHN. Few adverse events were reported in included studies, with fewer adverse events reported in participants who received acupuncture therapies compared with pharmacotherapy. Thus, acupuncture therapies appear to pose a low risk for people with PHN.

Acupuncture Therapies in Contemporary Literature and Clinical Studies

Similar to herpes zoster, acupuncture and moxibustion have been recommended in the contemporary literature (see Chapter 11) and

Table 17.2   Summary of Acupuncture Therapies

| Intervention | Clinical Guidelines and Textbooks (Chapter 11) | Clinical Studies (Chapter 15) | | | Combination Therapies (Chapter 16) |
		RCTs* (No. of Studies)	CCTs (No. of Studies)	Non-controlled Studies* (No. of Studies)	
Acupuncture (including electro-acupuncture)	Yes	8	0	7	12
Ear acupuncture	Yes	0	0	0	0
Scalp acupuncture	Yes	0	0	0	0
Moxibustion	Yes	2	0	0	3
Acupuncture-point magnetic therapy	Yes	0	0	0	0

*Some studies used more than one intervention e.g. acupuncture plus moxibustion. These are counted separately in this table.
Abbreviations: CCT, controlled clinical trial; RCT, randomised controlled trial.

were the most commonly evaluated interventions in clinical studies (see Table 17.2). Several interventions recommended in the textbooks and guidelines included in Chapter 11 were not evaluated in the clinical studies included in these analyses, such as ear acupuncture, scalp acupuncture, and acupuncture-point magnetic therapy. These interventions were also not evaluated in clinical studies for herpes zoster.

While consistency was seen for some interventions in clinical texts in Chapter 11 and clinical studies in Chapter 15, how this correlates with the treatment of PHN in ancient times remains uncertain. Based on the findings for herpes zoster, it is likely that acupuncture and moxibustion are techniques that may have been used to alleviate pain and improve other symptoms.

Implications for Practice

No guideline specifically detailing the CM management of PHN was identified in searches of the contemporary literature. There is a need for such a resource that describes the CM syndromes present in PHN as well as recommended treatments supported by evidence.

There is promising evidence for several CM therapies in the treatment of PHN. CHM as an adjunct to guideline-recommended pain management treatments reduced pain scores on the VAS. Herbs such as *dang gui* 当归, *gan cao* 甘草, *hong hua* 红花, *chai hu* 柴胡, *bai shao* 白芍, *chuan xiong* 川芎, and *tao ren* 桃仁 may have contributed to the positive effects demonstrated. Acupuncture was also observed to be similarly beneficial. Treatment approaches using *ashi* points 阿是穴 and EX-B2 *Huatuojiaji* points 夹脊穴 may have contributed to the positive effects seen in meta-analyses. Clinicians can consider using these treatments for PHN management.

Many people with PHN report that conventional pain management medications provide inadequate levels of pain control[3] and thus combinations of pain management therapies are often needed.[4] Polypharmacy may lead to undesirable drug interactions.[5] Achieving adequate pain relief for people with PHN is an unmet clinical need and CM therapies may prove to be a useful part of a patient's overall healthcare plan.

Implications for Research

There is promising evidence that CHM used as IM with guideline-recommended pain management treatments as well as acupuncture may alleviate pain for people with PHN. Many of the interventions suggested in key contemporary literature texts and guidelines lack evidence to support their use and clinicians should consider the appropriateness of interventions on a case-by-case basis.

Many of the areas for further research on herpes zoster (see Chapter 9) also apply for PHN. Improvements are needed in the scientific rigour of clinical studies, planning of interventions that reflect clinical practice, and reporting of study findings. As outlined above, there is a need for greater focus on PHN as a condition in its own right in CM contemporary literature. A clinical practice guideline for PHN would address this knowledge gap.

Findings from experimental studies suggest that many herbs act on herpes zoster and PHN through their anti-nociceptive and anti-inflammatory properties. Further research in this area is warranted to enhance the understanding of how CHM may contribute to pain modulation through *in vitro* and *in vivo* models. Identification of the most promising forms of CHM for pain modulation should direct future clinical research.

Future research must carefully consider the definition used for PHN. Many of the clinical studies reviewed for eligibility failed to clearly describe any definition of PHN, let alone one that would allow the reader to estimate the likelihood of participants actually having PHN and not simply generic pain as part of the healing process of herpes zoster. However, in the absence of a consensus on the definition of PHN, researchers should use the commonly accepted PHN definition of pain persisting for three or more months after the resolution of the rash.[6]

References

1. Johnson RW, Whitton TL. Management of herpes zoster (shingles) and postherpetic neuralgia. *Exp Opin Pharmacother.* 2004; **5**(3):551–9.
2. Rowbotham MC, Petersen KL. Zoster-associated pain and neural dysfunction. *Pain.* 2001; **93**(1):1–5.
3. Serpell M, Gater A, Carroll S, *et al.* Burden of post-herpetic neuralgia in a sample of UK residents aged 50 years or older: Findings from the Zoster Quality of Life (ZQOL) study. *Health Qual Life Outcomes.* 2014; **12**:92.
4. Dworkin RH, O'Connor AB, Audette J, *et al.* Recommendations for the pharmacological management of neuropathic pain: An overview and literature update. *Mayo Clin Proc.* 2010; **85**(3 Suppl):S3–14.
5. Gater A, Abetz-Webb L, Carroll S, Mannan A, Serpell M, Johnson R. Burden of herpes zoster in the UK: Findings from the zoster quality of life (ZQOL) study. *BMC Infect Dis.* 2014; **14**:402.
6. Dworkin RH, Portenoy RK. Pain and its persistence in herpes zoster. *Pain.* 1996; **67**(2–3):241–51.

Glossary

Terms	Acronym	Definition	Reference
95% confidence interval	95% CI	A measure of the uncertainty around the main finding of a statistical analysis. Estimates of unknown quantities, such as the odds ratio comparing an experimental intervention with a control, are usually presented as a point estimate and a 95% confidence interval. This means that if someone were to keep repeating a study in other samples from the same population, 95% of the confidence intervals from those studies would contain the true value of the unknown quantity. Alternatives to 95% confidence intervals, such as 90% and 99% confidence intervals, are sometimes used. Wider intervals indicate lower precision; narrow intervals, greater precision	https://training.cochrane.org/handbook
Acupressure	—	Application of pressure on acupuncture points	—

(Continued)

(Continued)

Terms	Acronym	Definition	Reference
Acupuncture	—	The insertion of needles into humans or animals for remedial purposes	WHO International Standard Terminologies of Traditional Medicine in the Western Pacific Region. World Health Organisation; 2007.
Allied and Complementary Medicine Database	AMED	Alternative medicine bibliographic database	https://www.ebscohost.com/products/research-databases/allied-and-complementary-medicine-database-amed
Australian New Zealand Clinical Trial Registry	ANZCTR	Clinical trial registry based in Australian	www.anzctr.org.au/
China National Knowledge Infrastructure	CNKI	Chinese language bibliographic database	www.cnki.net
Chinese Biomedical Literature database	CBM	Chinese language bibliographic database	www.imicams.ac.cn
Chinese Clinical Trial Registry	ChiCTR	Chinese clinical trial registry	http://www.chictr.org.cn/
Chinese herbal medicine	CHM	Chinese herbal medicine	—
Chinese medicine	CM	—	—
Chongqing VIP Information Company	CQVIP	Chinese language bibliographic database	www.cqvip.com
ClinicalTrials.gov	—	Clinical trial registry based in the United States of America	https://clinicaltrials.gov/
Cochrane Central Register of Controlled Trials	CENTRAL	Bibliographic database that provides a highly concentrated source of reports of controlled trials	https://community.cochrane.org/editorial-and-publishing-policy-resource/overview-cochrane-library-and-related-content/databases-included-cochrane-central-register-controlled-trials-central

(Continued)

(*Continued*)

Terms	Acronym	Definition	Reference
Combination therapies	—	Two or more Chinese medicines from different therapy groups (e.g., Chinese herbal medicine, acupuncture therapies, or other Chinese medicine therapies) administered together	—
Controlled clinical trials	CCT	A study in which people are allocated to different interventions using methods that are not random	95% CI
Convention on International Trade in Endangered Species of Wild Fauna and Flora	CITES	International convention aimed at preventing or regulating trade in treetend and endangered species of plants and animals	www.cites.org/eng/disc/text.php
Cumulative Index of Nursing and Allied Health Literature	CINAHL	Bibliographic database	https://www.ebscohost.com/nursing/products/cinahl-databases
Cupping therapy	—	Suction by using a vaccumised cup or jar	WHO International Standard Terminologies of Traditional Medicine in the Western Pacific Region. World Health Organisation; 2007.
Dermatology Life Quality Index	DLQI	A measure of quality of life related to dermatological conditions	Menter A, Gottlieb A, Feldman SR, Van Voorhees AS, Leonardi CL, Gordon KB, *et al.* Guidelines of care for the management of psoriasis and psoriatic arthritis: Section 1. Overview of psoriasis and guidelines of care for the treatment of psoriasis with biologics. J Am Acad Dermatol. 2008; 58(5):826–50.
Effect size	—	A generic term for the estimate of the; effect of a; treatment in a study	95% CI

(*Continued*)

(*Continued*)

Terms	Acronym	Definition	Reference
Effective rate	—	A measure of the proportion of participants who achieved an improvement as outlined in Chapter 4	—
Electro-acupuncture	—	Electric stimulation of the acupuncture needle following insertion	WHO International Standard Terminologies of Traditional Medicine in the Western Pacific Region. World Health Organisation; 2007.
EU Clinical Trials Register	EU-CTR	European clinical trial registry	www.clinicaltrialsregister.eu
Excerpta Medica dataBASE	Embase	Bibliographic database	www.elsevier.com/solutions/embase
Grading of Recommendations Assessment, Development, and Evaluation	GRADE	Approach used to grade the quality of evidence and strength of recommendations	www.gradeworkinggroup.org/
Health-related quality of life	HR-QoL	A conceptual or operational measurement that is commonly used in the healthcare setting as a means to assess the impact of disease on the person	Brooker C. Mosby's dictionary of medicine, nursing and health professions. Elsevier: United Kingdom; 2010
Heterogeneity	—	Used in a general sense to describe the variation in, or diversity of, participants, interventions, and measurement of outcomes across a set of studies, or the variation in internal validity of those studies. Used specifically, as statistical heterogeneity, to describe the degree of variation in the effect estimates from a set of studies. Also used to indicate the presence of variability among studies beyond the amount expected due solely to the play of chance	handbook.cochrane.org/

(*Continued*)

(Continued)

Terms	Acronym	Definition	Reference
Homogeneity	—	Used in a general sense to mean that the participants, interventions, and measurement of outcomes are similar across a set of studies. Used specifically to describe the effect estimates from a set of studies where they do not vary more than would be expected by chance	handbook.cochrane.org/
I^2	—	A measure of study heterogeneity which indicates the percentage of variance in a meta-analysis	95% Confidence Interval
Integrative medicine	—	Chinese herbal medicine combined with pharmacotherapy or other conventional therapy	
Mean difference	MD	In meta-analysis: A method used to combine measures on continuous scales, where the mean, standard deviation, and sample size in each group are known. The weight given to the difference in means from each study (e.g., how much influence each study has on the overall results of the meta-analysis) is determined by the precision of its estimate of effect; mathematically, this is equal to the inverse of the variance. This method assumes that all of the trials have measured the outcome on the same scale	95% Confidence Interval
Meta-analysis	—	The use of statistical techniques in a systematic review to integrate the results of included studies. Sometimes misused as a synonym for systematic reviews, where the review includes a meta-analysis	—

(Continued)

(Continued)

Terms	Acronym	Definition	Reference
Moxibustion	—	A therapeutic procedure involving ignited material (usually moxa) to apply heat to certain points or areas of the body surface for curing disease	WHO International Standard Terminologies of Traditional Medicine in the Western Pacific Region. World Health Organisation; 2007.
Non-controlled studies	—	Observations made on individuals, usually receiving the same intervention, before and after; the intervention but with no control group	95% Confidence Interval
Other Chinese medicine therapies	—	Other Chinese medicine therapies include all traditional therapies except Chinese herbal medicine and acupuncture moxibustion, such as *tai chi*, *qigong*, *tuina*, and cupping	
PubMed	PubMed	Bibliographic database	www.ncbi.nlm.nih.gov/pubmed
Qigong 气功	—	Physical exercises and breathing techniques	—
Randomised controlled trial	RCT	A clinical trial that uses a random method to allocate participants to treatment and control groups	—
Risk of bias	—	Assessment of clinical trials to indicate if results may overestimate or underestimate the true effect because of bias in study design or reporting	95% CI

(Continued)

(Continued)

Terms	Acronym	Definition	Reference
Risk ratio (relative risk)	RR	The ratio of risks in two groups. In intervention studies, it is the ratio of the risk in the intervention group to the risk in the control group. A risk ratio of one indicates no difference between comparison groups. For undesirable outcomes, a risk ratio that is less than one indicates that the intervention was effective in reducing the risk of that outcome	95% CI
Standardised mean difference	SMD	"Similar to mean difference (MD). Used when different instruments are used to measure the same construct. The SMD expresses the intervention effect in standard units rather than the original units of measurement. As a 'rule of thumb', an SMD of 0.2 represents a small effect, 0.5 a moderate effect, and 0.8 a large effect"	95% CI
Summary of findings	—	Presentation of results and rating the quality of evidence based on the GRADE approach	www.gradeworkinggroup. org/
Tai chi (taiji 推拿)	—	Physical exercises and breathing techniques	—
Transcutaneous electrical nerve stimulation	TENS	Application of transdermal electrical current to acupuncture points via conducting pads	—

(Continued)

(Continued)

Terms	Acronym	Definition	Reference
Tuina 推拿	—	Chinese massage: rubbing, kneading, or percussion of the soft tissues and joints of the body with the hands, usually performed by one person on another, especially to relieve tension or pain	WHO International Standard Terminologies of Traditional Medicine in the Western Pacific Region. World Health Organisation; 2007.
Tumour necrosis factor-alpha	TNF-α	A cytokine that is toxic to cancer cells and activates other leukocytes. It causes profound metabolic effects that include inflammatory responses, pyrexia, and weight loss leading to cachexia	Brooker C. Mosby's dictionary of medicine, nursing and health professions. Elsevier: United Kingdom; 2010
Wangfang database	Wanfang	Chinese language bibliographic database	www.wanfangdata.com
World Health Organisation	WHO	WHO is the directing and coordinating authority for health within the United Nations system. It is responsible for providing leadership on global health matters, shaping the health research agenda, setting norms and standards, articulating evidence-based policy options, providing technical support to countries, and monitoring and assessing health trends	www.who.int/about/en/

(Continued)

Terms	Acronym	Definition	Reference
Zhong Hua Yi Dian 中华医典	ZHYD	The Zhong Hua Yi Dian (ZHYD) 'Encyclopaedia of Traditional Chinese Medicine' is a comprehensive series of electronic books in CD-ROM format. The collection was put together by the Hunan electronic and audio-visual publishing house. It is the largest collection of Chinese electronic books and includes major Chinese ancient works, many of which are from rare manuscripts and are the only existing copies. These books cover the period from ancient times up to the period of the Republic of China (1911–1948)	Hu R, editor. Zhong Hua Yi Dian [Encyclopaedia of Traditional Chinese Medicine]. 4th ed. Chengsha: Hunan Electronic and Audio-Visual Publishing House; 2000.
Zhong Yi Fang Ji Da Ci Dian 中医方剂大辞典	ZYFJDCD	Compendium of Chinese herbal formulas with over 96,592 entries derived from classical Chinese books. The Nanjing Chinese Medicine Institute compiled the ZYFJDCD and first published it in 1993	Peng HR, editor Zhong Yi Fang, Ji Da Ci Dian [Great Compendium of Chinese Medical Formulae]. 1st ed. Beijing: People's Medical Publishing House, 1994

Appendix 1: References for Included Clinical Studies

Study No.	Reference
S1	叶田, 张剑, 邓永琼, 杨春艳. 喜炎平注射液治疗带状疱疹临床疗效观察[J]. 现代医药卫生, 2011,19:2908–2909.
S2	买建修. 中西医结合治疗带状疱疹34例[J]. 中医研究, 2009,07:51–52.
S3	赵梁, 赵季友, 谭达全. 五味消毒饮加减治疗带状疱疹39例总结[J]. 湖南中医杂志, 2013,10:53–54.
S4	王俊. 中西医结合治疗带状疱疹疗效观察[J]. 健康必读 (中旬刊), 2012, 11(12):233.
S5	肖云, 汪黔蜀, 李雁. 中西医结合治疗带状疱疹疗效观察[J]. 现代中西医结合杂志, 2007,28:4182–4183.
S6	史成和, 王秀娟. 凉血解毒通络中药治疗早期带状疱疹[J]. 中国实验方剂学杂志, 2010,11:197–199.
S7	周万伟. 辩证治疗带状疱疹及对后遗神经痛发生率的影响的观察[D]. 湖北中医药大学, 2011.
S8	刘成祥. 中药联合火针治疗肝经郁热型带状疱疹的临床观察[D]. 黑龙江中医药大学, 2014.
S9	黄志萍, 陈丽, 孙丽红. 中西医结合治疗带状疱疹34例疗效观察及临床护理[J]. 齐鲁护理杂志, 2014,05:91–92.
S10	马学伟, 苗文丽, 陈虎, 张培红, 刘京芳, 刘珊珊. 缬草清郁汤治疗老年带状疱疹40例[J]. 中国老年学杂志, 2012,08:1612–1613.
S11	王素梅, 吴玉敏, 赵浩. 带疱解毒汤联合泛昔洛韦和腺苷钴胺治疗老年带状疱疹临床观察[J]. 中华保健医学杂志, 2012,05:389–391.
S12	王万平. 加味龙胆泻肝汤联合泛昔洛韦治疗肝胆湿热型带状疱疹的临床疗效观察[J]. 中医临床研究, 2012,07:32–34.

(*Continued*)

(*Continued*)

Study No.	Reference
S13	杨爱霞, 冯永芳, 谢岱. 退热解毒灵颗粒辅助治疗带状疱疹30例[J]. 医药导报, 2010,06:725–726.
S14	张振汉. 西医常规治疗加中医辨证治疗带状疱疹疗效观察[J]. 广西中医药, 2011,05:14.
S15	贺芳, 蔡爱萍, 刘永胜. 中药治疗带状疱疹86例[J]. 中国中医急症, 2005,07: 638.
S16	庄志刚, 郭艳严, 丁飒爽. 神经阻滞加中药内服治疗带状疱疹神经痛疗效观察[J]. 中国实用神经疾病杂志, 2010,02:58–59.
S17	周淑桂, 高春秀. 薏苡竹叶散加味治疗脾经湿盛型蛇串疮疗效观察[J]. 北京中医药, 2008,05:369–370.
S18	江应政. 龙胆泻肝汤合川芎茶调散治疗带状疱疹110例[J]. 中国中医急症, 2010,08:1431–1432.
S19	施向红. 龙胆泻肝汤治疗带状疱疹60例[J]. 实用中医药杂志, 2001,10: 18–19.
S20	周海啸, 舒友廉, 许慧荣. 龙胆泻肝汤加味治疗带状疱疹临床疗效分析[J]. 中国中西医结合皮肤性病学杂志, 2004,02:99–100.
S21	卓堪培, 吴兆怀. 龙胆泻肝汤配合洗剂治疗老年性带状疱疹疗效观察[J]. 中国保健, 2010(10):122–123.
S22	杜耀战. 中西医结合治疗带状疱疹[J]. 光明中医, 2008,09:1289.
S23	廖兴隆, 张新强. 龙胆泻肝丸联合抗病毒药治疗带状疱疹30例临床观察[J]. 医学临床研究, 2014,(4):785–787.
S24	刘屹嵩, 樊开斌, 宋建强, 闫征斌. 中西医结合治疗带状疱疹的临床疗效观察[J]. 中国伤残医学, 2014,03:162–163.
S25	施桂泉, 李银元. 中西医结合治疗带状疱疹48例临床疗效观察[J]. 中国实用医药, 2013,03:177–178.
S26	吴丹. 中老年带状疱疹98例临床分析[J]. 医学美学美容 (中旬刊), 2013,(4):76.
S27	张传文. 中医辨证治疗带状疱疹的疗效观察[J]. 中国中医药咨讯, 2011, 3(16):431.
S28	蒋成章. 中医药治疗老年带状疱疹疼痛68例疗效观察[J]. 湖南中医药导报, 2002,09:553–554.
S29	宋振霞, 吕喜东. 中医辨证治疗带状疱疹的临床疗效[J]. 中国医药指南, 2011, 24:121–122.

(*Continued*)

Study No.	Reference
S30	曹周军. 中西医结合治疗带状疱疹42例[J]. 湖南中医杂志, 2010,05:83–84.
S31	孙毅刚. 龙胆泻肝汤加减治疗肝经郁热型带状疱疹的临床心得[J]. 当代医学, 2010,18:146–147.
S32	荆玉强. 清热利湿活血解毒法治疗带状疱疹临床疗效探讨[J]. 中医药信息, 2001,03:46.
S33	尹景霞, 梁连秀. 六神丸加阿昔洛韦治疗带状疱疹40例临床观察[J]. 吉林中医药, 2006,08:44.
S34	王翠连. 中西医结合治疗带状疱疹的疗效观察[J]. 内蒙古中医药, 2008,14:16–17.
S35	刘世贵, 徐桂萍, 侯茹. 拔毒涂膜剂的制备及临床观察[J]. 陕西中医学院学报, 2006,01:59–60.
S36	韩晓东, 许静, 吴范武. 傅青主火丹神方治疗带状疱疹37例临床观察[J]. 四川中医, 2007,04:91–92.
S37	高建刚. 中西医结合治疗带状疱疹的疗效观察[J]. 齐齐哈尔医学院学报, 2010,01:56.
S38	要武. 柴虎蚣蝎汤治疗带状疱疹80例[J]. 中国中西医结合杂志, 2002,10:788.
S39	冯永芳. 元通合剂联合伐昔洛韦治疗带状疱疹疗效观察[J]. 湖北中医杂志, 2010,03:55.
S40	田瑛瑜, 付索菊, 赵海燕. 消疹止痛汤加减治疗带状疱疹46例[J]. 河南中医, 2006,04:46.
S41	张惠芬, 丘秋香, 钟燕香. 草药七色花治疗带状疱疹的疗效观察与护理[J]. 护理实践与研究, 2013,06:63–64.
S42	张利君, 徐传华. 行气祛瘀汤联合阿昔洛韦治疗老年带状疱疹46例[J]. 中国中医药科技, 2013,04:430–431.
S43	高月平, 赵永辰, 罗金花. 青冰散外敷治疗带状疱疹疗效观察[J]. 中国皮肤性病学杂志, 2010,10:936.
S44	顾介礼, 单宝春. 中西医结合治疗带状疱疹42例. 中华当代医学[J], 2004, 2(9):67.
S45	王玉兰, 靳宝富, 张秀桃, 杨俊丽. 中西医结合治疗带状疱疹神经痛49例临床观察[J]. 临床医药实践, 2009,31:876–877.
S46	朱运喜, 王海涛, 丁丽君. 中药外敷治疗带状疱疹80例[J]. 中医杂志, 2007, 07:591.

(Continued)

(Continued)

Study No.	Reference
S47	钟捷, 余艳兰, 涂丽, 刘红娜. 西南文殊兰联合龙血竭治疗与护理带状疱疹的疗效观察[J]. 中医药导报, 2013,05:120–121.
S48	朱永辉. 局部外用板蓝根液治疗带状疱疹51例疗效观察[J]. 现代中西医结合杂志, 2004,06:732–733.
S49	梁天山, 吴艳华, 李其林. 中药薰蒸联合阿昔洛韦静脉滴注治疗带状疱疹40例疗效观察[J]. 皮肤性病诊疗学杂志, 2014,04:308–310.
S50	王明志, 王淑安, 赵莉等. 中西医结合治疗带状疱疹的疗效分析[J]. 中国伤残医学, 2014,(11):113–114.
S51	常玉山. 中药外敷联合阿西洛韦治疗带状疱疹疗效观察[J]. 中国民族民间医药, 2009,17:72.
S52	胡冰. 中药湿敷联合阿昔洛韦治疗带状疱疹临床观察[J]. 中国中医急症, 2013,07:1244–1245.
S53	杨建春, 徐鸿雁, 刘玉兰. 中西医结合治疗带状疱疹临床疗效观察[J]. 亚太传统医药, 2012,12:71–72.
S54	庄洪建, 渠鹏程, 揣瑞梅等. 阿昔洛韦联合中频交流电透入中药治疗带状疱疹疗效分析[C]. 山东中医药学会皮肤病专业委员会成立暨第一次学术会议论文集, 2005:133–134.
S55	黄东平. 中西医结合治疗带状疱疹42例临床分析[J]. 中医学报, 2014, 29(B07):88.
S56	张学权. 中药内外合治带状疱疹62例疗效观察[J]. 云南中医中药杂志, 2010,07:33.
S57	郎娜. 毒瘀并解方治疗带状疱疹毒瘀互结证的临床研究[D]. 中国中医科学院, 2007.
S58	王红. 龙血竭联合腺苷钴胺治疗中老年人带状疱疹疗效观察[J]. 中国基层医药, 2014(19):2963–2964.
S59	徐春凤, 张艳. 加味小柴胡汤治疗带状疱疹36例[J]. 国际中医中药杂志, 2014,36(7):662–663.
S60	徐翔, 梁东辉, 马红利. 新癀片治疗带状疱疹早期神经痛的序贯试验[J]. 药物流行病学杂志, 2011,08:385–387.
S61	郑玉莲, 赵善萍, 陈光林, 张畅, 王睿. 中西医结合治疗中老年患者带状疱疹急性期29例临床观察[J]. 江苏中医药, 2014,05:46–47.
S62	李应宏, 赵明芳. 伐昔洛韦联合中药治疗中老年带状疱疹50例[J]. 中医研究, 2012,05:24–26.

(Continued)

(Continued)

Study No.	Reference
S63	甄君. 紫草消疹汤联合神经阻滞治疗带状疱疹的疗效观察[J]. 中国中西医结合杂志, 2002,10:747.
S64	徐鸿雁. 解毒活血汤配合芦黄散治疗带状疱疹疗效观察[J]. 新中医, 2011,01:48–49.
S65	许德坚, 刘春辉. 中草药内外合用治疗蛇串疮的临床疗效观察[J]. 医药产业资讯, 2006,15:219.
S66	张晓军, 钱龙江. 清解化瘀组方治疗带状疱疹58例[J]. 河南中医, 2014,11:2227–2228.
S67	龚立军, 张娟红, 杜华, 柳文红, 徐凡翔. 独一味胶囊对带状疱疹患者的镇痛作用[J]. 西南军医, 2014,05:515–516.
S68	万桂芹. 三仁汤加减治疗蛇串疮45例临床观察[J]. 中国医药导报, 2010,16:109–110.
S69	毕春生, 孔连委, 马林. 疱疹颗粒剂治疗肝经郁热型带状疱疹60例临床疗效观察[J]. 黑龙江中医药, 2010,01:13.
S70	李启文. 胆草解毒汤治疗带状疱疹38例[J]. 中国医药学报, 2004,05:318.
S71	汤国华. 用通络凉血解毒汤治疗带状疱疹的临床疗效分析[J]. 当代医药论丛, 2014,02:154–155.
S72	钟萍. 和解清热法治疗带状疱疹热毒互结证的理论与临床研究[D]. 南京中医药大学, 2009.
S73	郜家平, 孙学东. 丹参酮胶囊防治老年带状疱疹后遗神经痛92例[J]. 中国麻风皮肤病杂志, 2007,06:547.
S74	李奇俊. 疏风解毒胶囊治疗带状疱疹的临床观察[J]. 河南中医, 2014,(B11):582–583.
S75	赵敏. 清开灵分散片联合伐昔洛韦治疗带状疱疹89例疗效观察[J]. 数理医药学杂志, 2013,01:78–79.
S76	李国泉, 陈明春. 盐酸万乃洛韦联合复方甘草酸苷治疗带状疱疹46例疗效分析[J]. 中国煤炭工业医学杂志, 2007,05:540–541.
S77	王鑫玺. 中西医结合治疗带状疱疹的疗效观察[J]. 大家健康(学术版), 2014,21:39–40.
S78	席建元, 陈达灿. 中西医结合治疗带状疱疹40例临床观察[J]. 中国中西医结合杂志, 2007,01:75.
S79	张伊平, 石娜. 百癣夏塔热片联合半导体激光治疗带状疱疹疗效观察[J]. 中国社区医师(医学专业), 2012,18:227.

(Continued)

(Continued)

Study No.	Reference
S80	周克伟, 宋顺鹏, 吕成志, 李波, 郑义宏. 加味小柴胡汤治疗头面部带状疱疹22例临床观察[J]. 中国保健营养, 2013,01:441.
S81	张晓军, 钱龙江. 中西医结合治疗带状疱疹疗效观察[J]. 中医学报, 2013, 28(B08):84.
S82	马文宇. 润燥止痒胶囊在治疗老年性带状疱疹患者中的应用[J]. 现代中医药, 2010,05:37.
S83	王恒明, 孙浩. 如意珍宝丸联合伐昔洛韦治疗带状疱疹疗效观察[J]. 山西中医, 2013,05:28–29.
S84	买建修. 胃苓汤合柴胡疏肝饮加减治疗带状疱疹临床观察[J]. 辽宁中医药大学学报, 2008,09:86.
S85	鲁飞. 阿昔洛韦配合中药治疗带状泡疹的疗效分析[J]. 中华现代临床医学杂志, 2003,1(3):244–245.
S86	王德霞. 中药拔毒膏外敷治疗带状疱疹32例疗效观察与护理干预[J]. 北方药学, 2013,04:188–189.
S87	程桂芝, 姜建德. 自拟方清疹止痛膏治疗带状疱疹30例临床疗效观察[J]. 中国医药指南, 2012,24:575–576.
S88	宋欢, 陈丽敏, 赵金涛. 中西医结合治疗带状疱疹急性期临床观察[J]. 实用中医药杂志, 2014,04:297–298.
S89	宋泽恩. 综合法治疗带状疱疹39例疗效观察[J]. 当代医学, 2012,09:150–151.
S90	郑改琴, 王迪. 三粉擦剂治疗带状疱疹40例[J]. 陕西中医, 2011,06:710–711.
S91	周书会. 伤科灵喷雾剂联合泛昔洛韦治疗带状疱疹疗效观察[J]. 当代医学, 2012,31:144–145.
S92	陆富永. 中药外治联合阿昔洛韦治疗带状疱疹[J]. 华夏医学, 2004,03:402–403.
S93	徐运安. 中西药不同方案治疗带状疱疹的成本-效果分析[J]. 中国药房, 2005,01:37–38.
S94	楼小慧. 疱疹散联合止痛汤治疗带状疱疹47例临床观察[J]. 甘肃中医学院学报, 2014,02:45–46.
S95	周光全, 徐文君. 伤科接骨片辅治中老年人带状疱疹神经痛30例疗效观察[J]. 临床合理用药杂志, 2012,22:101–102.
S96	陈长江, 汪雪晴, 尚政琴. 龙胆泻肝汤加减配金黄膏治疗带状疱疹92例[J]. 中国中医急症, 2011,12:2049.

(Continued)

Study No.	Reference
S97	李群康. 扶正祛邪中药治疗带状疱疹72例临床观察[J]. 健康之路, 2013, 12(5):328–329.
S98	梁洁利. 中西医结合治疗带状疱疹68例[J]. 医学理论与实践, 2002, 04:432.
S99	马国安, 王宝娟, 丁红炜. 自拟灭痛消疱汤联合泛昔洛韦和氦氖激光治疗带状疱疹疗效观察[J]. 中国中医药信息杂志, 2013,09:77–78.
S100	徐羹年, 沈培红, 林坚. 中西药物联合治疗中老年带状疱疹的疗效观察[J]. 浙江医学, 2008,03:280–282.
S101	郭静, 秦悦思, 刘瑶. 初探三焦辨证分部位治疗带状疱疹临床疗效[J]. 辽宁中医杂志, 2011,07:1385–1386.
S102	傅刚玉. 中西医结合治疗带状疱疹临床探讨[J]. 中国当代医药, 2009,03: 29–30.
S103	邝敏. 中西医结合治疗带状疱疹32例[J]. 实用中医药杂志, 2012,01:27.
S104	唐艺洪. 柴胡疏肝散治疗带状疱疹60例[J]. 中国中医药现代远程教育, 2010,09:47–48.
S105	严晓萍. 中西医结合辨治带状疱疹120例临床疗效分析[J]. 新医学导刊, 2008,7(3):23–24.
S106	陈建强. 任绪东主任医师治疗带状疱疹的经验[J]. 广西中医药, 2012,04: 36–37.
S107	崔炎, 代洪娜, 张榜, 刘兴涛, 刘宝辉. 崔公让治疗早期带状疱疹经验[J]. 辽宁中医杂志, 2012,10:1921–1922.
S108	杨正华. 中医辨证治疗带状疱疹2例报告[J]. 青岛医药卫生, 1994,03:40.
S109	郭家树. 加味龙胆泻肝汤治疗带状疱疹28例[J]. 云南中医中药杂志, 2009,09:81.
S110	林丽. 银紫解毒汤治疗带状疱疹36例疗效观察[J]. 云南中医中药杂志, 2004,03:14–15.
S111	武双智. 龙胆泻肝汤加减治疗带状疱疹80例[J]. 中华临床医药杂志(广州), 2003(62):95.
S112	陈艺娟. 带状疱疹临床诊治体会[J]. 云南中医中药杂志, 2007,10:16–17.
S113	于丽荣. 青黛治疗带状疱疹[J]. 中医杂志, 2005,12:894–895.
S114	李春明. 综合疗法治疗带状疱疹100例疗效观察[J]. 云南中医中药杂志, 2013,01:86.

(Continued)

(Continued)

Study No.	Reference
S115	李琴. 龙胆泻肝汤合二味膏治疗带状疱疹34例疗效观察[J]. 青海医药杂志, 1998,06:49.
S116	秦宗碧. 加味龙胆泻肝汤联合黄连膏外敷治疗带状疱疹38例临床观察[J]. 中国实用医药, 2012,11:154.
S117	李继端. 更昔洛韦联合龙胆泻肝汤治疗带状疱疹60例疗效观察[J]. 山西医药杂志(下半月刊), 2012,04: 401–402.
S118	杨长友. 中西医结合治疗带状疱疹42例临床总结[J]. 现代中医药, 2004,05:38.
S119	张跃营, 江韦宏, 艾儒棣. 中西医联合用药治疗带状疱疹35例[J]. 甘肃中医, 2010,12:47–48.
S120	黄丽敏. 中西医结合治疗带状疱疹16例[J]. 现代诊断与治疗, 2001,03:190.
S121	张磊. 中医药治疗带状疱疹临床观察[J]. 中华中西医学杂志, 2009,7(7): 42–43.
S122	孔文霞, 雷胜琪, 陈朝章. 内外合治带状疱疹[J]. 新中医, 2000,03:54.
S123	王文远, 朱毓生. 清上防风汤加减治疗头面部皮肤病[J]. 浙江中西医结合杂志, 2009,11:703–704.
S124	龙雄初, 龙枚飞, 李晓玲, 赵社海. 从"郁"论治——应用自拟方解郁清毒散治疗带状疱疹146例临床分析[J]. 临床和实验医学杂志, 2012,15: 1182–1183+1185.
S125	鲍正飞. 自拟消痰饮治疗带状疱疹93例[J]. 四川中医, 1998,07:41.
S126	陈文展. 老年人带状疱疹治验[A]. 中华中医药学会、重庆市中西医结合学会. 中华中医药学会皮肤科分会第七次学术年会、2010年重庆四川中西医结合皮肤性病学术年会、全国中西医结合诊疗皮肤性病新进展新技术学习班论文汇编[C]. 中华中医药学会、重庆市中西医结合学会, 2010:1.
S127	胡秀荣, 田晓晔. 应用雄黄油治疗带状疱疹116例[J]. 辽宁中医杂志, 2006,06:720.
S128	霍玉军. 虎甘散治疗带状疱疹46例[J]. 医学信息(上旬刊), 2011,04: 2050–2051.
S129	毛瑞源, 范丽, 王杰. 冰雄散外敷治疗带状疱疹32例[J]. 中国中医药信息杂志, 1999,11:19.
S130	牛鸿春. 大黄五倍子膏治疗带状疱疹40例[J]. 中医外治杂志, 2009,01:8.

(Continued)

(Continued)

Study No.	Reference
S131	唐燕. 芍药地黄汤加味治疗带状疱疹55例[J]. 实用中医药杂志, 2014,03:198.
S132	王艳艳. 三黄二香散治疗带状疱疹52例疗效观察与护理体会[J]. 中国保健营养, 2012,18:4037–4038.
S133	王正杰, 宁鸿珍. 复方雄黄软膏剂治疗带状疱疹58例临床疗效观察[J]. 今日健康, 2014,13(1):65–66.
S134	伊合帕尔·木拉提, 艾合买提·买买提, 米热古丽·卡米力. 维吾尔医治疗带状疱疹32例临床观察[A]. 内蒙古自治区中蒙医研究所、全国中医药信息工作委员会. 第四届全国民族医药学术交流暨《中国民族医药杂志》创刊10周年庆典大会论文集[C]. 内蒙古自治区中蒙医研究所、全国中医药信息工作委员会, 2005:1.
S135	戴国树. 龙芎汤治疗带状疱疹75例[J]. 河南中医学院学报, 2005,05:67–68.
S136	付玉玲. 中药内服加外敷治疗带状疱疹52例[J]. 中医外治杂志, 2007, 05:38.
S137	蒋薇, 辛大永. 黄连解毒汤加味治疗带状疱疹67例[J]. 实用中医内科杂志, 2002,04:227.
S138	孔松明. 清热解毒除湿汤治疗蛇串疮62例[J]. 内江科技, 2000,04:26.
S139	程立新, 史佩珍. 京万红治疗带状疱疹25例[J]. 解放军护理杂志, 2006,02:18.
S140	杜晓虹. 季德胜蛇药外敷治疗老年人带状疱疹疼痛40例疗效分析[J]. 内蒙古中医药, 2014,11:10.
S141	金鑫. 中西医结合治疗带状疱疹临床分析[J]. 中国医药指南, 2010,09:101–102.
S142	刘武, 廖红玲, 孙艳. 中西医结合治疗带状疱疹65例临床疗效观察[J]. 中华综合医学杂志(河北), 2004,6(1):29.
S143	龙云群. 连花清瘟胶囊治疗带状疱疹26例临床观察[J]. 浙江中医杂志, 2013,09:663.
S144	赵国萍. 中西医结合治疗带状疱疹48例疗效观察[J]. 当代医学, 2010, 32:144.
S145	郑直, 郑自忠. 带状疱疹28例疗效观察[J]. 医药与保健, 2014,(10):43.
S146	祝德超. 中西医结合治疗带状疱疹96例临床分析[J]. 现代中医药, 2005,01:39–40.

(Continued)

(*Continued*)

Study No.	Reference
S147	苗伟, 李如华, 缪新华, 王立平, 陈艳玲, 孙显军, 李明臣. 血府逐瘀汤联合云南白药热烘治疗带状疱疹临床研究[J]. 河北中医, 2010,12:1819–1820.
S148	苗伟, 李如华, 缪新华, 王立平, 孙翠玲, 高光鹏, 闫大方. 血府逐瘀汤热烘治疗带状疱疹126例临床观察[J]. 河北中医, 2010,11:1661.
S149	张向荣, 孟旭芳. 中药熏蒸治疗带状疱疹12例分析[J]. 实用中医内科杂志, 2004,05:468–469.
S150	赵明, 卢静. 云南白药治疗带状疱疹26例疗效分析[J]. 中华现代皮肤科学杂志, 2005,2(4):364.
S151	陈扬敏, 胡晶晶. 中药热敷联合紫外线照射治疗中老年带状疱疹45例[J]. 浙江中医杂志, 2013,03:217.
S152	王见良, 求晓恩. 艾炷灸治疗带状疱疹临床疗效观察[J]. 浙江中医药大学学报, 2010,03:402+404.
S153	张爱珍, 张强. 电针配合药物治疗带状疱疹疗效观察[J]. 实用中医药杂志, 2012,02:122–123.
S154	包峰峰. 针灸治疗带状疱疹32例[J]. 山东中医杂志, 2011,11:798–799.
S155	李雪薇. 不同针灸方法治疗带状疱疹多中心随机对照的临床研究[D]. 成都中医药大学, 2011.
S156	张争艳, 张申. 针灸联合刺络拔罐治疗带状疱疹的临床疗效观察[J]. 浙江中医药大学学报, 2014,12:1425–1427.
S157	周彩霞, 张鹏. 针刺结合半导体激光治疗仪治疗带状疱疹90例[J]. 陕西中医, 2013,03:353–354.
S158	刘银妮. 不同针灸方法治疗带状疱疹的临床研究[D]. 湖北中医药大学, 2010.
S159	郑新金, 李旅萍. 围针结合神经阻滞治疗带状疱疹神经痛40例临床疗效观察[J]. 亚太传统医药, 2010,09:43–44.
S160	李梦, 苟春雁, 唐国良, 王毅刚. 针刺加细灸条着肤灸治疗带状疱疹临床研究[J]. 中国中医急症, 2014,01:98–100.
S161	岳增辉, 何新群, 姜京明. 闪火灸法治疗带状疱疹的临床研究[J]. 湖南中医药大学学报, 2009,05:70–71+74.
S162	蔺莉莉. 带状疱疹的治疗研究[J]. 中国医药指南, 2010,35:223–224.
S163	卢爱文. 针灸对带状疱疹的临床观察[A]. 广东省针灸学会. 广东省针灸学会第九次学术交流会暨"针灸治疗痛症及特种针法"专题讲座论文汇编[C]. 广东省针灸学会:, 2004:3.

(*Continued*)

Study No.	Reference
S164	孙鹏颖. 针灸治疗带状疱疹的临床观察[J]. 中国社区医师, 2015,02:84+86.
S165	杨国辉. 毫针皮下扇形透刺配合艾灸治疗急性期带状疱疹29例[J]. 中国中医药现代远程教育, 2014,20:76–77.
S166	杨军雄, 向开维, 张玉学. 铺药棉灸法为主治疗带状疱疹:多中心随机对照研究[J]. 中国针灸, 2012,05:417–421.
S167	陈敏. 毫针皮下扇形针刺法加艾条治疗带状疱疹[J]. 中国保健营养(中旬刊), 2012,12:106.
S168	王敏. 针灸综合治疗带状疱疹的疗效观察[J]. 当代护士 (专科版), 2011,09: 135–136.
S169	林广华, 赵斌斌. 围刺为主配合悬灸治疗急性带状疱疹的疗效观察[J]. 针灸临床杂志, 2012,06:41–43.
S170	赵明, 汪月强, 漆军. 针刺联合阿昔洛韦治疗带状疱疹疗效观察[J]. 人民军医, 2010,12:934–935.
S171	张晓妮, 刘跃光. 针灸治疗带状疱疹的临床观察[J]. 四川中医, 2014,06: 149–150.
S172	罗胜平, 张进城. 针灸配合阿昔洛韦治疗带状疱疹40例临床观察[J]. 云南中医中药杂志, 2008,06:35.
S173	陈利远, 徐昭. 针刺疗法治疗带状疱疹46例疗效观察[J]. 航空航天医药, 2010,08:1530.
S174	邓宏. 泛昔洛韦联合梅花针治疗带状疱疹临床疗效评价[J]. 现代医药卫生, 2008,23:3505–3506.
S175	雷成业, 薛晓芳, 叶禹, 朱丽冰. 雷火灸治疗带状疱疹39例[J]. 中国中医药现代远程教育, 2013,13:56–57.
S176	杨润莲, 王俊富, 李春娥. 皮肤针叩刺配合治疗带状疱疹的疗效观察[J]. 护理研究, 2005,10:902.
S177	姜雪原, 胡永红. 艾灸治疗带状疱疹50例[J]. 陕西中医, 2010,08: 1050–1051.
S178	温萍, 詹巧莲, 陈敏, 李旭方, 陈建宁. 艾灸蜘蛛穴治疗带状疱疹的临床效果观察[J]. 社区医学杂志, 2014,21:41+46.
S179	刘金利. 口服伐昔洛韦加局部叩刺治疗带状疱疹66例疗效观察[J]. 海军医学杂志, 2010,04:343–344.
S180	赵南, 张玉洁, 张桂珍, 崔桂芬. 隔姜灸法治疗老年人带状疱疹36例[J]. 中国中医药科技, 2011,03:257.

(Continued)

(*Continued*)

Study No.	Reference
S181	李润芳, 巨萍莉, 全明. 针刺配合灯草灸治疗带状疱疹60例[J]. 陕西中医, 2004,12:1126–1127.
S182	史兴忠, 许建峰. 灯芯草灸治疗带状疱疹的临床观察[J]. 宁夏医学杂志, 2013,08:754–755.
S183	段天煜. 针灸局部围刺治疗肝胆火盛型带状疱疹30例临床观察[J]. 实用中医内科杂志, 2013,10:133–134.
S184	黄泳, 陈静. 欧阳群教授针灸医案选辑[J]. 时珍国医国药, 2007,11: 2850–2851.
S185	郭良才. 梅花针为主治疗带状疱疹100例[J]. 河南医药信息, 1995,08:35–36.
S186	白伟, 季奎, 许广里. 局部围刺治疗带状疱疹疗效观察[J]. 吉林中医药, 2007,02:44.
S187	陈晓梅. 针灸治疗带状疱疹53例疗效观察[J]. 云南中医中药杂志, 2004, 03:26–27.
S188	何睿, 丁丽玲. 围刺加艾熏治疗带状疱疹48例[J]. 云南中医中药杂志, 2012, 10:54.
S189	李瑾. 艾灸治疗带状疱疹24例[J]. 长春中医药大学学报, 2011,03:465.
S190	孙爱军, 张虚之. 围针浅刺法合夹脊穴治疗带状疱疹疗效观察[J]. 长春中医药大学学报, 2012,04:706–707.
S191	张国勇. 梅花针结合循经远刺治疗带状疱疹40例疗效观察[J]. 中外健康文摘, 2013,(26):210–211.
S192	刘洁石, 宫照敏, 叶昕. 中西医结合疗法治疗带状疱疹40例疗效观察[J]. 吉林医学, 2009,24:3323.
S193	姜占成. 针刺与TDP照射治疗带状疱疹26例观察[J]. 青海医药杂志, 2011, 01:77.
S194	李忠爽. 针刺配合紫外线照射治疗带状疱疹80例[J]. 实用中医药杂志, 2011, 12:850.
S195	孙燕. 华佗夹脊、局部围针加远红外照射治疗带状疱疹50例[J]. 陕西中医, 2009,10:1373–1374.
S196	王晓辉, 蒋云鹏. 沿皮围针配合TDP照射治疗带状疱疹护理体会[J]. 辽宁中医药大学学报, 2010,11:210–211.
S197	杨建花, 杨润成, 郑建平. 铺灸、围刺配合微波治疗带状疱疹疼痛40例临床观察[J]. 中国中医药科技, 2011,05:389.

(*Continued*)

(Continued)

Study No.	Reference
S198	岳延荣. 棉花灸结合超激光治疗带状疱疹27例[J]. 针灸临床杂志, 2011, 09:38–39.
S199	王明明, 杨颖. 火针为主治急性期带状疱疹的临床疗效[J]. 内蒙古中医药, 2014,30:53–54.
S200	魏巍, 张红星, 黄国付, 邹燃, 刘银妮. 电针夹脊穴配合刺络拔罐治疗带状疱疹的临床观察及其机制初探[J]. 湖北中医杂志, 2010,03:27–29.
S201	卢泽强. 针灸配合拔罐治疗带状疱疹疗效观察[J]. 上海针灸杂志, 2010,09: 601–602.
S202	杨加顺, 孙远征, 孟庆辉, 王瑾. 电围针结合叩刺治疗带状疱疹的对照研究[J]. 辽宁中医药大学学报, 2009,05:148–149.
S203	赵博华. 梅花针刺络拔罐法治疗带状疱疹急性期临床观察[J]. 北京中医药, 2013,05:371–372.
S204	杨晋翼. 电针拔罐配合壮医药线点灸治疗急性期带状疱疹的临床研究[D]. 广西中医药大学, 2014.
S205	谢倩, 徐佳, 杨榕青, 谢玉兰. 泛昔洛韦联合针刺拔罐放血疗法治疗带状疱疹疗效观察[J]. 临床医药实践, 2009,18:437–438.
S206	王智娟, 邹勇, 黄国琪. 电针夹脊穴配合中药治疗带状疱疹疗效观察(英文)[J]. Journal of Acupuncture and Tuina Science, 2012,05:313–317.
S207	杜艳, 徐鋆, 朱英. 传统外治法治疗早期带状疱疹的临床疗效评价[J]. 四川中医, 2007,11:84–85.
S208	刘亚军, 李若瑜. 生大黄粉外敷配合刺络拔罐放血治疗带状疱疹的临床观察[J]. 中国医药导报, 2013,14:110–111.
S209	任少杰, 孙钰. 齐刺配合放血拔罐治疗带状疱疹疗效观察[J]. 四川中医, 2014,06:153–155.
S210	周定伟. 皮下针、点灸及刺络拔罐治疗带状疱疹[J]. 中医临床研究, 2011,03:55–56.
S211	唐素元. 中西医结合治疗38例带状疱疹的效果[J]. 广西科学院学报, 2013,02:119–120.
S212	罗继红, 钟江. 龙胆泻肝汤联合壮医药线点灸治疗带状疱疹临床观察[J]. 广西中医药, 2013,02:21–22.
S213	刘铭, 邵欣, 余曙光. 针灸治疗带状疱疹65例疗效观察[J]. 针灸临床杂志, 2006,05:16–17.

(Continued)

(Continued)

Study No.	Reference
S214	惠小平, 姚峪岚, 袁民. 板蓝根合并针灸对照阿昔洛韦治疗带状疱疹分析[J]. 中华临床医药卫生杂志, 2005,3(9):48–49.
S215	徐雪怡. 针刺配合壮医药线点灸治疗带状疱疹的临床研究[D]. 广西中医学院, 2012.
S216	王小兰, 余鹏. 齐刺夹脊穴配合叩刺拔罐治疗带状疱疹60例临床观察[J]. 江苏中医药, 2010,12:60–61.
S217	吴红新. 齐刺夹脊穴配合叩刺拔罐治疗带状疱疹的临床效果观察[J]. 中国医药指南, 2011,29:337–339.
S218	姬素梅. 针灸加火罐治疗带状疱疹30例[J]. 中国社区医师(医学专业), 2012,09:221.
S219	喻元元, 夏锴. 药物配合梅花针叩刺拔罐治疗带状疱疹的临床观察及护理[J]. 中国保健营养(中旬刊), 2014,(7):4468.
S220	张玲. 中西医治疗急性期带状疱疹疗效比较[J]. 光明中医, 2013,02: 337–338.
S221	刘志国. 带状疱疹的中西医治疗疗效对比[J]. 家庭心理医生, 2014,10(5): 94.
S222	牟淑兰. 中西医结合治疗带状疱疹34例疗效观察[J]. 中国中医药信息杂志, 2010,11:72.
S223	岳全, 谭艳梅, 孙云芳, 李娟, 李学丽. 隔板蓝根注射液灸治疗带状疱疹的护理观察[J]. 光明中医, 2011,06:1246–1247.
S224	张益辉. 针刺拔罐为主治疗带状疱疹30例[J]. 上海针灸杂志, 2007,09:36.
S225	杨励. 通络解毒汤配合局部拔罐治疗带状疱疹240例疗效观察[J]. 中医临床研究, 2012,18:21–22.
S226	吴银, 杜忠. 梅花针叩刺拔罐结合云南白药外敷治疗带状疱疹35例[J]. 中国医学创新, 2009,6(17):94–95.
S227	陈玮, 刘桂珍, 姚秋红. 刺络拔罐治疗急性期带状疱疹临床疗效观察[J]. 上海针灸杂志, 2014,12:1132–1134.
S228	姜晓君. 梅花针叩刺治疗带状疱疹70例疗效观察[J]. 中国医药导报, 2010,16:108+112.
S229	朱炯, 吴怡峰. 刺络拔罐配合悬灸治疗带状疱疹疗效观察[J]. 上海针灸杂志, 2007,11:22–24.
S230	龙雄初, 龙枚飞, 赵社海, 李晓玲. 自拟解郁清毒散治疗带状疱疹后遗神经痛42例临床疗效观察[J]. 世界中西医结合杂志, 2013,11:1142–1144.

(Continued)

(Continued)

Study No.	Reference
S231	程靖. 祛瘀镇痛汤加减治疗带状疱疹后遗神经痛临床疗效观察[D]. 湖北中医学院, 2009.
S232	方玉甫, 刘爱民. 疏肝活血止痛方治疗带状疱疹后遗神经痛30例疗效观察[J]. 新中医, 2009,11:56–57.
S233	冯培民, 陈蕾. 六神丸治疗带状疱疹后遗神经痛的临床研究[J]. 中成药, 2008,06:799–801.
S234	梁俊梅. 带状疱疹后遗神经痛治疗方案优选研究[D]. 山东中医药大学, 2011.
S235	查锦东. 身痛逐瘀汤联合多虑平治疗带状疱疹后遗神经痛临床疗效观察[D]. 湖北中医药大学, 2013.
S236	张庆华. 益气活血化痰汤为主治疗带状疱疹后神经痛疗效观察[J]. 上海中医药杂志, 2011,12:61–62.
S237	赵继华. 中西医结合治疗带状疱疹后遗神经痛临床观察[J]. 医学理论与实践, 2013,05:619–620.
S238	孙春秋, 温为伟, 陈圣丽, 楼小航, 徐田红. 中西药结合治疗带状疱疹后遗神经痛疗效观察[J]. 中国中西医结合皮肤性病学杂志, 2012,02:98–99.
S239	徐舰, 陈伟星. 祛痛方治疗带状疱疹后遗神经痛20例——附西药治疗20例对照观察[J]. 浙江中医杂志, 2000,05:21.
S240	张媚霞, 王海涛, 孙树华. 血府逐瘀汤联合加巴喷丁治疗带状疱疹后遗神经痛34例[J]. 中国中医药现代远程教育, 2014,04:47–48.
S241	黄俊青, 陈长丽, 张丽珠. 中药祛痛汤结合多虑平治疗带状疱疹后遗神经痛疗效观察[J]. 检验医学与临床, 2014,09:1165–1166.
S242	崔鸿, 张池金. 疏肝解痛汤治疗带状疱疹后遗神经痛34例[J]. 吉林中医药, 2011,02:153+172.
S243	蒋蓝. 身痛逐瘀汤治疗带状疱疹后遗神经痛31例[J]. 中外健康文摘, 2013, (21):201.
S244	田红霞. 中药蒸汽浴联合治疗带状疱疹后遗神经痛30例[J]. 中医外治杂志, 2013,01:49.
S245	王热闹, 钱爱云. 益气活血汤治疗带状疱疹后遗神经痛21例[J]. 中国民间疗法, 2003,02:43–44.
S246	谢辉. 复方丹参饮治疗带状疱疹后遗神经痛30例临床观察[J]. 医学信息, 2013,(14):500–501.
S247	段小素. 膈下逐瘀汤联合神经阻滞治疗老年人头面部带状疱疹后遗神经痛疗效观察[J]. 中国中医药现代远程教育, 2012,13:76–77.

(Continued)

(Continued)

Study No.	Reference
S248	王天舒, 杜健儿, 朱全刚, 王景阳, 熊源长. 中药三七和利多卡因巴布贴剂用于带状疱疹后神经痛的治疗[J]. 实用疼痛学杂志, 2005,04:225–227.
S249	Nakanishi M, Arimitse J, Kageyama M, *et al.* Efficacy of traditional Japanese herbal medicines-Keishikajutsubuto (TJ-18) and Bushi-matsu (TJ-3022)-against postherpetic neuralgia aggravated by self-reported cold stimulation: a case series. *J Altern Complement Med* 2012;18(7):686–92.
S250	林辰, 杨建萍, 陈攀. 标准化壮医药线点灸治疗带状疱疹后遗神经痛的疗效及安全性研究[J]. 河北中医, 2011,08:1189–1190+1251.
S251	冯启廷, 何彬, 陈小丽, 李荣华. 冯氏排针法治疗带状疱疹后遗肋间神经痛疗效观察[J]. 实用中医药杂志, 2015,01:51–52.
S252	张淑杰, 邹艳红. 针刺夹脊穴配合围刺治疗带状疱疹后遗神经痛[J]. 针灸临床杂志, 2009,02:4–6.
S253	谭健忠. 火针治疗带状疱疹后遗症随机平行对照研究[J]. 实用中医内科杂志, 2013,03:139–140.
S254	胡春兰, 陈训军, 杜华平等. 针刺联合加巴喷丁治疗带状疱疹后遗神经痛疗效观察[J]. 中外健康文摘, 2013,(29):172–173.
S255	张岱权, 唐礴. 电针联合芬太尼透皮贴剂治疗老年胸腰段带状疱疹后遗神经痛疗效观察[J]. 中国中医急症, 2009,07:1080+1084.
S256	王文娟, 赵梓纲, 李恒进. 电针联合普瑞巴林治疗带状疱疹后神经痛的疗效观察[J]. 中华保健医学杂志, 2013,02:146–148.
S257	陈晓英, 杨强, 李明波. 浮针联合加巴喷丁治疗带状疱疹后遗神经痛36例疗效分析[J]. 中国医药科学, 2012,18:88–89.
S258	李菊莲. 阶梯针刺法治疗带状疱疹后遗神经痛临床观察[J]. 针灸临床杂志, 2010,09:43–44.
S259	热孜完·亚生. 围刺配合TDP照射治疗带状疱疹后遗神经痛45例疗效观察[J]. 中国保健营养, 2013,08:1796–1797.
S260	沙德花, 买文菊, 郑贵芝, 李春香, 丁勇. 电针治疗带状疱疹后遗神经痛87例临床分析[J]. 现代医药卫生, 2014,02:287.
S261	洪东方. 电针结合TDP照射扶他林软膏外用治疗带状疱疹后遗神经痛56例[J]. 中国中医急症, 2013,05:780–781.

(Continued)

(Continued)

Study No.	Reference
S262	Valaskatgis P, Macklin EA, Schachter SC, Wayne PM. Possible effects of acupuncture on atrial fibrillation and post-herpetic neuralgia — a case report. *Acupunct Med.* 2008;26(1):51–6.
S263	Liu DDJ, Childs GV, Raji MA. Possible Role of Acupuncture in the Treatment of Post-Zoster Limb Pain and Paresis: Case Report and Literature Review. *J Neuropathic Pain Symptom Palliation.* 2005; 1(3):45–9.
S264	卜召飞. 针药合用治疗带状疱疹后遗神经痛41例[J]. 河南中医, 2013,11:1955–1956.
S265	李文娜, 蔡国良, 王玉珍. 电针夹脊穴配合刺络拔罐治疗30例带状疱疹后遗神经痛的临床疗效观察[J]. 现代诊断与治疗, 2014,07:1506–1507.
S266	李清萍, 马骏. 益气养阴活血汤配合热敏灸治疗带状疱疹后遗神经痛的临床研究[J]. 光明中医, 2014,07:1470–1472.
S267	张思为, 邓世芳, 苏峥, 郭少军, 邓茜, 蒋红玉. 芪棱汤配合针刺治疗带状疱疹后遗神经痛30例临床研究[J]. 亚太传统医药, 2011,07:112–114.
S268	张慧玲. 中医综合治疗带状疱疹后遗神经痛临床研究[J]. 中国临床研究, 2012,01:76–77.
S269	嘉士健, 黄翠华, 嘉雁苓, 何继原, 罗斌. 络病理论指导治疗顽固性带状疱疹后遗神经痛[J]. 长春中医药大学学报, 2014,03:514–517.
S270	范永龙, 蔡卉. 加巴喷丁联合针灸、通络活血止痛汤治疗带状疱疹后遗神经痛疗效观察[J]. 江西医药, 2011,06:561–562.
S271	嘉士健. 刺血疗法配合丹栀逍遥散治疗PHN30例临床观察[J]. 中国医药导刊, 2013,11:1839–1840.
S272	梁俊梅. 带状疱疹后遗神经痛治疗方案优选研究[D]. 山东中医药大学, 2011.
S273	肖卫敏, 李振民, 范淑凤. 中西医结合治疗带状疱疹后神经痛80例[J]. 四川中医, 2014,03:102–104.

(Continued)

Index